12 CHAPTERS ON NUCLEAR MEDICINE

Edited by **Ali Gholamrezanezhad**

12 Chapters on Nuclear Medicine
Edited by Ali Gholamrezanezhad

Published by InTech

Janeza Trdine 9, 51000 Rijeka, Croatia

Publishing Process Manager Molly Kaliman

Technical Editor Teodora Smiljanic

Cover Designer InTech Design Team

Additional hard copies can be obtained from orders@intechopen.com

12 Chapters on Nuclear Medicine, Edited by Ali Gholamrezanezhad
p. cm.
ISBN 978-953-307-802-1

For EU product safety concerns:
IN TECH d.o.o., Prolaz Marije Krucifikse Kozulić 3, 51000 Rijeka, Croatia,
info@intechopen.com or visit our website at intechopen.com.

Meet the editor

Ali Gholamrezanezhad, MD, specialist of nuclear medicine and molecular imaging from Tehran University of Medical Sciences and Fellow of the European Board on Nuclear Medicine (FEBNM) is the author of more than 60 publications in the field of nuclear medicine. He currently is involved in research activities in department of nuclear medicine at Johns Hopkins University. He has published in almost all nuclear medicine journals, including Journal of Nuclear Medicine, European Journal of Nuclear Medicine, Clinical Nuclear Medicine, Journal of Nuclear Cardiology, Journal of Nuclear Medicine technology, Nuclear Medicine Communications, Nucklearmedizine, Annals of Nuclear Medicine, Hellenic Journal of Nuclear Medicine, Nuclear Medicine and Biology, Revista Espanola de Medicina Nucleare, and Iranian Journal of Nuclear Medicine. He serves as a reviewer or member of editorial board for a number of international journals, such as Rare Tumors, Clinical Neurology and Neurosurgery, Anatolian Journal of Cardiology.

Contents

Preface

Nuclear Medicine is a collection of 12 chapters providing a comprehesnive overview of the nuclear medicine, with insights into both its historical and contemporary practices. I hope that readers enjoy the chapters greatly and find it informative, practical and educational in the presented discussions.

I would like to convey my respects and thanks to the authors for their efforts and contribution. Collaboration has always been important in academic environment. I am very happy to see that the publication and chapters are the result of fruitful international collaboration involving more than 20 leading scientists and investigators from all over the world. I hope the "12 Chapters on Nuclear Medicine" encourage continued close cooperation and collaboration among its authors.

Best regards,

Ali Gholamrezanezhad, MD, FEBNM

1

Physiologic and False Positive Pathologic Uptakes on Radioiodine Whole Body Scan

Byeong-Cheol Ahn
Kyungpook National University School of Medicine and Hospital, South Korea

1. Introduction

A radioiodine whole body scan relies on the fact that differentiated thyroid cancer is more efficient at trapping circulating radioiodine than any other tissues.(Hyer, Newbold et al. 2010) Therefore, when I-131 is administered it accumulates in the thyroid cancer tissues and a radioiodine whole body scan plays an important role in the management of patients with differentiated thyroid cancer. Uptake of iodine by the cancer is related to the expression of sodium iodide symporter (NIS), which actively transports iodide into the cancer cells. Extrathyroidal tissues, such as stomach, salivary glands and breast, are known to have the NIS expression and the organs can physiologically take up iodine.(Riesco-Eizaguirre and Santisteban 2006)

On a whole body scan with diagnostic or therapeutic doses of I-131, except for the physiological radioiodine uptake in the salivary glands, stomach, gastrointestinal and urinary tracts, the lesions with radioiodine uptake can be considered as metastatic lesions in thyroid cancer patients who previously underwent total thyroidectomy.

However, a variety of unusual lesions may cause a false positive result on the radioiodine whole body scan and so careful evaluation of an abnormal scan is imperative to appropriately manage patients with differentiated thyroid cancer.(Mitchell, Pratt et al. 2000; Shapiro, Rufini et al. 2000; Carlisle, Lu et al. 2003; Ahn, Lee et al. 2011) The decision to administer radioiodine treatment is mainly based on the diagnostic scan, and misinterpretation of physiological or other causes of radioiodine uptake as metastatic thyroid cancer could lead to the decision to perform unnecessary surgical removal or to administer a high dose of I-131, which results in fruitless radiation exposure. Therefore, correct interpretation of the diagnostic scan is critical for the proper management.

Physiologic iodine uptake, pathologic iodine uptakes that are not related to thyroid cancer and contamination by physiologic excretion of tracer on the whole body scan are presented and discussed in this chapter. The purpose of this chapter is to make readers consider the possibility of physiologic or pathologic false positive uptake as a reason for the tracer uptake seen on the radioiodine whole body scan.

2. Iodine and the thyroid gland

Iodine is an element with a high atomic number 53, it is purple in colour and it is represented by the symbol I, and the iodine is an essential component of the hormones

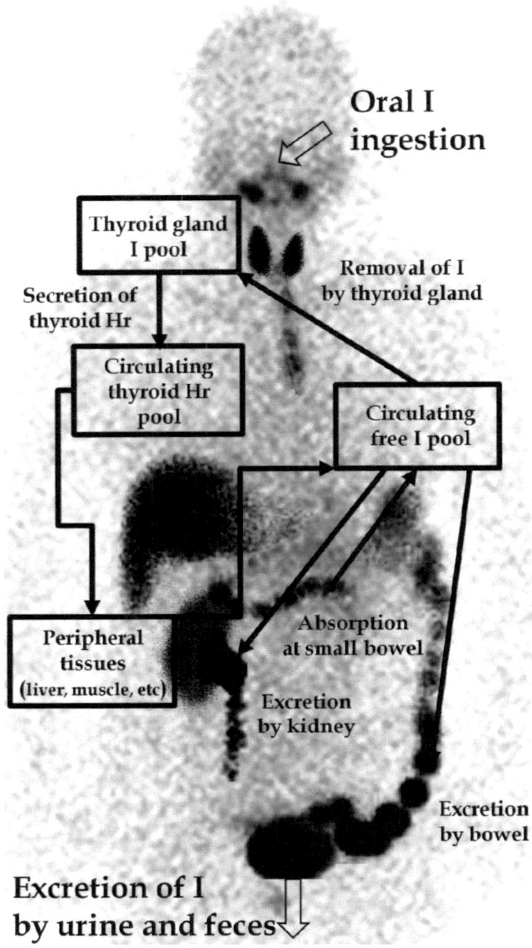

Fig. 1. Simplified diagram of the metabolic circuit of iodine. Iodine (I) ingested orally is absorbed from the small bowel into the circulating iodine pool. About one fifth of the iodine in the pool is removed by the thyroid gland and surplus iodine is rapidly excreted by the kidney and bowel. In the thyroid gland, iodine is used to produce thyroid hormones (Hr), which act in peripheral tissues. Iodine released from thyroid hormones re-enter into the circulating iodine pool.

produced by the thyroid gland. The thyroid hormones are essential for the health and well-being for mammals. Iodine comprises about 60% of the weights of thyroid hormones. The body of an adult contains 15~20mg of iodine, of which 70~80% is in the thyroid gland.(Ahad and Ganie 2010) To produce a normal quantity of thyroid hormone, about 50 mg of ingested iodine in the form of iodides are required each year. Oceans are the world's main repositories of iodine and very little iodine is found in the soil.(Ahad and Ganie 2010) The major dietary sources of iodine are bread and milk in the US and Europe, but the main source is seaweed in some Asian countries.(Zimmermann and Crill; Ahad and Ganie 2010; Hall 2011) Iodine is found in various forms in nature such as inorganic sodium or potassium salts (sodium iodide or potassium iodide), inorganic diatomic iodine or organic monoatomic iodine. (Ahad and Ganie 2010) Iodide, represented by I^-, is the ion of iodine and it combines with another element or elements to form a compound. Although the iodine content of iodised salt may vary from country to country, common table salt has a small portion of sodium iodide to prevent iodine deficiency.(Hall 2011)

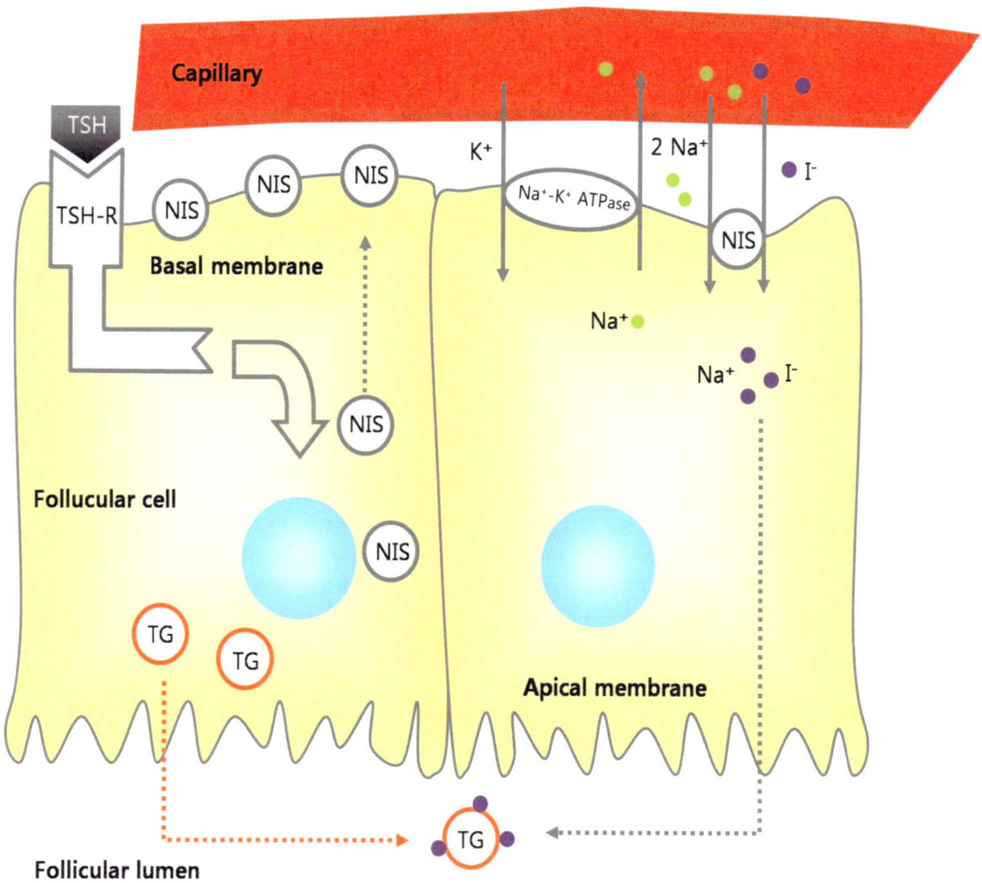

Fig. 2. Cellular mechanism for iodine uptake in thyroid follicular cells. This commences with the uptake of iodide from the capillary into the follicular cell of the thyroid gland. This process occurs against chemical and electrical gradients via the sodium iodide symporter (NIS) located in the basal membrane of the follicular cell. Increased intracellular sodium is pumped out by the action of Na^+/K^+ ATPase. The iodide within the follicular cell moves towards the apical membrane to enter into the follicular lumen and then it is oxidized to iodine by peroxidase. Organification of the iodine follows the oxidation by iodination of the tyrosine residues present within the thyroglobulin (TG) molecule, and the iodine stays in the follicle before it is released into the circulation as thyroid hormones. Thyroid stimulating hormone (TSH) activates the follicular cell via TSH receptor (TSH-R) and increases the expression of the NIS and the TG.

2.1 Iodine absorption and metabolism

Ingested iodides are rapidly and nearly completely absorbed (>90%) from the duodenum into the blood and most of the iodides are excreted by kidneys. Sodium iodide symporter (NIS) on the apical membrane of enterocytes mediates active iodide uptake. Normally about one fifth of absorbed iodides are taken up by thyroid follicular cells and this is used for thyroid hormone synthesis, yet the clearance of circulating iodide varies with iodine intake. In the condition of an adequate iodine supply, ≤10% of absorbed iodides are taken up by the thyroid and in chronic iodine deficiency, this fraction can exceed 80%.(Zimmermann and Crill) The basal membrane of the thyroid follicular cell is able to actively transport iodide to the interior of the cell against a concentration gradient by the action of the NIS, which co-transports one iodide ion along with two sodium ions. The process of concentrating iodide in the thyroid follicular cells is called iodide trapping and presence of the NIS is essential for the process.(Hall 2011) Thyroid hormones are produced by oxidation, organification and coupling processes in the thyroid gland and they are finally released into the blood stream for their action.

2.2 Sodium iodide symporter

The rat NIS gene and the human NIS gene were cloned in 1996.(Dai, Levy et al. 1996; Smanik, Liu et al. 1996) NIS is a 13 transmembrane domain protein with an extracellular amino- and intracellular carboxyl-terminus and the expression of the NIS gene is mainly regulated by thyroid stimulating hormone (TSH). Binding of TSH to its receptor activates the NIS gene transcription and controls translocation and retention of NIS at the plasma membrane, and so this increases iodide uptake.

In addition to its expression in the thyroid follicular cells, NIS is detectable and active in some extrathyroidal tissues such as the salivary glands, gastric mucosa, lactating mammary glands, etc. Therefore, these tissues are able to take up iodide by the action of the NIS. However, contrary to thyroid follicular cells, there are no long-term retention of iodide and TSH dependency. (Baril, Martin-Duque et al. 2010) The physiologic function of the NIS in the extrathyroidal tissues is not yet clear.

3. Procedures for radioiodine whole body imaging

3.1 Patients preparation

Thyroid hormone replacement must be withheld for a sufficient time to permit an adequate rise of TSH (>30 uIU/mL). This is at least 2 weeks for triiodothyronine (T3) and 3–4 weeks for thyroxine (T4). This is also achieved by the administration of recombinant human TSH (rhTSH, Thyrogen®, given as two injections of 0.9 mg intramuscularly on each of two consecutive days) without stopping thyroid hormone replacement. rhTSH must be used in patients who may not have an elevation of TSH to the adequate level due to a large residual volume of functioning thyroid tissue or pituitary abnormalities, which precludes elevation of TSH. rhTSH might be used to prevent severe hypothyroidism related to the stopping of thyroid hormone replacement.(Silberstein, Alavi et al. 2005; Silberstein, Alavi et al. 2006)

All patients must discontinue eating/using iodide-containing foods or preparations, and other medications that could potentially affect the ability of thyroid cancer tissue to accumulate iodide for a sufficient time before radioiodine administration. A low-iodine diet is followed for 7–14 days before the radioiodine is given, as it significantly increases the uptake of radioiodine by the well differentiated thyroid cancer tissue. The avoided or permitted food items are summarized in table 1. The recommended time interval of drug withdrawal is summarized in table 2. Imaging should be delayed for a long enough period to eliminate the effects of these interfering factors. The goal of a low iodine diet and the drug withdrawal is to make a 24-hour urine iodine output of about 50 ug.(Silberstein, Alavi et al. 2006).

	Allowed	Not-allowed
Salts	Non -iodized salt	Iodized salt Sea salt
Fruits and vegetables	Fresh fruits and juices	Rhubarb Fruit or juice with red dye # 3 Canned or preserved
Seafood and sea products	None	Fish Shellfishs Seaweeds Seaweed tableets Agar-agar
Dairy products	None	Milk Cheese Yogurt Butter Ice cream Chocholate (has milk content)
Paultries and Meats	Fresh unsalted	Canned and processed
Egg	Whites of eggs	Egg yolks Whole eggs
Grain products	breads, cereal and crackers without salt unsalted pasta, rice, rice cakes, and popcorn	Breads, cereals or crackers made with salt Salted pasta, rice or popcorn
drinks	Cola, diet cola, lemonade Coffee or tea without milk or cream Fruit juice without red dye#3 Fruit smoothies made without dairy or soy products Beer, wine and spirits	Milk, cream or drinks made with dairy Fruit juice and soft drinks with red dye#3

Table 1. Food guide for a low iodine diet. Some items on the allowed list may not be low in iodine in some forms or merchandise brands. The labels must be checked to be sure that the items meet the requirements of the low-iodine diet. (Amin, Junco et al.; Nostrand, Bloom et al. 2004)

3.2 Types of radioiodine

3.2.1 I-131

I-131 is produced in a nuclear reactor by neutron bombardment of natural tellurium (Te-127) and decays by beta emission with a half-life of 8.02 days to xenon-133 (Xe-133) and it emits gamma emission as well. It most often (89% of the time) expends its 971 keV of decay energy by transforming into the stable Xe-131 in two steps, with gamma decay following rapidly after beta decay. The primary emissions of I-131 decay are beta particles with a maximal energy of 606 keV (89% abundance, others 248–807 keV) and 364 keV gamma rays (81% abundance, others 723 keV).

I-131 is administered orally with activities of 1–5 mCi or less, with many preferring a range of 1–2 mCi because of the data suggesting that stunning (decreased uptake of the therapy dose of I-131 by the residual functioning thyroid tissue or tumour due to cell death or dysfunction caused by the activity administered for diagnostic imaging) is less likely at the lower activity range. However, detection of more iodine concentrating tissue has been reported with higher dosages.(Silberstein, Alavi et al. 2006)

Type of medication	Recommended time interval of withdrawal
Natural synthetic thyroid hormone Thyroxine (T4) Triiodothyroinine (T3)	 3 to 4 weeks 10 to 14 days
Amiodarone	3 to 6 months
Multivitamine	6 weeks
Lugol's solution, potassium iodide solution (SSKI)	6 weeks
Topical iodine	6 weeks
Radiographic contrast agents	3 to 6 months, depending on iodide content
Iodinated eyedrops and antiseptics	6 weeks
Iodine containing expectorants and anti-tussives	2 to 4 weeks

Table 2. Recommended time intervals of withdrawal for drugs affecting radioiodine uptake. The time interval can be changed by the administered doses of the medications. The amount of iodine for the drug must also be considered.(Nostrand, Bloom et al. 2004; Silberstein, Alavi et al. 2005; Luster, Clarke et al. 2008)

3.2.2 I-123

I-123 is produced in a cyclotron by proton irradiation of enriched Xe-124 in a capsule and I-123 decays by electron capture with a half-life of 13.22 hours to Te-123 and it emits gamma radiation with predominant energies of 159 keV (the gamma ray primarily used for imaging) and 127 keV.

I-123 is mainly a gamma emitter with a high counting rate compared with I-131, and I-123 provides a higher lesion-to-background signal, thereby improving the sensitivity and imaging quality. Moreover, with the same administered activity, I-123 delivers an absorbed radiation dose that is approximately one-fifth that of I-131 to the thyroid tissue, thereby lessening the likelihood of stunning from imaging. I-123 is administered orally with activities of 0.4–5.0 mCi, which may avoid stunning.(Ma, Kuang et al. 2005; Silberstein, Alavi et al. 2006)

3.2.3 I-124

I-124 is a proton-rich isotope of iodine produced in a cyclotron by numerous nuclear reactions and it decays to Te-124 with a half-life of 4.18 days. Its modes of decay are: 74.4%

electron capture and 25.6% positron emission. It emits gamma radiation with energies of 511 and 602 keV.(Rault, Vandenberghe et al. 2007)
I-124 is administered intravenously with activities of 0.5–2.0 mCi for detection of metastatic lesions or assessment of the radiation dose related to I-131 therapy.

Types	Advantages	Disadvantages
I-131	• Cheap • Readily available • Allows longer delayed image	• Potential stunning • Requirement of possible radiation safety precautions for family and caregivers
I-123	• No stunning • Good image quality	• Limited availablity • Expensive
I-124	• Superior image quality • Tomographic image • Allows intermediate delayed image • Fusion image with CT or MR	• Very limited availability • Very expensive

Table 3. Advantages and disadvantages according to the types of radioiodine.(Nostrand, Bloom et al. 2004)

3.3 Planar, SPECT and PET imaging

3.3.1 Planar imaging

Planar gamma camera imaging can be obtained with gamma emitting I-123 or I-131 for the detection of thyroid cancer tissue expressing the NIS gene which takes up iodine. The main emission energy peak of I-131 is approximately 364 keV, so it requires the use of a high-energy all-purpose collimator for imaging acquisition. The peak of the I-123 is 159 keV, which is close to the 140 keV from Tc-99m for which the gamma camera's design has traditionally been optimized. I-123 can be imaged with a low-energy high-resolution collimator, which is optimized for image acquisition with Tc-99m. (Rault, Vandenberghe et al. 2007)
With radioiodine's avidity for differentiated thyroid cancer tissues, planar radioiodine whole body image has been mainly used for the detection of metastatic thyroid cancer lesions. However, the limited resolution of planar imaging together with the background activity in the radioiodine images can give false-negative results for small lesions. Physiologic uptake of radioiodine is not always easily differentiable from pathologic uptake and it can give false-positive results. (Spanu, Solinas et al. 2009) Therefore, the sensitivity and specificity of planar images for the diagnosis of metastatic thyroid cancer may be limited. (Oh, Byun et al. 2011)

3.3.2 SPECT (Single Photon Emission Computed Tomography) or SPECT/CT imaging

Although a radioiodine whole body scan is one of the excellent imaging tools for the detection of thyroid cancer, false negative results may be observed in cases with small recurrent lesions in an area of rather high background activity or in cases with poorly differentiated cancer tissues, which have low uptake ability for radioiodine (due to dedifferentiation).(Geerlings, van Zuijlen et al.) SPECT, which can provide cross-sectional scintigraphic images, has been proposed as a way to overcome the limitations of planar imaging and it is known to have higher sensitivity and better contrast resolution than planar imaging. Radioiodine SPECT has higher performance for detecting recurrent lesion compared to planar imaging in thyroidectomized thyroid cancer patients and it also changes the patients' management.

Radioiodine SPECT has excellent capability to detect thyroid cancer tissues, yet the anatomic evaluation of lesion sites with radioiodine uptake remains difficult due to the minimal background uptake of the radioiodine. The performance of SPECT with radioiodine may be further improved by fusing the SPECT and CT images or by using an integrated SPECT/CT system that permits simultaneous anatomic mapping and functional imaging.(Geerlings, van Zuijlen et al.; Spanu, Solinas et al. 2009) The fusion imaging modality can synergistically and significantly improve the diagnostic process and its outcome when compared to a single diagnostic technique. (Von Schulthess and Hany 2008) Therefore, SPECT/CT with radioiodine can demonstrate a higher number of radioiodine uptake lesions, and it can more correctly differentiate between physiologic and pathologic uptakes, and so it permits a more appropriate therapeutic approach to be chosen.(Spanu, Solinas et al. 2009) Despite its many advantages, SPECT/CT cannot be applied for routine use or whole body imaging due to the long scanning time and the additional radiation burden, and so the fusion image should be selected on a personalized basis for those who clinically need the imaging. (Oh, Byun et al. 2011)

3.3.3 PET (Positron Emission Tomography) or PET/CT imaging

PET detects a pair of gamma rays produced by annihilation of a positron which is introduced by a positron emitting radionuclide and this produces three-dimensional image. Owing to its electronic collimation, I-124 PET gives better efficiency and resolution than in I-123 or I-131 SPECT, and so it offers the best image quality. (Rault, Vandenberghe et al. 2007) A fusion imaging modality with I-124 PET and CT can improve the diagnostic efficacy when compared to I-124 PET imaging by the same reasons of SPECT/CT over SEPCT only. I-124 PET/CT has superiority due to the better spatial resolution and faster imaging speed compared to I-123 or I-131 SPECT/CT.(Van Nostrand, Moreau et al. 2010) PET fused with MR is recently being used for research and in clinic fields and it will allow state of art imaging in the near future.

4. Physiologic radioiodine uptake

Following thyroid ablation, physiologic activity is expected in the salivary glands, stomach, breast, oropharynx, nasopharynx, oesophagus, gastrointestinal tract and genitourinary tract.(Ozguven, Ilgan et al. 2004) Physiologic radioiodine accumulation is related to the expression of the NIS and metabolism related to or the retention of excreted iodine. (Bakheet, Hammami et al. 2000; Ahn, Lee et al. 2011) Uptake of radioiodine in the thyroid tissue, salivary gland, stomach, lacrimal sac, nasolacrimal duct and choroid plexus is related to the NIS expression of the cells of the organs.(Morgenstern, Vadysirisack et al. 2005) Ectopic thyroid tissues are found by a variety of embryological maldevelopments of the thyroid gland such as lingual or sublingual thyroid (by failure of migration), a thyroglossal duct (by functioning thyroid tissue in the migration route) and a mediastinal thyroid gland (by excessive migration). Other abnormal migration may produce widely divergent ectopic thyroid tissue in many organs such as liver, oesophagus, trachea, etc. In addition, normal thyroid tissue can be in the ovary (Struma ovarii. It can be classified as uptake in a pathologic lesion.). (Shapiro, Rufini et al. 2000) Ectopic gastric mucosa can be located in the small bowel (Meckel's diverticulum) or terminal oesophagus (Barrett's oesophagus). (Ma, Kuang et al. 2005) The ectopic thyroid and gastric mucosal tissues are able to take up radioiodine.

Uptake of iodine in the liver after radioiodine administration is related to the metabolism of radioiodinated thyroglobulin and thyroid hormones in the organ. The gall bladder also may occasionally be depicted with the biliary excretion of the radioiodine. (Shapiro, Rufini et al. 2000; Carlisle, Lu et al. 2003) A simultaneous hepatobiliary scan with Tc-99m DISIDA (Diisopropyl Iminodiacetic Acid) or mebrofenin is useful for characterizing the gall bladder uptake. Tracer accumulation in the oropharynx, nasopharynx and oesophagus is related to retention of salivary excretion of administered radioiodine.

Visualization of the oesophagus is extremely common and vertical linear uptake in the thorax that is removed by drinking water is characteristic of oesophageal uptake by swallowing of radioactive saliva. The oesophageal activity may also arise from gastric reflux. (Carlisle, Lu et al. 2003) Image acquisition after a drink of water is able to distinguish the activity from mediastinal node metastasis. (Shapiro, Rufini et al. 2000)

Urinary or gastrointestinal anomalies can be responsible for false positive radioiodine uptake. (Ma, Kuang et al. 2005) Visualization of kidney and bladder after radioiodine administration is possible and this is known to be related to the urinary excretion of radioiodine into the urinary collecting system. Administered radioiodine is excreted mainly by the urinary system, and so all dilations, diverticuli and fistulae of the kidney, ureter and bladder may produce radioiodine retention.(Shapiro, Rufini et al. 2000) Visualizing the location of the renal pelvis of ectopic, horseshoe and transplanted kidneys is not usual and radioiodine at the pelvis may lead to misinterpretation. In fact, the renal pelvis and ureter are usually not visualized due to the rapid transit time of the radioiodine. (Bakheet, Hammami et al. 1996) A simultaneous renal scan with Tc-99m DTPA (Diethylene Triamine Pentaacetic Acid) or MAG3 (Mercapto Acetyl Triglycine) is useful for characterizing the urinary tract uptakes. (Shapiro, Rufini et al. 2000) Although the incidence is very uncommon, renal cysts are known to produce radioiodine uptake. The proposed mechanisms for the renal cyst uptake are a communication between the cyst and the urinary tract and radioiodine secretion by the lining epithelium of the cyst. (Shapiro, Rufini et al. 2000)

Tracer accumulation in the colon is very common. Incomplete absorption of the oral radioiodine administration is not considered as the reason of colonic activity due to the lack of colonic activity seen on the early images. Tracer accumulation is probably due to transport of radioiodine into the intestine from the mesenteric circulation and biliary excretion of the metabolites of radioiodinated thyroglobulin. (Hays 1993) Appropriate use of laxatives can be a simple remedy for the activity. (Shapiro, Rufini et al. 2000)

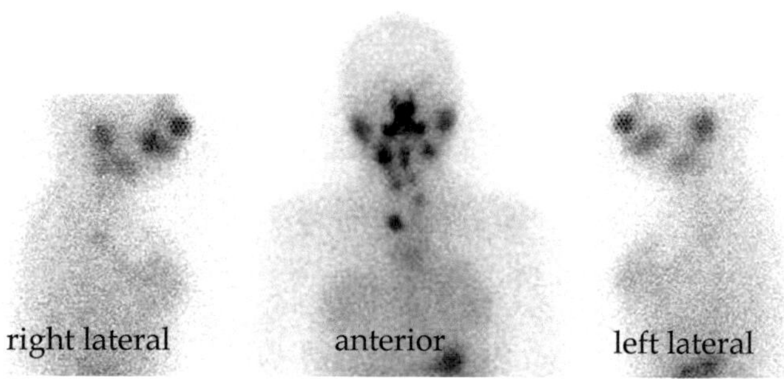

Fig. 3. Physiologic uptake of radioiodine in the nasal cavity, the so called "hot nose". Intense tracer uptake was noted at the thyroid bed area (due to residual thyroid tissue), breast and salivary gland (by the NIS expression of the glands).

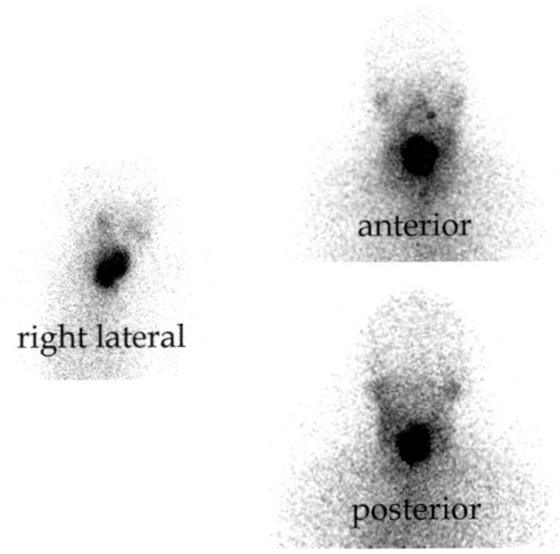

Fig. 4. Physiologic uptake of radioiodine in residual thyroid tissue. Intense tracer uptake was noted at the thyroid bed area due to residual thyroid tissue.

Lactating mammary glands express the NIS, and so the lactating breast shows intense radioiodine uptake that might persist for months after cessation of lactation. Mild to moderate uptake is also seen in non-lactating breast tissue, which can be asymmetrical, presumably owing to the same mechanism that operates in lactation.(Shapiro, Rufini et al. 2000; Tazebay, Wapnir et al. 2000)

Uptake of radioiodine can occur in a residual normal thymus or in thymic hyperplasia and the suggested mechanisms for the uptake are the expression of the NIS in thymic tissues and the iodine concentration by the Hassal's bodies that are present in the thymic tissue, which resemble the follicular cells of the thyroid. Thymic radioiodine uptake is more common in young patients compared to older patients. Even though the incidence is very rare, an intrathymic ectopic thyroid tissue or thyroid cancer metastases to the thymus can be a possible cause of uptake. (Mello, Flamini et al. 2009)

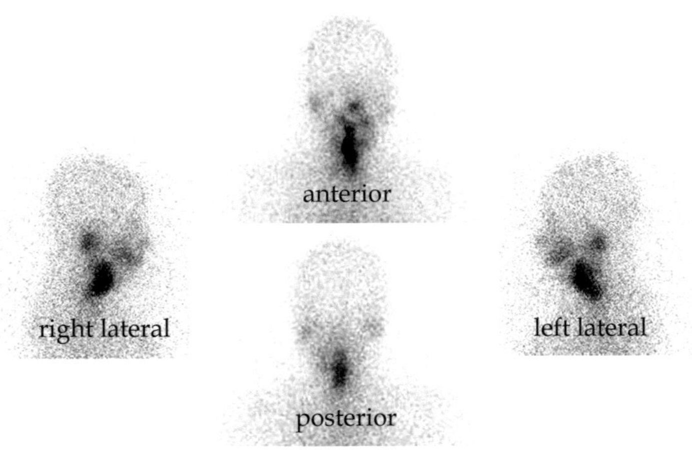

Fig. 5. Physiologic uptake of radioiodine in residual thyroid tissue. Intense tracer uptake was noted at the midline of the upper neck due to residual thyroid tissue in the thyroglossal duct. Mild tracer uptake of the salivary gland (by the NIS expression of the glands) was also noted.

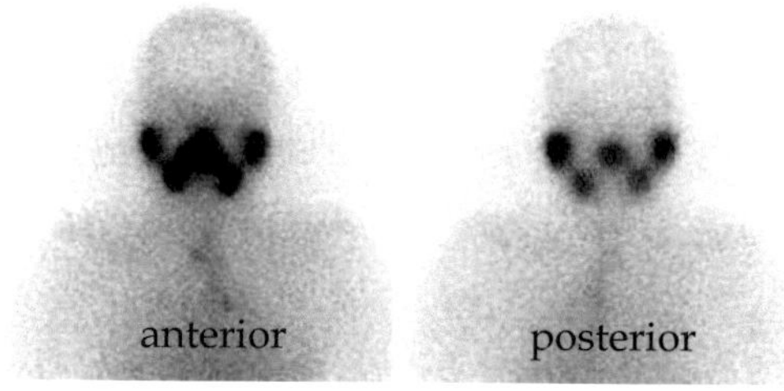

Fig. 6. Physiologic uptake of radioiodine in both the parotid and submandibular salivary glands. Intense activity in the oral and nasal cavities (by saliva and nasal secretion) was also noted.

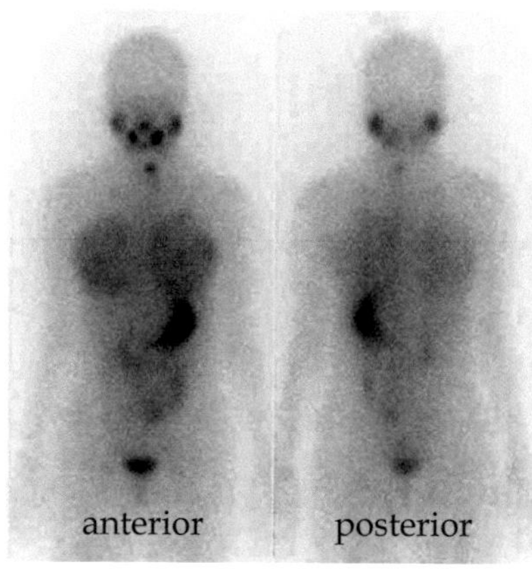

Fig. 7. Physiologic uptake of radioiodine in the breast. Diffuse, moderate radioactivity in the breast was noted. There was also noted physiologic tracer uptake in the thyroid bed (suggesting remnant thyroid tissue, which has the NIS expression), salivary glands (by the NIS expression of the glands), stomach (by the NIS expression of the glands), bowel (by secretion of radioiodine into the intestine or biliary excretion of the metabolites of radioiodinated proteins) and urinary bladder (by urine activity).

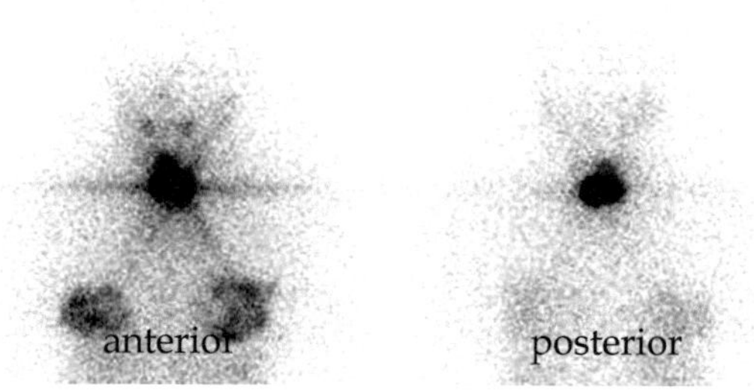

Fig. 8. Physiologic uptake of radioiodine in the breast. Intense tracer accumulation was noted in both breasts. Physiologic tracer uptake was also noted in the thyroid bed (suggesting remnant thyroid tissue, which has the NIS expression).

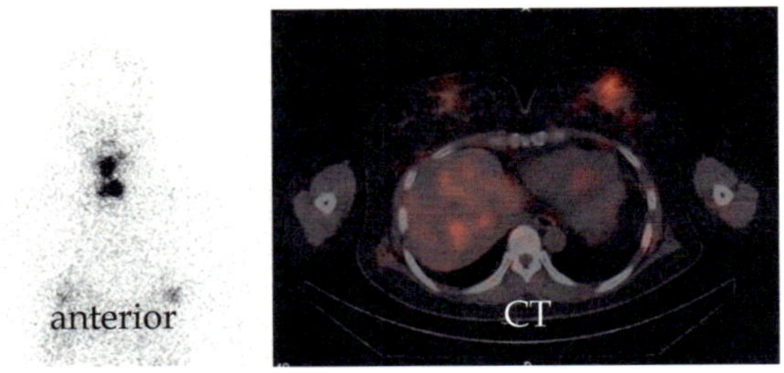

Fig. 9. Physiologic uptake of radioiodine in the breast. Focal tracer uptake in the breast was noted. SPECT/CT revealed the accurate location of the breast uptake. Physiologic intense tracer uptake was noted in the thyroid bed (suggesting remnant thyroid tissue, which has the NIS expression) and mild tracer uptake in the liver (by metabolism of radioiodinated thyroglobulin and thyroid hormones).

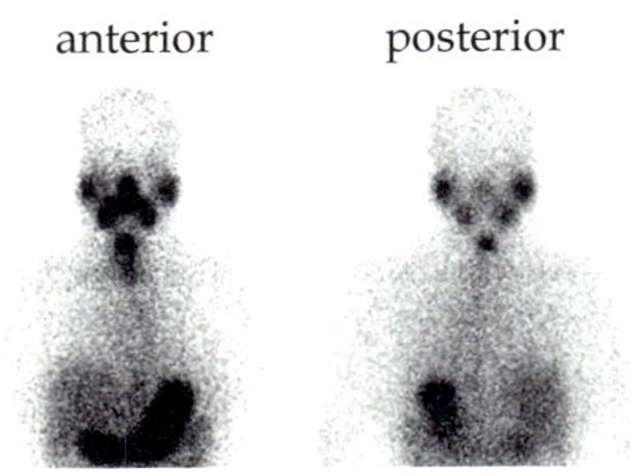

Fig. 10. Physiologic uptake of radioiodine in the oesophagus. Vertical linear radioactivity in the chest was noted by stagnation of swallowed saliva containing radioiodine. There was also noted physiologic tracer uptake in the thyroid bed area (by residual thyroid tissue) and salivary glands (by the NIS expression of the glands).

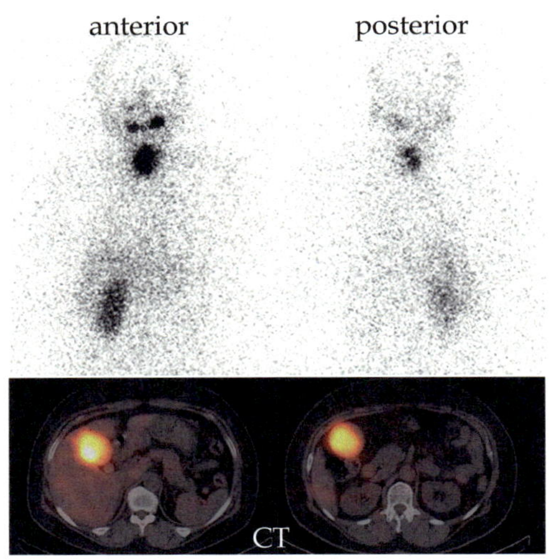

Fig. 11. Physiologic uptake of radioiodine in the gall bladder. Intense tracer accumulation was noted at the GB fossa area on the whole body scan and SPECT/CT revealed accurate localization of the uptake. There was also noted physiologic tracer uptake in the thyroid bed area by residual thyroid tissue.

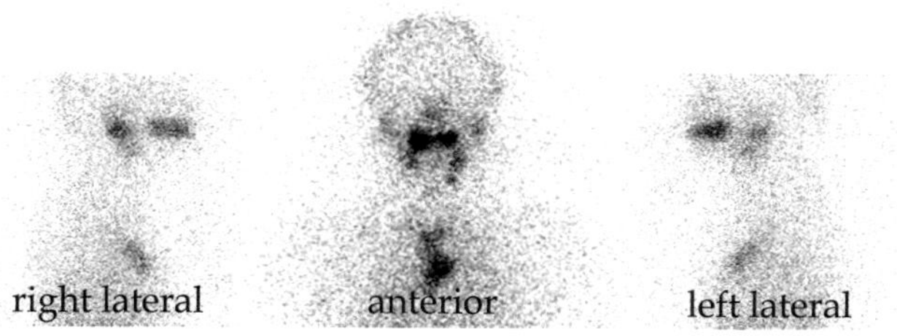

Fig. 12. Physiologic uptake of radioiodine in the thymus. Diffuse, mild radioactivity in the mid-thorax was noted. There was also noted physiologic tracer uptake in the salivary glands (by the NIS expression of the glands) and oral cavity (by saliva containing radioiodine).

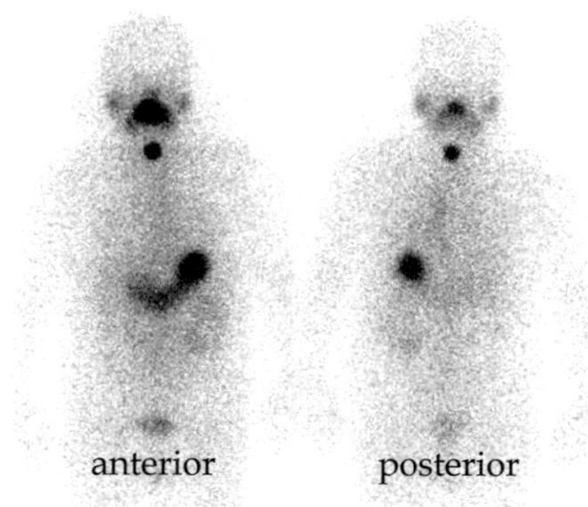

Fig. 13. Physiologic uptake of radioiodine in the stomach. Intense tracer uptake was noted at the left upper quadrant of abdomen due to stomach uptake of the tracer. There was also noted tracer uptake in the oral cavity (radioactivity of secreted saliva), salivary gland (by the NIS expression of the glands), thyroid bed (suggesting remnant thyroid tissue, which has the NIS expression) and urinary bladder (by urine activity).

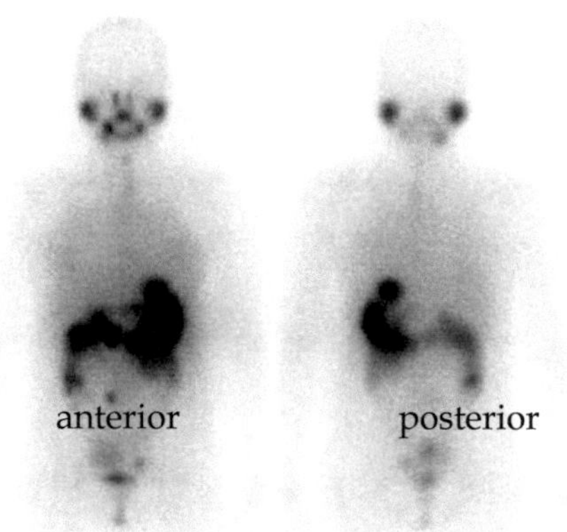

Fig. 14. Focal radioiodine uptake was noted at the center of the abdomen. The uptake might be related to ectopic gastric mucosa in the Meckel's diverticulum. There was also noted tracer uptake in the stomach (by the NIS expression of the gastric mucosa), oral cavity (radioactivity of the secreted saliva) and salivary gland (by the NIS expression of the glands).

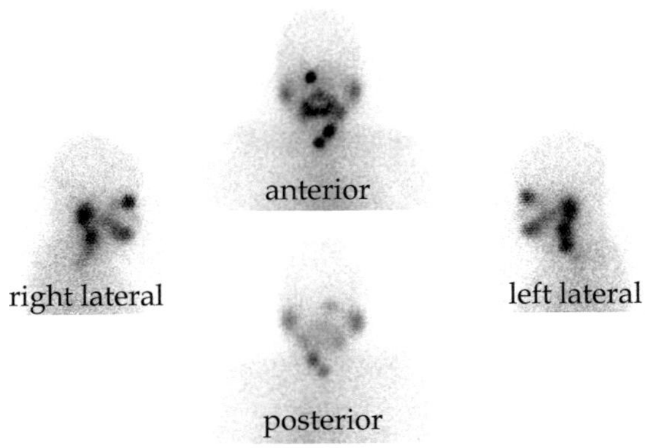

Fig. 15. Physiologic uptake of radioiodine in the lacrimal sac. The uptake is known to be related to active iodine transport by the NIS at the lining epithelium of the sac. There was also noted intense tracer accumulation in the thyroid bed (by remnant tissue of the thyroid, which has the NIS expression) and oral cavity (by the radioactivity of secreted saliva) and minimal tracer uptake in the salivary glands (by the NIS expression of the glands).

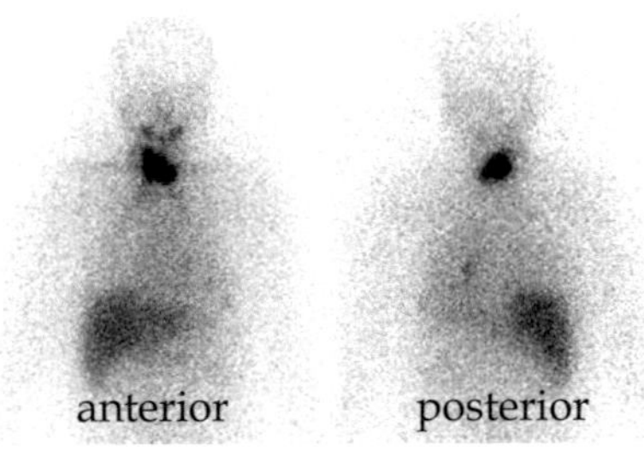

Fig. 16. Physiologic uptake of radioiodine in the liver. The uptake is known to be related to metabolism of radioiodinated thyroglobulin and thyroid hormones in the liver. There was also noted intense tracer accumulation in the thyroid bed (by the remnant tissue of the thyroid).

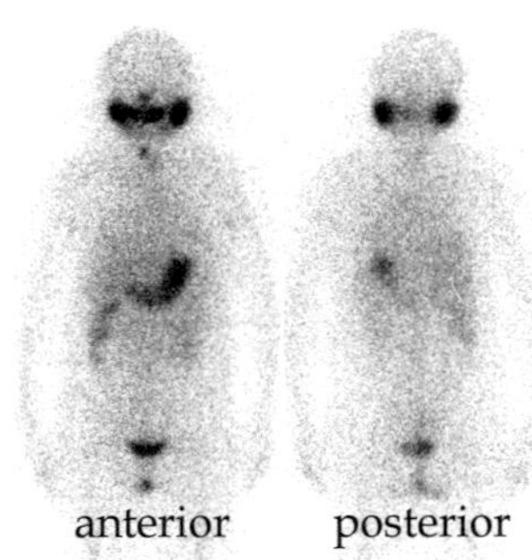

Fig. 17. Physiologic uptake of radioiodine in the urinary bladder. Intense tracer uptake was noted at the suprapubic area by radioactive urine in the bladder. Tracer uptake was noted in the salivary glands (by the NIS expression of the glands) and perineal area (due to urine contamination).

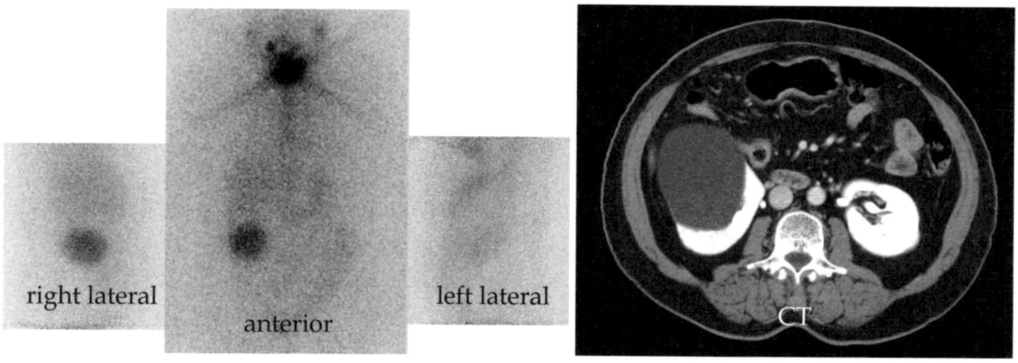

Fig. 18. Physiologic uptake of radioiodine in a simple cyst of the right kidney. Focal tracer uptake was noted at the right side abdomen. The proposed mechanisms are communication between the cyst and the urinary tract and radioiodine secretion by the lining epithelium of the cyst. There was intense tracer uptake noted in the thyroid bed area (by the remnant tissue of the gland) and mild tracer uptake in the salivary gland (by the NIS expression of the glands).

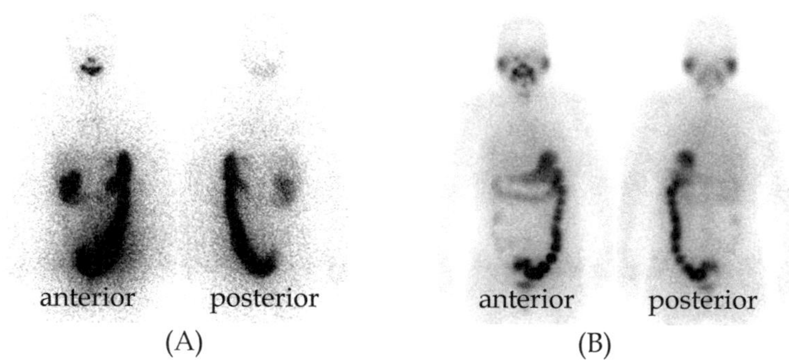

Fig. 19. Physiologic uptake of radioiodine in the colon. Intense tracer uptake was noted at the colon. The suggested mechanisms for the uptake are transportation of radioiodine into the intestine from the mesenteric circulation and biliary excretion of the metabolites of radioiodinated thyroglobulin or thyroid hormones. There was also noted tracer uptake in (A) the oral cavity (by the radioactivity of secreted saliva), (B) the salivary glands (by the NIS expression of the glands) and stomach (by the NIS expression of the gastric mucosa).

5. Pathologic lesions might show false positive radioiodine uptake

A variety of pathologic lesions producing a false positive radioiodine whole body scan have been reported and contrary to the physiologic uptakes that usually do not create diagnostic confusion, they might be tricky enough to cause some patients to undergo unnecessary fruitless invasive surgical or high dose radioiodine treatment.(Mitchell, Pratt et al. 2000)
The not uncommon pathologic lesions showing radioiodine uptake are cystic, inflammatory, non-thyroidal neoplastic diseases. Cystic lesions in various organs can accumulate radioiodine and the mechanism of the uptake is passive diffusion of the tracer into the cysts. Radioiodine accumulation in ovarian, breast and pleuropericardial cysts has been reported.

(Shapiro, Rufini et al. 2000) Effusion of the pleural, pericardial and peritoneal cavities can also have radioiodine uptake by the same mechanism.(Shapiro, Rufini et al. 2000)
A variety of inflammatory and infectious disease can have radioiodine accumulation by increased blood flow that delivers increased levels of radioiodine to the site, and enhanced permeability of the capillary that increases diffusion of the tracer to the extracellular water space.(Shapiro, Rufini et al. 2000) Radioiodine accumulation in bronchiectasis, pulmonary aspergilloma, skin wound, arthritis, paranasal sinusitis, skin infection, myocardial infarction and dacryocystitis has been reported.(Shapiro, Rufini et al. 2000; Ahn, Lee et al. 2011)
Even though only a minority of such lesions accumulate the tracer, a variety of non-thyroidal neoplasms are also known to take up radioiodine. The suggested mechanisms are i) a tumour expression of the NIS, which actively accumulates the tracer and ii) increased vascularity and enhanced capillary permeability that might be secondary to the inflammatory response associated with the neoplasm.(Mitchell, Pratt et al. 2000; Shapiro, Rufini et al. 2000) Radioiodine accumulation in breast cancer, gastric adenocarcinoma, bronchial adenocarcinoma, bronchial squamous carcinoma, salivary adenocarcinoma, teratoma, ovarian adenocarcinoma and meningioma has been reported.(Shapiro, Rufini et al. 2000)
Fortunately, false positive uptake on a radioiodine whole body scan can be interpreted with using the serum thyroglobulin value, which is very sensitive marker for residual or recurrent thyroid cancer. Therefore, the false positive uptake usually does not cause a diagnostic dilemma for experienced practitioners. The clinical features and other imaging studies can also help to distinguish the false positive pathologic lesions from true positive metastatic thyroid cancer lesions.(Mitchell, Pratt et al. 2000; Ahn, Lee et al. 2011)

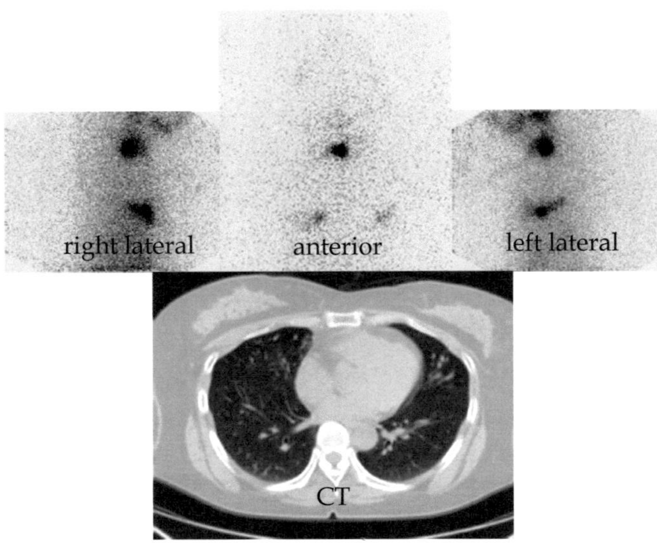

Fig. 20. Pathologic uptake of radioiodine in the bronchectatic lesions of both lungs. There was also noted intense tracer uptake in the thyroid bed area (by the remnant tissue of the gland).

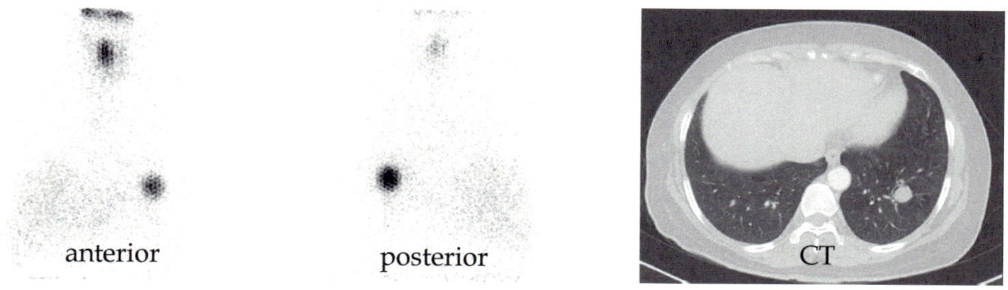

Fig. 21. Pathologic uptake of radioiodine in a pulmonary fungus ball. There was also noted tracer uptake in the thyroid bed area (by the remnant tissue of the gland) and the liver (by metabolism of the radioiodinated thyroglobulin and thyroid hormones).

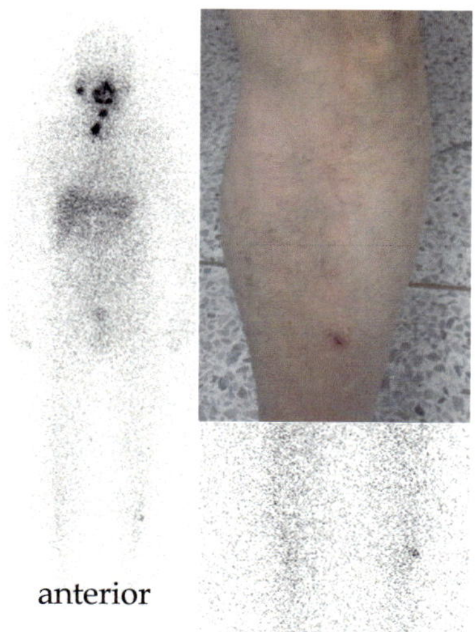

Fig. 22. Pathologic uptake of radioiodine in a skin wound. There was tracer uptake in the left lower leg where the skin wound was located. There was tracer uptake in the salivary gland (by the NIS expression of the glands), thyroid bed (by the remnant tissue of the gland) and the liver (by metabolism of the radioiodinated thyroglobulin and thyroid hormones).

6. Contaminations by physiological secretions

External contamination by physiological or pathological body secretions or excretions can cause positive radioiodine uptake and this mimics metastatic involvement of differentiated thyroid cancer.(Bakheet, Hammami et al. 2000) Sweat, breast milk, urine, vomitus and nasal, tracheobronchial, lacrimal, salivary secretions and faeces contain radioiodine and their contamination on the hair, skin or clothes can be misinterpreted as metastasis of thyroid cancer.(Shapiro, Rufini et al. 2000) Any focus of radioiodine uptake that cannot be explained by physiological or pathological causation must also be suspected as arising from contamination by secretions. Fortunately, the contaminations are usually easily recognized by their pattern and acquiring images after removing the contamination with decontaminating procedures and with taking the stained clothes off. However, unusual patterns of contamination might occur and suspecting uptake lesions as contamination would be difficult.

Patients' peculiar physical characteristics or odd habits produce extraordinary contamination patterns. Uptake in the scalp or a wig has been reported in patient with excessive sweating, and contamination of a wig was reported in patient with a bizarre habit of styling hair with sputum.(Bakheet, Hammami et al. 2000) False positive scans due to contamination can be kept to a minimum by careful preparation of patients, such as image acquisition in a clean gown after taking a shower.
Contaminations are almost always superficial, (Carlisle, Lu et al. 2003), therefore, the use of lateral and/or oblique views to give a third dimension to the scan may help to identify the contamination. Furthermore, the SPECT image alone or the SPECT image fused with the anatomical image, which provides detailed information about the anatomic location of the radiotracer uptake sites, can be the best way to correctly determine that contamination is the reason for the uptakes.

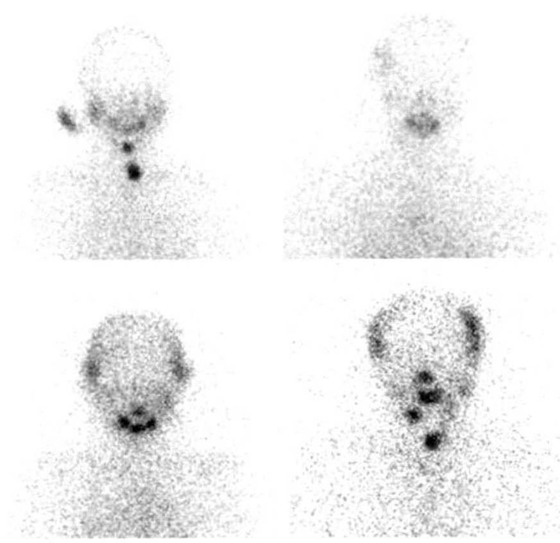

Fig. 23. Cases with contaminations at the hair and scalp. A case with unilateral hair contamination by saliva and cases with uni- or bilateral scalp contamination by excessive perspiration are demonstrated.

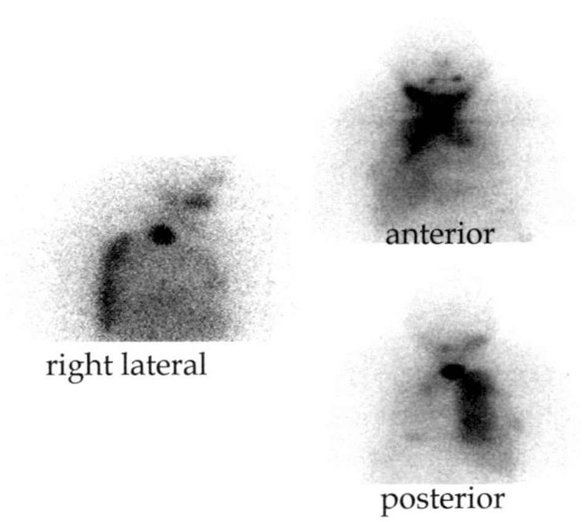

Fig. 24. Contamination at the right posterior chest wall by excessive perspiration. There was also noted intense tracer accumulation in the thyroid bed (by remnant tissue of the thyroid and edema of the cervical soft tissue).

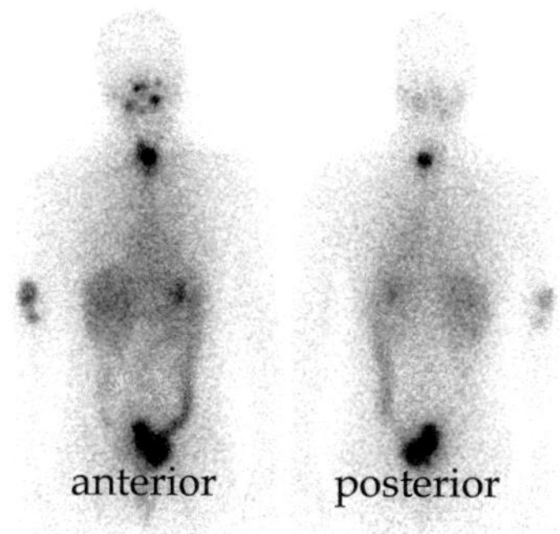

Fig. 25. Contamination at the skin of the right upper arm. There was also noted intense tracer accumulation in the rectum and moderate tracer accumulation in the descending colon and the liver.

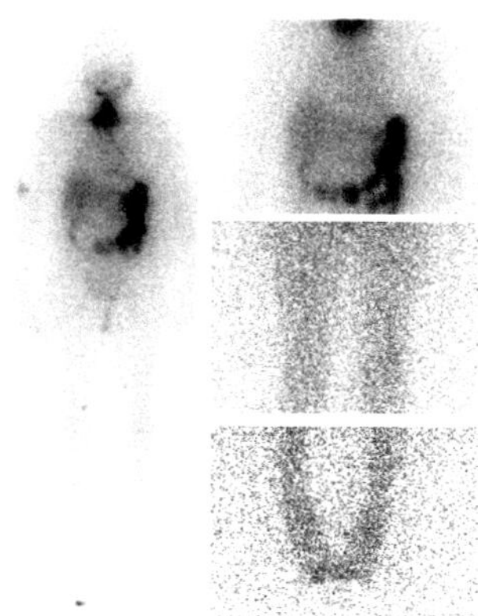

Fig. 26. Vanishing contaminations after cleansing the right forearm, both thighs and right foot. There was also noted intense tracer accumulation in the thyroid bed area and colon and moderate tracer accumulation in the liver.

	Sites of uptake	Mechamism of radioiodine uptake
	Physiologic	
Residual thyroid tissue	thyroid bed	Active radioiodine uptake by expression of the NIS
Ectopic normal thyroid tissues	Lingual thyroid mediatinal thyroid Intratracheal thyroid Paracardiac thyroid Intraheaptic thyroid	Active radioiodine uptake by the expression of the NIS
Salivary gland	Parotid and submandibular salivary glands	Active radioiodine uptake by the expression of the NIS
Lacrimal sac/nasolacrimal duct Lacrimal gland*	Ocular and periocular area	Active radioiodine uptake by the expression of the NIS **controversial*

	Sites of uptake	Mechamism of radioiodine uptake
By excreted or swallowed saiva	Oral cavity Oesophagus Oesophageal diverticulum Oesophageal stricture or scarring Achalasia	Focal accumulated saliva with radioiodine activity from the salivary glands
By nasal secretion	Nose "hot nose"	Focal accumulated nasal secretion with radioiodine
By excreted urine	Renal pelvis Ureter Urinary bladder Urinary tract diverticulum Urinary tract fistula Renal cyst*	Accumulated urine radioiodine activity excreted by the kidneys * *Active radioiodine uptake by the expression of the NIS can be another mechanism*
Choroid plexus	Brain	Active radioiodine uptake by the expression of the NIS
Thymic uptake	Thymus	Expression of the NIS in thymic tissues and/or iodine concentration by Hassal's bodies
Gastric mucosa	Stomach Gastric duplication cyst Meckel's diverticulum Barrett esophagus	Active radioiodine uptake by the expression of the NIS
By excreted gastric secretion	Oesophageal uptake Bowel uptake	Gastroesophagel reflux Translocation of excreted gastric secretion into the bowel
Metabolism of radioiodinated proteins	Liver Biliary tract Gall bladder Bowels	Metabolism of radioiodinated thyroid hormones or thyroglobulin and their excretion into the gall bladder and bowels via the biliary tract
Breast	Breast, especially lactating	Active radioiodine uptake by the expression of the NIS
Colon	Diffuse and/or focal (any part of colon)	Transport of radioiodine into the intestine from the mesenteric circulation and biliary excretion of the metabolites of radioiodinated thyroglobulin.
Pathologic		
Heterotopic thyroid tissue	Struma ovarii	Active radioiodine uptake by the expression of the NIS
Inflammations associated with/without infection	Pericarditis Skin burn Dental disease Arthritis Cholecystitis Folliculitis Paranasal sinusitis Dacryocystitis Bronchiectasis Fungal infection (eg, aspergilloma)	Increased perfusion and vasodilation, and enhanced capillary permeability by the inflammation

	Sites of uptake	Mechamism of radioiodine uptake
	Pleural and pericardial effusions	
Non-thyroidal neoplasm	Gastric adenocarcinoma Salivary adenocarcinoma Lung adenocarcinoma Fibroadenoma Meningioma Nurilemoma Teratoma	Active radioiodine uptake by the NIS of the tumor and/or incresed blood flow and enhanced capillary permeability in the tumor
Trauma	Biopsy site Tracheostomy site	Increased perfusion and vasodilation, and enhanced capillary permeability by the tissue trauma
Contaminations		
Tear	Skin of any part of the body, hair, wig, cloth, etc	Contamination by physiological or pathological body secretions or excretions
Saliva		
Sweat		
Vomitus		
Breast milk		
Urine		
Feces		

Table 4. Causes of radioiodine uptake not related to thyroid cancer on the radioiodine whole body scan.

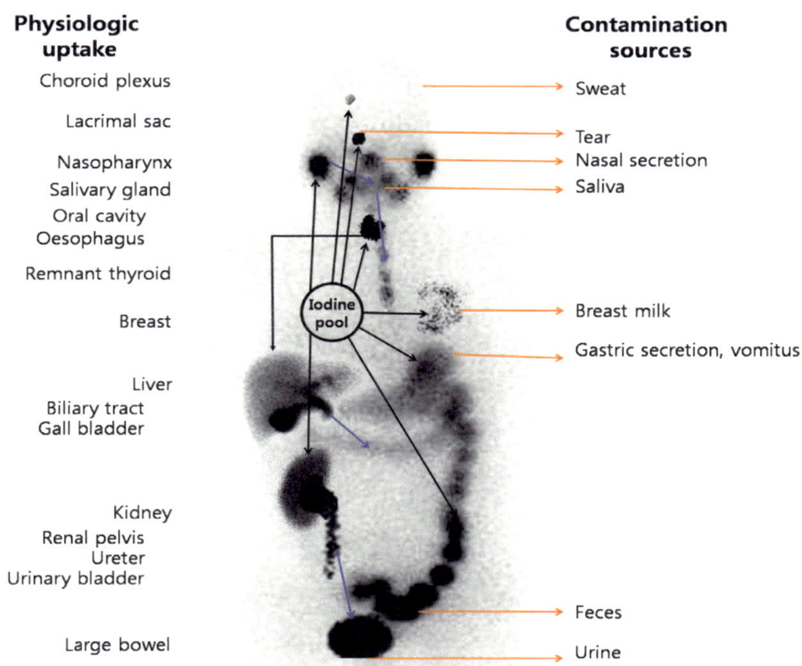

Fig. 27. Schematic presentation for the locations of physiologic uptake and possible contamination sources the radioiodine whole body scans.

7. Conclusion

A whole body scan obtained with the administration of a diagnostic or therapeutic dose of radioiodine has a definite role in the management of patients with well differentiated thyroid cancer after total thyroidectomy. Accurate interpretation of the scan requires a thorough knowledge and understanding of potential confounding factors for uptakes on the scan, and recognition of the variable causes of false positive uptake will provide correct prognostic inferences and prevent inappropriate therapeutic interventions. In addition, the cause of radioiodine uptake on the scan is always evaluated in conjunction with the serum thyroglobulin level and the clinico-radiological results in order to lessen the chance of an incorrect conclusion about the uptakes.

This chapter was written to make readers consider a broad variety of diseases as the causes of the uptake on the radioiodine whole body scan and I have demonstrated a wide variety of causes of false positive uptakes on these scans.

8. Acknowledgment

The author thanks Doctor Do-Hoon Kim for gathering the radioiodine whole body images.

9. References

Ahad, F. and S. A. Ganie (2010). "Iodine, Iodine metabolism and Iodine deficiency disorders revisited." Indian J Endocrinol Metab 14(1): 13-7.

Ahn, B. C., S. W. Lee, et al. (2011). "Pulmonary Aspergilloma Mimicking Metastasis from Papillary Thyroid Cancer." Thyroid 21(5): 555-8.

Amin, N. P., R. Junco, et al. "A short-term diet to Prepare for radioactive Iodine treatment or scan." from http://www.entrustmd.com/low-iodine-diet-entrust-medical-group-orange-ca.html.

Bakheet, S. M., M. M. Hammami, et al. (1996). "False-positive radioiodine uptake in the abdomen and the pelvis: radioiodine retention in the kidneys and review of the literature." Clin Nucl Med 21(12): 932-7.

Bakheet, S. M., M. M. Hammami, et al. (2000). "Radioiodine uptake in the head and neck." Endocr Pract 6(1): 37-41.

Baril, P., P. Martin-Duque, et al. (2010). "Visualization of gene expression in the live subject using the Na/I symporter as a reporter gene: applications in biotherapy." Br J Pharmacol 159(4): 761-71.

Carlisle, M. R., C. Lu, et al. (2003). "The interpretation of 131I scans in the evaluation of thyroid cancer, with an emphasis on false positive findings." Nucl Med Commun 24(6): 715-35.

Dai, G., O. Levy, et al. (1996). "Cloning and characterization of the thyroid iodide transporter." Nature 379(6564): 458-60.

Geerlings, J. A., A. van Zuijlen, et al. "The value of I-131 SPECT in the detection of recurrent differentiated thyroid cancer." Nucl Med Commun 31(5): 417-22.

Hall, J. E. (2011). Textbook of medical physiology. Philadelphia, Saunders Elsevier.

Hays, M. T. (1993). "Colonic excretion of iodide in normal human subjects." Thyroid 3(1): 31-5.

Hyer, S. L., K. Newbold, et al. (2010). "Early and late toxicity of radioiodine therapy: detection and management." Endocr Pract 16(6): 1064-70.

Luster, M., S. E. Clarke, et al. (2008). "Guidelines for radioiodine therapy of differentiated thyroid cancer." Eur J Nucl Med Mol Imaging 35(10): 1941-59.

Ma, C., A. Kuang, et al. (2005). "Possible explanations for patients with discordant findings of serum thyroglobulin and 131I whole-body scanning." J Nucl Med 46(9): 1473-80.

Mitchell, G., B. E. Pratt, et al. (2000). "False positive 131I whole body scans in thyroid cancer." Br J Radiol 73(870): 627-35.

Morgenstern, K. E., D. D. Vadysirisack, et al. (2005). "Expression of sodium iodide symporter in the lacrimal drainage system: implication for the mechanism underlying nasolacrimal duct obstruction in I(131)-treated patients." Ophthal Plast Reconstr Surg 21(5): 337-44.

Nostrand, D. V., G. Bloom, et al. (2004). Thyroid cancer; A guide for patients. Baltimore, Keystone Press, Inc.

Oh, J. R., B. H. Byun, et al. (2011). "Comparison of (131)I whole-body imaging, (131)I SPECT/CT, and (18)F-FDG PET/CT in the detection of metastatic thyroid cancer." Eur J Nucl Med Mol Imaging.

Ozguven, M., S. Ilgan, et al. (2004). "Unusual patterns of I-131 contamination." Ann Nucl Med 18(3): 271-4.

Rault, E., S. Vandenberghe, et al. (2007). "Comparison of image quality of different iodine isotopes (I-123, I-124, and I-131)." Cancer Biother Radiopharm 22(3): 423-30.

Riesco-Eizaguirre, G. and P. Santisteban (2006). "A perspective view of sodium iodide symporter research and its clinical implications." Eur J Endocrinol 155(4): 495-512.

Shapiro, B., V. Rufini, et al. (2000). "Artifacts, anatomical and physiological variants, and unrelated diseases that might cause false-positive whole-body 131-I scans in patients with thyroid cancer." Semin Nucl Med 30(2): 115-32.

Silberstein, E. B., A. Alavi, et al. (2006). "Society of Nuclear Medicine Procedure Guideline for Scintigraphy for Differentiated Papillary and Follicular Thyroid Cancer."

Silberstein, E. B., A. Alavi, et al. (2005). "Society of Nuclear Medicine Procedure Guideline for Therapy of Thyroid Disease with Iodine-131 (Sodium Iodide) Version 2.0."

Smanik, P. A., Q. Liu, et al. (1996). "Cloning of the human sodium lodide symporter." Biochem Biophys Res Commun 226(2): 339-45.

Spanu, A., M. E. Solinas, et al. (2009). "131I SPECT/CT in the follow-up of differentiated thyroid carcinoma: incremental value versus planar imaging." J Nucl Med 50(2): 184-90.

Tazebay, U. H., I. L. Wapnir, et al. (2000). "The mammary gland iodide transporter is expressed during lactation and in breast cancer." Nat Med 6(8): 871-8.

Van Nostrand, D., S. Moreau, et al. (2010). "(124)I positron emission tomography versus (131)I planar imaging in the identification of residual thyroid tissue and/or metastasis in patients who have well-differentiated thyroid cancer." Thyroid 20(8): 879-83.

Von Schulthess, G. K. and T. F. Hany (2008). "Imaging and PET-PET/CT imaging." J Radiol 89(3 Pt 2): 438-47; quiz 448.

Zimmermann, M. B. and C. M. Crill "Iodine in enteral and parenteral nutrition." Best Pract Res Clin Endocrinol Metab 24(1): 143-58.

2

Internal Radiation Dosimetry: Models and Applications

Ernesto Amato, Alfredo Campennì, Astrid Herberg, Fabio Minutoli and Sergio Baldari
University of Messina, Department of Radiological Sciences, Nuclear Medicine Unit, Italy

1. Introduction

Internal radiation dosimetry has a fundamental and growing role in planning nuclear medicine therapies with radionuclides.

The principle of nuclear medicine therapy is to destroy pathologic tissues through the irradiation with the ionizing radiation emitted by properly chosen radionuclides, while preserving other organs and tissues from unnecessary exposure to the same radiation.

In order to realize this result, proper pharmaceuticals are chosen with a biodistribution targeted on target tissues, and labelled with a suitably chosen radionuclide. The choice of the best radionuclide is carried on with the aim of maximizing radiation energy deposition in the target tissue during the desired treatment time. Beta-emitters are the best choice in most cases, because beta radiation has a mean range in tissue from few millimetres to few centimetres. Also used are alpha- and Auger-emitters, for millimetre and sub-millimetre ranges.

The absorbed dose to the target tissues as well as to other organs and tissues depends from the biokinetics of the radiopharmaceutical and from the physical decay scheme of the radionuclide employed. While the physical properties of each nuclide are well known from experimental data, the biodistribution of the radiopharmaceutical within the patient's body depends on the dynamic biologic pathway that in turns is governed by the role of the molecule, by the characteristics of the patient, by the type and stage of the disease, and by the route of administration.

The distribution of radioactivity within the human body must be sampled several times post-administration, by means of planar or tomographic (SPECT or PET) imaging techniques. Tomographic techniques are rapidly substituting planar whole body imaging, since, thanks also to the accurate attenuation correction and image co-registration brought by a simultaneous CT scan, they reach a spatial resolution and an accuracy in activity quantification unprecedented.

After a general introduction on dosimetric quantities and their relationships, we focus on the dosimetric anthropomorphic models. We introduce also 3D techniques based on voxel dose factors, convolution of dose point-kernels and direct Monte Carlo computation, focusing on the contribution of Monte Carlo simulation to the development of new and more accurate dosimetric and microdosimetric models for internal dosimetry.

We describe the application of such dosimetric approaches in the main nuclear medicine therapies such as the ^{131}I therapy of thyroid diseases, the therapy of neuroendocrine tumours (NET) with somatostatin analogues labelled with beta- or Auger-emitters, and the palliation of painful bone metastases, focusing on dose-efficacy relationships and on the limiting of side effects to other potentially critical organs.

2. Definitions

If we consider a radioactive volume containing, at the time t, N radioactive nuclei, we know that the activity $A(t)$, representing the number of decays per second, is proportional to N through the decay constant λ:

$$A(t) = \frac{dN}{dt} = -\lambda N \tag{1}$$

Equation 1 can be integrated, leading to the exponential decay law for the number of radio-atoms present at the time t in a radioactive sample:

$$N = N_0 e^{-\lambda t} \tag{2}$$

The decay constant λ is related to the decay time τ and to the half-life $T_{1/2}$ by the relationships:

$$T_{1/2} = \frac{\ln 2}{\lambda} = \tau \ln 2 \tag{3}$$

The SI unit of activity is the *Becquerel* (Bq), defined as one disintegration per second:

$$1Bq = 1dis \cdot s^{-1}, \tag{4}$$

while the old unit of activity was the *Curie* (Ci):

$$1Ci = 3.7 \times 10^{10} Bq \tag{5}$$

The radiation absorbed dose, commonly intended as dose, is defined as the average energy imparted by the radiation per unit mass of the irradiated volume:

$$D = \frac{d\overline{E}}{dm} \tag{6}$$

In the SI system, the dose is expressed in joules per kilogram or Gray (Gy); the older unit, no longer employed but often encountered in aged texts, was the Rad (1 erg/g). The conversion is such that 1 Gy = 100 Rad.

In internal dosimetry, the dose to an organ or tissue accumulating a radiopharmaceutical can be evaluated following the MIRD approach (Snyder et al., 1975).

The dose imparted to a target volume k from a single source volume h, can be calculated as:

$$D(r_k \leftarrow r_h) = \tilde{A}_h S(r_k \leftarrow r_h) \tag{7}$$

where $\tilde{A}_h$ is the cumulated activity in the source organ and S is the average dose absorbed by the target per unit cumulated activity in the source. The cumulated activity in h is defined as the total number of disintegrations in that organ, i.e. the integral of the activity A over the time:

$$\tilde{A}_h = \int_0^{\infty} A_h(t)dt \ , \tag{8}$$

The definition of the S factor appearing in Equation 7 is:

$$S(r_k \leftarrow r_h) = \frac{\sum_i \Delta_i \varphi_i (r_k \leftarrow r_h)}{m_k} \tag{9}$$

where Δ_i is the average energy emitted per transition as i-th radiation, φ_i is the "absorbed fraction", i.e. the fraction of the energy emitted in the source volume r_h which was absorbed in the target volume r_k, and m_k is the mass of the target.
In general, if several organs accumulate the radiopharmaceutical, the overall dose to the target volume (organ or tissue) k is obtained by summing up all the contributions coming from the various regions h:

$$D(r_k) = \sum_h \tilde{A}_h \sum_i \Delta_i \Phi_i (r_k \leftarrow r_h) / m_h \tag{10}$$

Another usually employed quantity is the residence time, defined as the ratio between the cumulated activity in h and the administered activity A_0:

$$\tau_h = \frac{\tilde{A}_h}{A_0} \tag{11}$$

Even if the residence time has the physical dimensions of a time and it is often indicated with the same Greek letter, it must not be confused with the decay time of a radionuclide. In fact, while the decay time is the time necessary to reduce by 1/e = 0.37 the activity of an isolated sample, the residence time is the length of time an activity A_0 would have to reside in the volume to give that cumulated activity.

3. Radiobiological models of the radiation effects

The estimation of the effect of the radiation absorbed dose in biological tissues can not neglect biological models accounting for the ability of tissues and cells to repair in some degree the radiation-induced injury. (Cremonesi, 2011; Strigari, 2011)
The radiation damage can vary due to the different tissue properties (the "five Rs" of radiobiology: *repair, repopulation, reoxigenation, redistribution* and *intrinsic radiosensitivity*) in tumours and in healthy tissues, and due to the difference in possible irradiation regimes (type and energy of the radiation, dose rate, repetition or fractionation of treatments).
In nuclear medicine therapies with radiopharmaceuticals, the radiation dose is often imparted by beta or Auger electrons, even if the role of alpha emitters as therapeutic agents is increasing again.

Thus, the dose and the dose rate in the single treatment are governed by the biokinetics of the radiopharmaceutical and by the administered activity and route of administration.
The biological effect of such irradiation in tumours and in healthy tissues will depend firstly on the *repair* ability of the sub-lethal damage with related repair time T_{rep}, which is due to the mechanisms that counteract all the natural damages to the DNA. This is the fastest mechanism influencing the response to irradiation, since its effects are detectable in external irradiations already after 30 minutes.
The cell life cycle is divided in four consecutive steps: G1, S, G2 and M. The two gaps of apparent inactivity, G1 and G2, divide the two active phases, the DNA synthesis S and the mitosis M. Radiobiology studies demonstrated that the highest cell radiosensitivity belongs to G2 and M phases. After an irradiation, the survival fraction will be higher for cells in the G1 or S phases; thus a *redistribution* of population is initiated, with a synchronization of cell life cycles.
This effect could, in principle, play a certain role in external irradiations repeated at the times of higher sensitivity, but no clear evidence of efficacy has been demonstrated yet.
Cells surviving to an exposure to radiations will continue to proliferate; such a repopulation has a detrimental effect on therapeutic results. On the other hand, tumour cell death leads to tumour tissue shrinkage and, consequently, can improve the *reoxigenation* of the residual hypoxic cells. Since hypoxic cells are more radio-resistant than the oxygenated ones, repeated cycles of irradiation are useful to improve therapeutic outcomes.
As a consequence of these mechanisms, the effect of a radiation therapy depends not only on the radiation absorbed dose, but also on the dose rate and on the fractionation regime.
The most widely applied radiobiological model describing cell survival after irradiations is the linear-quadratic model, in which the effect E, in logarithmic relation with the surviving fraction SF, is a function of the dose D and the dose squared:

$$E = -\log(SF) = \alpha D + \beta D^2 \tag{12}$$

The linear component accounts for the lethal cell damage given by a single radiation producing, for example, double-strand breaks of the DNA helix, while the quadratic component accounts for the lethal damage obtained by summing up the effects of two consecutive ionizing radiations. It should be noticed that the parameter α has dimensions of Gy^{-1}, while β of Gy^{-2}. The dose in correspondence of which the linear contribution L equals the quadratic one Q (see Fig. 1), is given by $D= \alpha/\beta$ (Gy). This value expresses the *intrinsic radiosensitivity* of the tissue, and external as well as internal radiation therapies exploit the higher radiosensitivity of cancer cells with respect to normal tissue cells.
When the radiation dose is imparted in a time T comparable or even longer than the repair time of the sub-lethal damage, T_{rep}, Eq. 12 must be corrected in order to account for the competition between radiation-induced damage and cell repair rate:

$$E = -\log(SF) = \alpha D + g(T)\beta D^2 \tag{13}$$

where $g(T)$ is a properly chosen function of the irradiation time. When $T \gg T_{rep}$, as in the case of targeted radionuclide therapies, it was demonstrated that a good approximation is:

$$g = \frac{T_{rep}}{T_{rep} + T_{eff}} \tag{14}$$

where T_{eff} is the effective half-life of the radionuclide in the target tissue.

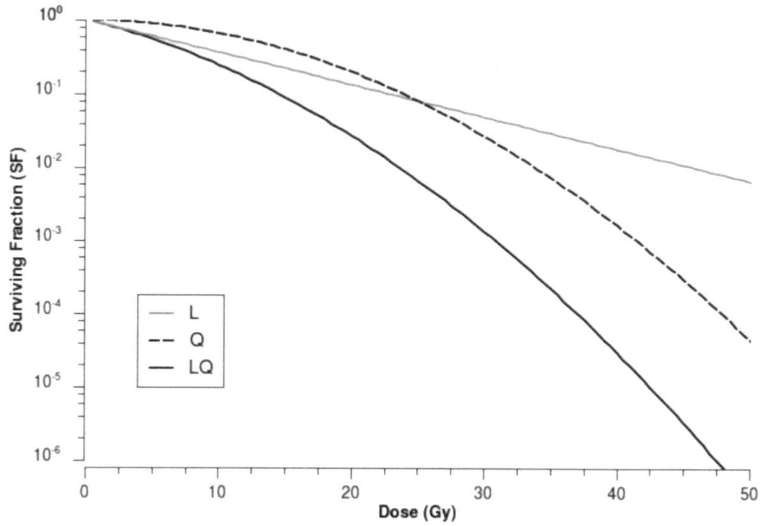

Fig. 1. Cell surviving fraction as a function of the radiation dose, following the linear-quadratic (LQ) model. Linear (L) and quadratic (Q) part of the equation are represented, too. In the proposed example, $\alpha/\beta = 25$ Gy.

The Biologically Effective Dose (*BED*) is defined in a way such that the effect *E* is linearly related to *BED* through the parameter α:

$$E = \alpha BED \tag{15}$$

From Eq. 13, *BED* is related to the cell surviving fraction and to the dose with the relationships:

$$BED = -\frac{1}{\alpha}\log(SF) = D + \frac{\beta}{\alpha}g(T)D^2 \tag{16}$$

For radionuclide therapies, Eq. 14 holds for the correction factor *g*, resulting, for a single irradiation imparting a radiation dose *D*:

$$BED = D + \frac{\beta}{\alpha}\frac{T_{rep}}{T_{rep} + T_{eff}}D^2 \tag{17}$$

In the case of repeated irradiations, each one imparting a dose D_i, the total *BED* can be calculated as:

$$BED = \sum D_i + \frac{\beta}{\alpha}\frac{T_{rep}}{T_{rep} + T_{eff}}\sum D_i^2 \tag{18}$$

In the next Sections, we will see how BED is related to the impairment of kidneys after repeated cycles of peptide radio-receptor therapies (PRRT) with somatostatin analogues labelled with beta-emitting radioisotopes. In such evaluations, it is usually assumed α/β = 2.4 Gy and for T_{rep} a value of 2.8 hours.

4. Time sampling and determination of the cumulated activity

In Section 2, the main equations of internal dosimetry were introduced, and the role played by the cumulated activity, i.e. the total number of disintegrations in the considered target, was taken in evidence.

In general, the biokinetics of a radiopharmaceutical within the human body will be influenced by the type of the carrier molecule and its physiologic and pathologic pathway, by the route of administration and by the preparation and clinical state of the patient. Clinical studies and trials give information about the average residence times of groups of patients, but, in order to plan the single treatment, only an accurate individualized dosimetry can be usefully employed.

In order to calculate the cumulated activity, the activity up-taken in each organ or region of interest must be properly sampled after administration. In principle, more measurements allow a more accurate fit of the A=A(t) curve, and, consequently, a better estimation of the total number of disintegrations.

However, we must remember that each measurement is carried out through planar scintigraphic or emission computed tomography (ECT) techniques, which are time consuming for both patient and hospital personnel.

Even in the case of non-imaging techniques, such as thyroid uptake measurements with a scintillation probe, the patient must come back to the nuclear medicine department for each measurement.

Hence the need to optimize dosimetric protocols in order to the number and timing of the acquisitions. The optimal choice will depend on the expected biokinetics of the radiopharmaceutical in the organs of interest, which can be assumed from previous clinical studies.

The simplest model applies when the uptake phase, i.e. the phase in which the radiopharmaceutical is accumulating in the organ and its radioactivity rises with time, is short enough to be considered instantaneous. Consequently, immediately after administration, the washout phase begins.

If, in the simplest assumption, the radiopharmaceutical is washed out with a mono-exponential rate, the variation of N with time follows a law analogous to Eq. 1:

$$\frac{dN}{dt} = \lambda_{eff} N \tag{19}$$

where the effective decay constant $\lambda_{eff} = \lambda + \lambda_{bio}$ is given by the sum of the physical decay constant introduced in Eq. 1 and the biological decay constant, characteristic of the biological wash-out of the radiopharmaceutical from the organ. In analogy with Eq. 3, the effective decay time τ_{eff} and the effective half-life T_{eff} can be defined as:

$$T_{eff} = \frac{\ln 2}{\lambda_{eff}} = \tau_{eff} \ln 2 \tag{20}$$

and the cumulated activity will be:

$$\tilde{A} = A\int_0^\infty e^{-\lambda_{eff}t}dt = \frac{A}{\lambda_{eff}} \tag{21}$$

In more complex cases, the uptake phase can require a certain amount of time and, consequently, the assumption of instantaneous uptake must be released and the uptake phase can be usually described by an exponential growth. Furthermore, the washout phase can be not accurately described by a simple mono-exponential decay. For example, a bi-exponential curve can fit better to a biokinetical behaviour composed by a first phase of rapid clearance in which the biologic half-life is much smaller than the physical half-life, followed by a slower retention phase in which, on the contrary, it is the physical half-life that governs the overall effective half-life.

In Figure 2, an example of near-instantaneous uptake, followed by a washout phase described by a bi-exponential decay, is shown. The renal uptake of a diagnostic dose of ^{111}In-DTPA-Octreotide, a somatostatin analogue used for the diagnosis of neuroendocrine tumours, was imaged at 1, 6, 24 and 48 hours post-injection.

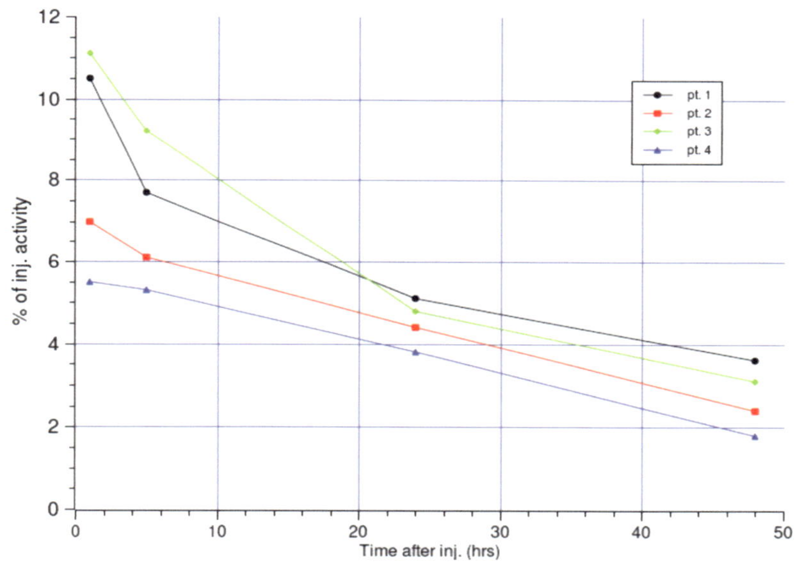

Fig. 2. Uptake curves for kidneys in four patients after ^{111}In-DTPA-Octreotide intravenous administration.

In Figure 3 we present three examples of ^{131}I uptake curves for hyperthyroid patients (pt. 1 and 2 affected by toxic nodular goitre, TNG, and the third by Basedow disease), acquired by means of a scintillation probe at six times after oral administration of a diagnostic activity of 1.8 MBq.

In these cases, the uptake phase is expected to last up to one day, followed by a decay phase with a characteristic half-life of 100-200 hours, deriving from both physical (eight days) and biological decay.

Thanks to the simplicity and rapidity of thyroid uptake measurements with a gamma probe, it is possible to sample properly in time these patients. Usually, two measurements during the first day, 3 and 6 hours after oral administration, properly characterize the uptake phase.

Measurements can proceed at 24, 48, 72 (or 96, or 120) and 168 hours, in order to detect the maximum uptake and the decay phase.
Points can be then fitted with the function:

$$U(t) = \frac{\lambda_{in} U_{max}}{\lambda_{out} - \lambda_{in}} \left(e^{-\lambda_{in} t} - e^{-\lambda_{out} t} \right) \tag{22}$$

where the uptake and washout constants λ_{in} and λ_{out} depend upon the rapidity of the increase and decrease in uptake, respectively.
Even if the maximum uptake is expected, on average, around 24 hours, this is not a rigid rule, of course. Patient 3, for example, reached the maximum uptake already at the sixth hour, and the fit of patient 1 data show its maximum earlier than 24 hours; cases of late maxima are observed, too.
In order to evaluate properly the effective half-time of the washout phase, measurements should extend at least up to 120 hours, better up to 168 hours. In fact, since each point is affected by statistical fluctuations and by minor biases due to the practical procedure, repeated measurements help in reducing errors in fit.
As an example, in Figure 3 we represent, together with the fits of the whole data series (solid lines), the fits obtained by considering only the first four points, i.e. 3, 6, 24 and 48 hours (dashed lines).
It is apparent from figure the underestimation of the decay time for the first patient, and, on the contrary, the overestimation for the second one.
Such outcome is confirmed numerically by the results reported in Table 1, where the effective half-time of the washout, T_{eff}, is calculated from the decay constants obtained from the complete fit and from the 3-48 hours data. Results from incomplete data give a 24% shorter half-time for the first patient, while for the second one an overestimation as high as 91% comes from a dosimetric protocol limited to 48 hours.

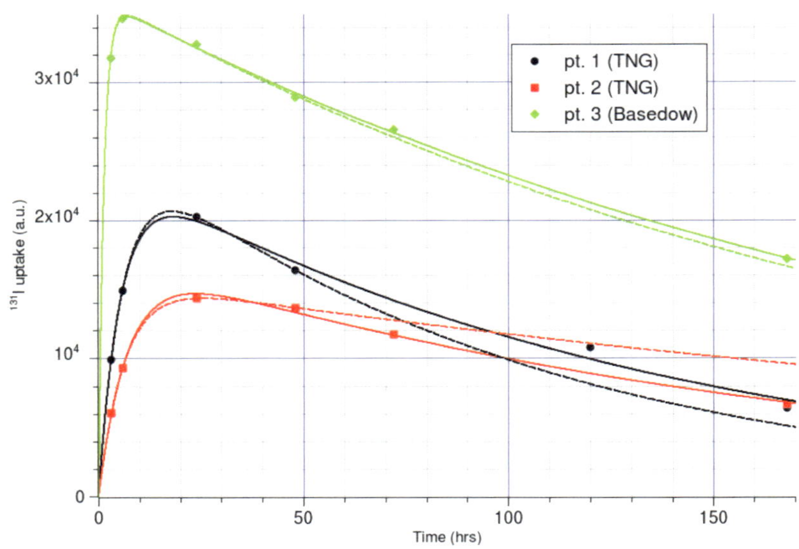

Fig. 3. ^{131}I uptake curves for the three patients. Solid curves represent the analytical fits of complete data series with Eq. 22, dashed lines represent fits of 3-48 hours data.

Pt. no.	U_{max}	λ_{in}	λ_{out}	λ_{out}(48h)	T_{eff}	T_{eff}(48h)	error
1 (TNG)	23184	0.184	7.41E-3	9.72E-3	93	71	-24%
2 (TNG)	16755	0.142	5.62E-3	2.95E-3	123	235	+91%
3 (Bas.)	35920	0.740	4.42E-3	4.66E-3	157	148	-6%

Table 1. Fit parameters for the complete data series, and for the first four points. Relative error in T_{eff} determination are reported.

5. Anthropomorphic models for internal dosimetry

In the past decades, several schematic anthropomorphic models were proposed in order to standardize and simplify dose calculation both in medical applications of radionuclides and in internal contamination evaluations for radiological protection purposes.

Among these, a common approach to internal dosimetry is based on standardized phantoms and S factors pre-calculated for couples of Source-Target organs and for various radionuclides (Snyder et al., 1975).

Organ S factors were calculated through Monte Carlo simulations and are currently available in a tabular form. As a consequence, once calculated the cumulated activity in the source organ with the methods described in the previous Section, the dose to the target organ is calculated with Equation 7, using the proper S factor accounting for the radionuclide emission and for the geometry of the source-target couple.

An advantage of this method is the simplicity of measurements and the standardization of the dosimetric procedure, allowing easier comparisons between results. However, the simplified organ models, described by fixed geometrical shapes and volumes, do not account properly for the anatomy of the single patient. Furthermore, each organ is treated as a whole, neglecting inhomogeneity in the uptake within each organ or tissue.

In real cases, the shape and size of an organ can be varied by a disease, and pathologic tissues, which are the target of the treatment, are not present in standard models of healthy humans.

A sphere model is often employed in order to represent small target tissues such as tumours or pathologic lymph-nodes. Recently, we developed a model to calculate the absorbed fractions in ellipsoidal shapes uptaking beta-gamma emitting radionuclides (Amato et al. 2009, 2011).

Considering a radionuclide which emits mono-energetic and beta electrons, and gamma photons, the average dose to the target volume is given by:

$$\overline{D} = D_\beta + D_e + D_\gamma = \frac{\tilde{A}}{m}\left[\int \frac{dn(E)}{dE} E\varphi(E)dE + \sum_i \left(n_{e,i}E_{e,i}\varphi_{e,i} + n_{\gamma,i}E_{\gamma,i}\varphi_{\gamma,i}\right)\right], \qquad (23)$$

where n_e and n_γ are the mono-energetic electron and gamma photon emission probabilities, respectively, of energies E_e and $E\gamma$, φ_e and φ_γ are the electron and photon absorbed fractions. These absorbed fractions can be derived from the equation:

$$\varphi(\rho) = \left(1 + \frac{\rho_0}{\rho^s}\right)^{-1} \qquad (24)$$

where ρ is the "generalized radius", defined as:

$$\rho = 3\frac{V}{S} \tag{25}$$

where V and S are the volume and surface of the ellipsoid. The parameters ρ_0 and s in Equation 24 depend on the nature (electron or photon) and energy of the radiation, and can be derived from proper parametric functions described in (Amato et al. 2009, 2011).

In Figure 4, the absorbed fraction as a function of the generalized radius is reported for photons and electrons uniformly emitted in ellipsoids of various shapes. These data are calculated by means of a Monte Carlo simulation in Geant4.

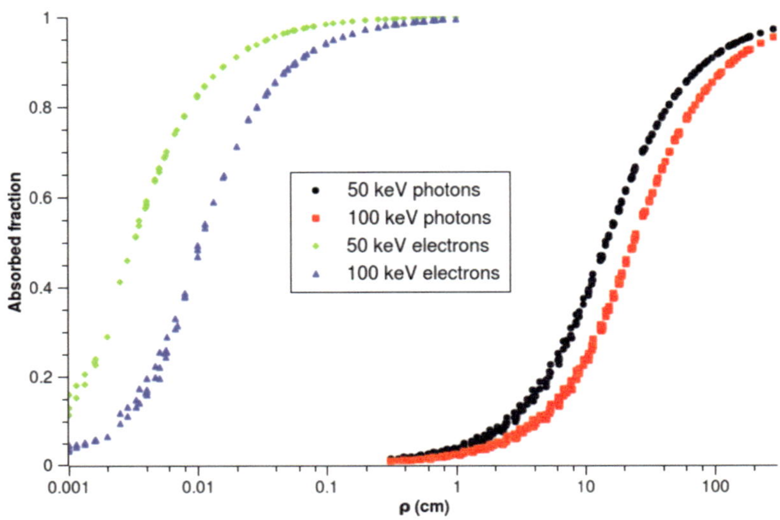

Fig. 4. Electron and photon absorbed fraction in ellipsoidal volumes, as a function of the generalized radius (Amato et al. 2009, 2011).

6. Three-dimensional dosimetry

Traditional approaches to internal dosimetry employ anatomic models to obtain mean organ doses. With the diffusion of SPECT-CT and PET-CT tomographs, dosimetric methods which can utilize non-uniform activity distributions to derive dose distributions within organs become increasingly important.

This result can be obtained either with dose point-kernel convolution methods, or by means of a direct Monte Carlo simulation, or exploiting the voxel S factor approach.

The voxel S factor approach, introduced in (Bolch et al., 1999), has been used more widely than dose point-kernel and direct Monte Carlo computation approaches, due to its recognized simplicity.

Following this approach, the average dose to the k-th voxel can be calculated as:

$$\bar{D}_k = \sum \tilde{A}_h \cdot S_{k \leftarrow h} \tag{26}$$

where $\tilde{A}_h$ is the cumulated activity in the generic h-th voxel and $S_{k \leftarrow h}$ is the voxel S factor, defined as:

$$S_{k\leftarrow h} = \sum \Delta_i \cdot \frac{\varphi_i(k \leftarrow h)}{m_k} \tag{27}$$

where Δ_i is the mean energy emitted as radiation i per decay, φ_i is the absorbed fraction in k of the radiation i emitted in h, and m_k is the mass of the k-th voxel.
In (Bolch et al., 1999), voxel S factors were tabulated for five radionuclides and two cubic voxel sizes. Recently, Dieudonnè et al. (2010) presented a generalization of this approach to variable voxel sizes, which allows to obtain S factors for a generic voxel size for nine radionuclides by means of a resampling method.
The dose point-kernel gives the dose per decay event at a given distance from a point source located inside an infinite and homogeneous absorbing medium. Dose point-kernels for electrons and photons were calculated by means of Monte Carlo simulations, and are available either in tabular form or as analytical functions obtained fitting the simulative data (Mainegra-Hing et al., 2005) (Maigne et al., 2011).
By convolving the dose point-kernels evaluated for the actual radionuclide spectrum in the three-dimensional distribution obtained from the volume distribution of cumulated activity, obtained from SPECT-CT or PET-CT images, one can retrieve the volume distribution of the absorbed dose. In order to speed up calculations, fast Fourier or fast Hartley transformations can be employed.
Finally, the Monte Carlo approach is the most demanding in terms of computational power, but it is the only one which can account accurately for tissue inhomogeneity. Known the three-dimensional map of tissue density and composition from CT scan and the volume distribution of the cumulated activity through SPECT or PET emission tomography, it is possible to generate a fixed number of decay events statistically distributed in space according to emission tomography data within the patient's body reconstructed from CT and track all the emitted secondaries in order to calculate the geometrical distribution of energy deposition, i.e. the three-dimensional map of absorbed dose, and finally to rescale the results to the actual values of cumulated activity (Furhang et al., 1997).

7. ^{131}I therapy of hyperthyroidism

Hyperthyroidism is a consequence of an excess in free-thyroid hormone action on the tissues. The most frequent causes of hyperthyroidism are: Graves' Disease (GD), Toxic Adenoma (TA) or Toxic Multinodular Goiter (TMG). In any cases, hyperthyroidism can be caused by sub-acute thyroiditis or silent thyroiditis.
The treatment of GD, TA and TMG can be symptomatic with anti-thyroid drugs (often used as first line therapy) or definitive: radioiodine therapy (RaIT) or surgery (total or near-total thyroidectomy).
RaIT is a well established method for the treatment of hyperthyroidism; aim of the RaIT is to achieve an euthyroid or hypothyroid (such as in the Graves patients) status.
Presently, the optimal ^{131}I activity to be administered is still matter of debate.
Many authors evaluated the effectiveness of different dosimetric methodologies. The results were variable and often controversial, in order to the frequency of recurrence and hypothyroidism (Regalbuto et al., 2009) (Giovannella, 2000).
In order to determine the ^{131}I activity to be administered for the treatment of hyperthyroidism, fixed activity and adjusted activity approaches are currently employed. In

both cases it is necessary, if possible, to suspend anti-thyroid drugs treatment 4-6 days before RaIT or thyroid scintigraphy.

The ^{131}I "fixed"activity for RaIT is usually about 555 MBq. In such case, the thyroid scintigraphy with or without radioiodine thyroid uptake (RTU) curve can be not necessary.

In the adjusted activity approach, a dosimetric procedure is employed which requires two diagnostic steps: a) thyroid ultrasonography to calculate the volume of the gland, or the hot thyroid nodule(s), assuming for them an ellipsoidal shape; b) thyroid scintigraphy and RTU measurements after ^{131}I tracer activity administration (1.8 MBq).

The dosimetric method most frequently employed was proposed by the MIRD commission (Snyder et al., 1975). In this approach, RTU measurements are usually conducted between 3 and 120 hours after administration. Multiple RTU measurements allow to calculate the effective half-life of the radioiodine into the hot nodules or in the whole gland (Figure 3).

In TMG and TA patients, the effective volume of the hot nodule(s) was calculated taking into account the presence of involving area(s) (whole nodule volume - involving area volume).

The radiation doses to be imparted to the gland (GD) or to the nodule(s) (TA and TMG) are up to 200 and 300 Gy, respectively.

In GD with ophtalmopathy, the radiation dose to be imparted must be adjusted, up to a maximum value of 250 Gy. In these patients, it is useful to administer anti-inflammatory drugs for a time duration ranging from 4 to 12 weeks after RaIT.

In all patients, the choice of the therapeutic dose will be determined also in function of: sex and age, type of hyperthyroidism (overt or sub-clinical) and its temporal duration, concomitant Hashimoto thyroiditis, anti-thyroid drugs therapy and its temporal duration.

Basing on the above considerations, the activity to be administered can be calculated as:

$$A = 5.829 \frac{Dm}{U_{max} T_{1/2eff}} \tag{28}$$

where A is the activity to be administered in MBq in order to impart a dose D in cGy to the target (nodule or gland) of mass m in g, U_{max} is the maximum per cent radioiodine uptake (usually measured at 24 hours) and $T_{1/2eff}$ is the effective half-time in hours.

Recently, Amato et al. (2011) proposed an improved calculation method for the activity to be administered during the radioiodine treatment of hyperthyroidism. In this approach, a Monte Carlo simulation had been employed to derive the radiation dose in nodules or in the whole gland within an anthropomorphic phantom, taking into account the ellipsoidal shape of the target volumes.

As a result, the activity to be administered can be calculated with the formula:

$$A = \frac{Dm}{U_{max} T_{1/2eff}} \cdot \frac{32.31\rho + 1}{\rho(0.2625\rho + 5.1819)} \tag{29}$$

where we recall the definition of generalized radius, $\rho=3V/S$, stated in Equation 12, and here expressed in cm. The volume and the surface of the ellipsoidal target (nodule or thyroid lobe) can be calculated from the semiaxes measured through ultrasonography as:

$$V = \frac{4}{3}\pi abc , \qquad S = 4\pi \left(\frac{(ab)^p + (bc)^p + (ac)^p}{3} \right)^{1/p} \tag{30}$$

8. ^{131}I therapy of differentiated thyroid carcinoma

Differentiated thyroid cancer (DTC) is the most common cancer of the endocrine system.
The first line therapy is represented by total or near-total thyroidectomy (with dissect of the sixth lymph nodes level and, if necessary, of the lateral-cervical lymph nodes of the same side respect to primary lesion).
After Total or near-Total Thyroidectomy (nTT) it is useful to ablate the thyroid remnant with 131-radioiodine therapy (RaIT). In fact, several Authors, such as Mazzaferri et al. (1997) demonstrated that the *prognosis quod vitam* and the survival curve of the DTC-patients significantly improve if RaIT follows TT or NTT.
In addition, the ablation of thyroid remnant (TRA) allows a better management of the follow-up of these patients.
In fact, in the patients treated with TT or NTT and TRA, the Thyroglobulin (hTg) serum levels should be undetectable. Thus, any enhancement of hTg serum (both under L-T4 suppressive therapy or after exogenous TSH stimulation -rhTSH-) can be considered as a relapse of disease.
RaIT can be carried out in hypothyroidism state (TSH>=30) or after rhTSH stimulation.
Post dose whole body scan and static images of the head, neck and thorax acquired 4-8 days after RIT allow to identify the thyroid remnant and metastases (loco-regional and/or distant).
For the RaIT of TRA, fixed activities are employed more frequently: 1110, 2220 or 3700 MBq.
In the patients treated after rhTSH stimulation it is necessary to employ a medium-to-high activity of radioiodine (2220 and 3700 MBq, respectively), because in this condition the effective half-life of radioiodine in the thyroid remnant is shorter than in the state of hypothyroidism.
However, the TRA activity can be adjusted through a dosimetric approach (Lassmann, 2010), which requires a pre-therapeutic scintigraphy with ^{131}I or ^{124}I PET. The dose to the thyroid remnant can be calculated using ^{131}I post-therapy whole body scan, too.
Both methods show advantages and disadvantages. The main disadvantage of the pre-therapeutic scintigraphic method is correlated to the stunning or mass change effects that could be determined by a diagnostic activity of ^{131}I.
On the other hand, the main disadvantage of the post-therapeutic scintigraphic method is correlated to technical difficulties such as the limitations deriving from the gamma-camera dead time.
The clinical evidence demonstrated that the dosimetry adjusted activities do not differ significantly from the fixed values. Thus, in the clinical practice, the dosimetric approach is not employed frequently. However, the dosimetric approach is useful for the treatment of loco-regional and/or distant metastases.
Dosimetry is particularly useful in patients with lung and/or bone metastases, where standard activities can lead to a radiation dose imparted to the lesions lower than the necessary. In such cases, it is necessary to acquire some whole scans starting from 6-7 hours after radio-iodine therapy. (Eschmann et al., 2002) (Sgouros et al., 2004).

9. Usefulness of radiopharmaceuticals for the palliation of painful bone metastases

The development of bone metastases is commonly related to a serious reduction in quality of patient life because of pain occurrence and side effects of analgesics intake, especially opiates (Silberstein, 2001). Therapeutic options for pain palliation include systemic therapy with cytotoxic agents, diphosphonate therapy, external beam radiotherapy and radionuclide therapy. Diphosphonate therapy has become a possible option for the treatment of patients affected by bone metastases since a new generation of diphosphonate has been developed; using zoledronic acid, indeed, the clinical benefits of diphosphonate (skeletal complications reduction and analgesic effects on bone pain), previously limited to patients with bone metastases from breast cancer or lesions due to multiple myeloma, have been extended to patients with bone metastases secondary to a broad range of solid tumors (Berenson, 2005). However, diphosphonates achieve only a modest analgesic effect and are associated with some non-renal adverse effects (Hillner, 2003; Lewington, 1996). External beam radiotherapy is the therapy of choice in cases of a single site of pain. However, when multiple painful metastases have been developed, local field radiotherapy is less effective and hemibody radiotherapy is associated with a significant morbidity (Lewington, 1996). Furthermore, external beam radiotherapy is often not suitable for repeated treatments. On the other hand, bone-seeking beta-emitting radiopharmaceuticals represent an effective tool for pain palliation in patients with multifocal bone disease, and make it possible to perform multiple administrations (Lam, 2004; Daformou, 2001; Englaro, 1992; Maini, 2003). Pain arises from both umoral and mechanical effects, including bone invasion, micro-fractures, increased intramedullary pressure and periosteal stretching (Lewington, 2005). Unlike opiates, which affect the entire nervous system, radionuclides exert their action mainly on cells at the peripheral nerve endings, where inflammatory, immune and malignant cells accumulate and release chemicals that modulate pain at the site of malignant invasion (Krishnamurthy, 2000). Furthermore, early response gene induction and a psychological-placebo component could account for the pain alleviation effect (Lewington, 1996; Leondi, 2004; Roche, 1994; Hellmann, 1994).

The goals of therapy are to alleviate pain, improve quality of life and mobility, reduce dependence on narcotic and non-narcotic analgesics, and improve performance status and possibly survival (Minutoli, 2006; Hindorf, 2011).

Bone tumours can be divided into osteolytic and sclerotic tumours. Sclerotic tumours are more suitable for targeted radionuclide therapy because of higher uptake of the radiopharmaceutical within the lesions. The majority of bone metastases from prostate cancer are sclerotic whilst metastases of breast cancer generally are mixed osteolytic/sclerotic. Also patients with bone metastases from tumours other than prostate and breast cancer and increased ^{99m}Tc-MDP uptake on bone scan can benefit from targeted radionuclide therapy (Leondi, 2004; Minutoli, 2006).

Two radiopharmaceuticals for the treatment of bone tumours are currently approved by the European Medicines Agency (EMEA): ^{153}Sm-EDTMP (Quadramet®) and ^{89}Sr-Cl_2 (Metastron®). Other radiopharmaceuticals are at different stages of research, or are approved in some European Countries. These include ^{186}Re-HEDP, ^{117m}Sn-DTPA and ^{223}Ra-Cl_2 (Alpharadin®). The use of ^{32}P is now considered to be obsolete.

Strontium-89 was suggested for the treatment of bone tumours during the 1940s. It is naturally taken up in bone and is a pure β^- emitter with a long half-life (50.53 days). Pharmacokinetic and dosimetry studies have been based on imaging of ^{85}Sr-Cl (Blake, 1986, 1987, 1998; Breen, 1992), although imaging based on bremsstrahlung photons from ^{89}Sr has also been performed (ICRP, 1997). Tumour dosimetry is generally performed under the assumption that the activity uptake is five times higher than for normal bone. Strontium leaves the blood quickly after an intravenous injection. The kidneys are the main route of excretion, but the gut has been seen in scintillation camera images and IRCP report assumes 4:1 ratio for urinary to faecal excretion.

Tin-117m labelled DTPA is investigated for the treatment of bone pain from metastases. Tin-117m can be imaged via the 156 keV gamma photons and the main energy deposition is performed by the corresponding conversion electrons. The conclusion from a phase I/II clinical study was that ^{117m}Sn-DTPA is an effective and safe radiopharmaceutical for the treatment of bone metastases (Krishnamurthy, 1997; Srivastava, 1998).

^{153}Sm-EDTMP is a therapeutic agent consisting of radioactive samarium and a tetraphosphonate chelator, ethylenediaminetetramethylenephosphonic acid (EDTMP). It is formulated as a sterile, non-pyrogenic, clear, colorless to light amber isotonic solution of samarium-153 lexidronam for intravenous administration (37 MBq/kg body weight) (Bodei, 2008). Onset of pain relief comes within one week, lasting from four weeks up to four months. The highest absorbed dose is received by bone marrow and bone surfaces. Imaging is commonly performed three hours after injection to verify the activity uptake. All activity not taken up in bone is excreted via urine and no further activity is excreted 24 hours after the injection. Dosimetry can therefore be performed from one scintillation camera imaging acquired 24h after injection or from one single probe measurement. The activity uptake in bone has been reported to increase with an increase in number of bone tumors (Farhangi, 1992; Brenner, 2001).

Renium-186 is a beta minus emitter with a maximum beta energy of 1.07 MeV. The physical half-life is 89 hours. The radiopharmaceutical is taken up in bone via the phosphor complex HEDP (hydroxyethylidene diphosphonate). Quantitative imaging for pharmacokinetics and dosimetry is possible via the emission of 137 keV photons with a 9.47% probability. Excretion is predominantly through the kidneys.

Radium-223-chloride is taken up in bone by natural affinity. It decays in six steps into stable ^{207}Pb. The injected activity has been reported as 46-250 kBq per kg of whole body weight (Nilsson, 2005, 2007). A clinical phase II study showed an improved survival without severe toxicity after four weekly injections of 50 kBq per kg of whole body weight compared to placebo injections (Nilsson, 2007). The photon emissions at 81.1 keV and 83.8 keV show the highest emission probabilities and offer the best opportunity to perform quantitative imaging during the treatment, which enables pharmacokinetic and dosimetric studies to be performed. The main route of excretion is via faeces (Hindorf, 2008).

Contraindications for radionuclide therapy are a life expectancy shorter than four weeks, severe renal insufficiency, and low blood counts due to a compromised bone marrow function. The absorbed dose to the tumour is the factor that determines the effectiveness of the therapy while the absorbed dose to the bone marrow correlates to the toxic effects received. The bone marrow is the dose limiting organ when bone-seeking radiopharmaceuticals are used (Lewington, 1993). Radionuclide therapy for pain palliation from bone metastases is currently performed based on a pre-set injected activity. The patients will, therefore, receive a range of absorbed doses due to individual differences in the pharmacokinetics. Voxel based, patient specific dosimetry automatically takes into account individual differences in pharmacokinetics and macroscopic anatomy. Furthermore, Monte Carlo simulations also take into account different cross sectional interaction data for all materials present in the body, which is, therefore, more accurate than convolution with a dose point kernel as this is based on an assumption of infinite, uniform medium.

Radionuclide therapy as a palliative treatment of bone pain is efficient, although improved dosimetry methods could help to improve the treatment further.

10. Peptide radio-receptor therapy of neuroendocrine tumours

Neuroendocrine tumours (NETs) derive from the neuroendocrine cell system, which is widely distributed in the body, and are a heterogeneous group of neoplasms characterized by embryological, biological and histo-pathological differences. The most frequent sites of NETs are the gastrointestinal tract (70%) and the bronco-pulmonary system (25%), followed by the skin, the adrenal glands, the thyroid and the genital tract.

Present classification is based on tumour biology and patho-histological features (cellular grading, primary tumour size and site, cell proliferation markers, local or vascular invasivity and the production of biologically active substances), which are crucial to guide the diagnostic work-up and therapeutic planning.

The great majority are benign (well-differentiated neuroendocrine tumours) or slow-growing neoplasms with a low grade of malignancy. Poorly differentiated endocrine carcinomas have a high grade of malignancy and a poor prognosis. Furthermore, a few moderately differentiated tumours with cellular and structural types intermediate between well and poorly differentiated NETs have also been found.

A typical feature of differentiated NETs is the expression of several specific receptors on the cell membrane and in particular of somatostatin receptors (SSTR) which can be visualized by somatostatin receptor imaging with radiolabelled somatostatin analogues (^{111}In-OCTREOSCAN, ^{68}Ga-DOTANOC). These radiopharmaceuticals bind with high affinity to subtypes 2, 5 and 3 of SSTR and provide an approximation of somatostatin receptor density, having a positive predictive value of the therapeutic efficacy of the somatostatin analogues.

Peptide receptor radionuclide therapy (PRRT) is an effective tool for the treatment of tumours with a high somatostatin receptor density.

This approach is based on the administration of a therapeutic activity of radiolabelled somatostatin analogues. Radiopharmaceutical with various radionuclides and peptides are currently available.

High activities of ^{111}In-DTPA-octreotide (OCTREOSCAN®), the same radiopharmaceutical used for imaging, have been used in pilot trials and in some experiences (Herberg, 2009, 2011). Besides the gamma radiation of ^{111}In used for scintigraphic scans (γ photons of 172 and 245 keV), its therapeutic effect is due to the emission of Auger and conversion electrons with a medium-to-short tissue penetration range (0.02-10 and 200-500 μm, respectively). Its potential effect depends on the preservation of mechanism of octreotide-receptor complex internalization (through endocytosis) and its translocation to the nuclear compartment, where short path-length Auger or conversion electrons are able to reach the target (DNA). In clinical trials, ^{111}In-DTPA-octreotide showed a low rate of tumour regression: the most accredited explanation is that ^{111}In electrons fail to reach the DNA helix, possibly due to the lack of nuclear receptors that were never definitely demonstrated (Kwekkeboom, 2005).

The radiopeptides for PRRT that have been studied most extensively are ^{90}Y-DOTATOC and ^{177}Lu-DOTATATE. These beta-emitting radiolabelled peptides are preferred for their advantageous physical properties.

^{90}Y (E_{max} = 2.28 MeV, R_{max} = 11 mm, $\langle E \rangle$ = 0.935 MeV; half-life 2.67 days) has a pure beta emission with long range particles that, besides the direct action, lead to irradiation also of no-receptor expressing tumour-cell (cross-fire effect). For these reasons ^{90}Y-peptides are preferred especially for the treatment of larger and inhomogeneous lesions. In figure 5, the comparison between electron paths within small and large inhomogeneous lesions is represented through a Monte Carlo simulation in Geant4, in which radiations emitted from ^{177}Lu and ^{90}Y are compared.

^{177}Lu has a longer half-life (6.7 days) and lower energy beta-emission (E_{max} = 0.497 MeV; R_{max} = 2 mm) that allows to concentrate all the energy inside smaller tumours; moreover the gamma-emission of ^{177}Lu (113 keV and 208 keV) is suitable for scintigraphy and dosimetry during PRRT.

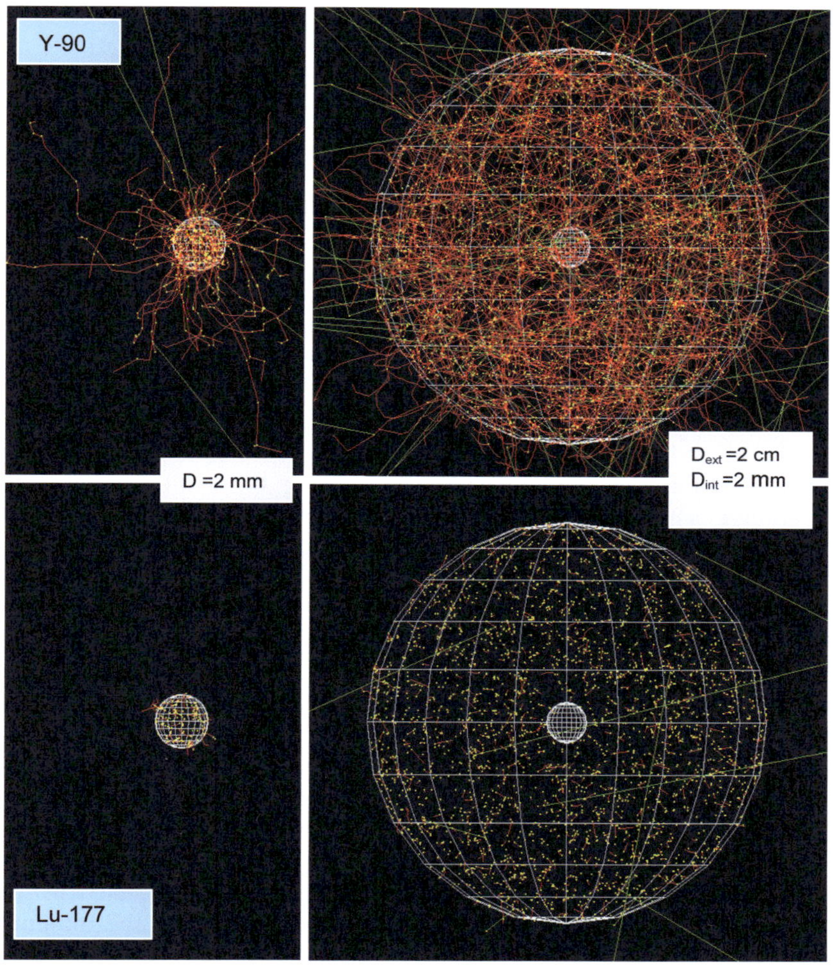

Fig. 5. Comparison between the high-energy electron tracks (red) of ^{90}Y and the ones of the lower-energy electrons from ^{177}Lu. Photons originating from gamma ray emission or bremsstrahlung are represented in green.

Concerning peptides, several new somatostatin analogues have been introduced for therapeutic and diagnostic purposes, including the agonists DOTA-(1-NaI3)octreotide (DOTANOC) and DOTA-(BzThi3)octreotide (DOTABOC).

These compounds have a broader somatostatin receptor affinity profile than DOTATATE and DOTATOC because of a higher affinity for sst3 and sst5 in addition to their high affinity for sst2. This could increase the number of tumours that could benefit from PRRT in the future.

Recently, peptides targeting all the sst receptors (pansomatostatins) have shown high affinity of ^{90}Y-DOTA-cyclo(D-diaminobutyric acid-Arg–Phe–Phe-D-Trp–Lys–Thr–Phe) (^{90}Y-KE88) for all 5 sst receptors and, in future, they could improve the therapeutic potential of sst-targeted PRRT.

To date, the therapy administration protocols rely essentially on empirical criteria with injection of standard activities, as derived from escalation studies or clinical experience, at variable time intervals (6-12 weeks).

For therapy optimization and prevention of toxicity, dosimetry represent a precious guide, providing evaluation of biodistribution, pharmacokinetics, radiation doses and biological effective doses to healthy organs and tumours.

The gamma-emission of ^{111}In and ^{177}Lu-peptide enable imaging, dosimetry and therapy with the same compound. In the case of ^{90}Y-peptide, for the lack of gamma emission, the same analogue radiolabeled with ^{111}In or positron emitters as ^{86}Y or ^{68}Ga can be used as surrogates for dosimetric imaging. Some recent studies have been published for ^{90}Y-peptide dosimetry with bremsstrahlung images through SPECT-TC systems, or exploiting the rare positron decay of ^{90}Y imaged by new generation PET-CT scanners.

A dosimetric protocol consists in the acquisition of multiple planar whole-body (WB) scan to obtain biokinetics data over the time (at least 4-5 acquisitions at different times), complementary SPECT imaging to evaluate intra-organ activity distribution (especially at the level of the kidneys and in tumour lesion), WB transmission imaging for attenuation correction, blood and urine samples. Anatomical imaging (CT or ultrasonographic) provide important parameters for organ mass evaluation (Cremonesi, 2011).

Dose calculation can be performed in the framework of the MIRD formalism, in order to obtain average dose estimates at the organ level assuming standard phantom models, with possible organ mass adjustments according to patient data. Voxel dosimetry method or direct Monte Carlo simulation can provide more reliable dose estimates.

Pharmacokinetic studies have shown fast blood clearance and urinary elimination. The higher uptake has been noticed in the spleen, kidneys and liver and no uptake is visible in the bone marrow in normal conditions. Pharmacokinetic data of different radiopeptides are similar but not identical: as the peptide influences biokinetics, for the single patient the data need to be assessed specifically with regard to the radiopharmaceutical.

Furthermore, dosimetric data should be collected during therapeutic cycles because many factors can influence the results.

The adsorbed doses, especially with regards to the tumour, are affected by wide intra-patient variation between treatment cycles. The adsorbed dose to the tumour is higher during the first two cycles with a gradually reduced uptake in the following treatments, probably due to saturation or down-regulation of peptide receptors. Tumour adsorbed dose should exceed 100 Gy to obtain a therapeutic effect, with better results for higher doses (about 230 Gy).

Nephrotoxicity is the dose-limiting factor, due to renal reabsorption and retention of radiolabeled peptides that results in high kidney radiation doses.

The renal adsorbed dose is influenced by the radionuclide emission: using a microdosimetry model, Konijnenberg et al. (2004) found that ^{111}In- and ^{177}Lu-labelled somatostatin analogues are likely to have higher renal toxicity thresholds than ^{90}Y, whose emitted electrons have a path length of 12 mm.

Renal doses can be reduced by co-administration of basic amino acids, bovine gelatine-containing solution Gelofusine or albumin fragments, which interfere with the radiopeptide reabsorption pathway to achieve kidney protection. Amino acids, in particular, are already commonly used in the clinical setting during PRRT, being able to reduce the kidney adsorbed dose consistently (25-65% with respect to baseline data). The dose fraction markedly influences the total tolerated dose.

The dose to kidneys should not exceed a limit value of 28 Gy, established for external beam radiotherapy, which results in a 50% probability of developing severe late renal failure. Nevertheless, for the difference between the two radiation therapy modalities, this recommendation has been questioned and the biological effective dose (BED) is considered a more accurate quantity, with a good correlation with the loss of kidney function.

BED for a given organ or tissue was defined in Equation 18. We recall that BED is a function of the doses imparted in each PRRT cycle, and depends upon the effective half-time of the radiopeptide in the organ and upon its intrinsic radiosensitivity.

Data in literature show that patients with risk factors, such as hypertension and diabetes, should not receive a BED higher than 28 Gy, while patients with no risk factors might have a renal BED threshold of 40 Gy (Bodei, 2008).

The risk of bone marrow toxicity increases with increasing therapeutic dose. Studies aimed to increase the therapeutic dose (more cycles, higher dose per cycle, improvement in specific activity of the compound) to the tumour in a renoprotective (and bone marrow-protective) regimen are needed to further improve PRRT with somatostatin analogues in the future.

11. References

Amato, E. et al. (2009). Absorbed fractions for photons in ellipsoidal volumes. *Phys Med Biol,* 54, N479-487.

Amato, E. et al. (2009). Absorbed fractions in ellipsoidal volumes for $\beta-$ radionuclides employed in internal radiotherapy. *Phys Med Biol,* 54, 4171-4180.

Amato, E. et al. (2011). Absorbed fractions for electrons in ellipsoidal volumes. *Phys Med Biol,* 56, 357-365.

Amato, E. et al. (2011). An analytical model for improving absorbed dose calculation accuracy in non spherical autonomous functioning thyroid nodule. *Quart. J. Nucl. Med. Mol. Imag.* EPUB 18-01-2011 PMID: 21242948.

Berenson, J. R. (2005). Recomendations for zoledronic acid treatment of patients with bone metastases. *Oncologist,* 10, 52-62.

Blake, G. et al. (1998). Strontium-89 therapy: measurements of absorbed dose to skeletal metastases. *J Nucl Med,* 29, 549-557.

Blake, G. M. et al. (1986). Sr-89 therapy: strontium kinetics in disseminated carcinoma of the prostate. *Eur J Nucl Med,* 12, 447-454.

Blake, G. M. et al. (1987). 89Sr radionuclide therapy: dosimetry and haematological toxicity in two patients with metastasising prostatic carcinoma. *Eur J Nucl Med,* 13, 41-46.

Bodei, L. et al. (2008). Long-term evaluation of renal toxicity after peptide receptor radionuclide therapy with 90Y-DOTATOC and 177Lu-DOTATATE: the role of associated risk factors. *Eur. J. Nucl. Med.* 35, 1847.

Bodei, L. et al. (2008). EANM procedure guideline for treatment of refractory metastatic bone pain. *Eur J Nucl Med Mol Imaging,* 35, 1934-1940.

Bolch, W.E. et al. MIRD Pamphlet No. 17: the dosimetry of nonuniform activity distributions - radionuclide S values at the voxel level. *J Nucl Med,* 40, 11S-36S.

Breen, S. L. et al. (1992). Dose estimation in strontium-89 radiotherapy of metastatic prostatic carcinoma. *J Nucl Med,* 33, 1316-1323.

Brenner, W. et al. (2001). Skeletal uptake and soft-tissue retention of 186Re-HEDP and 153Sm-EDTMP in patients with metastatic bone disease. *J Nucl Med,* 42, 230-236.

Cremonesi, M. et al. (2011). Recent issues on dosimetry and radiobiology for peptide receptor radionuclide therapy. *Quart. J. Nucl. Med. Mol. Imag,* 55(2), 155-167.

Dafermou, A. et al. (2001). A multicentre observational study of radionuclide therapy in patients with painful bone metastases of prostate cancer. *Eur J Nucl Med Mol Imaging,* 28, 788-798.

Dieudonnè, A. et al. (2010). Fine-resolution voxel S values for constructing absorbed dose distributions at variable voxel size. *J Nucl Med,* 51, 1600-1607.

Englaro, E.E. et al. (1992). Safety and efficacy of repeated sequential administrations of Re186(Sn)HEDP as palliative therapy for painful skeletal metastases. Initial case reports of two patients. *Clin Nucl Med,* 17, 41-44.

Eschmann, S. M. et al. (2002). Evaluation of dosimetry of radioiodine therapy in benign and malignant thyroid disorders by means of iodine-124 and PET. *Eur. J. Nucl. Med. Mol. Imaging,* 29, 760-767.

Farhangi, M. et al. (1992). Samarium-153-EDTMP: pharmacokinetic, toxicity and pain response using escalation doses schedule in treatment of metastatic bone cancer. *J Nucl Med,* 33, 1451-1458.

Furhang, E. E. et al. (1997). Implementation of a Monte Carlo dosimetry method for patient-specific internal emitter therapy. *Med. Phys,* 24, 1163-1172.

Giovannella (2000). *Radiol. Med.,* 105, 12

Hellmann, S. and Weichsellbaum, R. R. (1994). Radiation oncology. *JAMA,* 271, 1712-1714.

Herberg, A. et al. (2009). 90Y-DOTATOC and/or 111In-Pentetreotide in the treatment of somatostatin receptors-expressing tumors (SSTR): our experience. *Eur J Nucl Med Mol Imaging,* 36 S.2, S418.

Herberg, A. et al. (2011). 111In-Pentetreotide for the treatment of neuroendocrine tumours: an alternative therapeutic option in particular cases. *Quart J Nucl Med Mol Imaging,* 52 S.1, 131.

Hillner, B.E. et al. (2003). American Society of Clinical Oncology 2003 update on the role of bisphosphonates and bone health issues in women with breast cancer. *J Clin Oncol,* 21, 4042-4057.

Hindorf, C. et al. (2008). A biodistribution and dosimetry study of therapeutic 223RA-chloride (Alpharadin) in patientts with osteoblastic skeletal metastases secondary to hormone refractory prostate cancer. *J Nucl Med,* 49, 145P.

Hindorf, C. et al. (2008). Quantitative imaging of 223Ra during radionuclide therapy of bone metastases. *J Nucl Med,* 49, 326P.

Hindorf, C. et al. (2011). Clinical dosimetry in the treatment of bone tumors: old and new agents. *Q J Nucl Med Mol Imaging,* 55, 198-204.

ICRP, (1987). International Commission on Radiological Protection. Radiation dose to patients from radiopharmaceuticals. Oxford, UK; Pergamon Press.

Konijnenberg, M. W. et al. (2004). A stylized computational model of the rat for organ dosimetry in support of preclinical evaluations of peptide receptor radionuclide therapy with (90)Y, (111)In, or (177)Lu. *J Nucl Med,* 45, 1260–1269.

Kraeber-Bodere, F. et al. (2000). Treatment of bone metastases of prostate cancer with strontium-89chloride: efficacy in relation to degree of bone involvement. *Eur J Nucl Med* 27, 1487-1493.

Krishnamurthy, G. T. et al. (1997). Tin-117m(4+)DTPA: pharmacokinetics and imaging characteristics in patients with metastatic bone pain. *J Nucl Med,* 38, 230-237.

Krishnamurthy, G. T. et al. (2000). Radionuclides for metastatic bone pain palliation:a need for rational re-evaluation in the new millenium. *J Nucl Med,* 41, 688-691.

Kwekkeboom, D. J. et al. (2005).
Overview of Results of Peptide Receptor Radionuclide Therapy with 3 Radiolabeled Somatostatin Analogs
. *J. Nucl. Med.* 46, 62S.

Lam, M. J. E. H. et al. (2004). 186Re-HEDP for metastatic bone pain in breast cancer patients. *Eur J Nucl Med Mol Imaging,* 31, S162-S170.

Lassmann, M. (2010). *Dosimetry Concepts of radioiodine therapy for the Treatment of differentiated thyroid cancer,* EANM Dosimetry Committee

Leondi, A. H. et al. (2004). Palliative treatment of painful disseminated bone metastases with 186Rhenium-HEDP in patients with lung cancer. *Q J Nucl Med,* 48, 211-219.

Lewington, V. J. (1993). Targeted radionuclide therapy for bone metastases. *Eur J Nucl Med,* 20, 66-74.

Lewington, V. J. (2005). Bone-seeking radionuclides for therapy. *J Nucl Med,* 46, 38S-47S.

Lewington, V.J. (1996). Cancer therapy using bone-seeking isotopes. *Phys Med Biol,* 41, 2027-2042.

Maigne, L. et al. (2011). Comparison of GATE/GEANT4 with EGSnrc and MCNP for electron dose calculations at energies between 15 keV and 20 MeV. *Phys. Med. Biol,* 56, 811.

Mainegra-Hing, E. et al. (2005). Calculation of photon energy deposition kernels and electron dose point kernels in water. *Med. Phys,* 32, 685-699.

Maini, C. L. et al. (2003). Radionuclide therapy with bone seeking radionuclides in palliation of painful bone metastases. *J Exp Clin Cancer Res,* 22, 71-74.

Maini, C. L. et al. (2004). 153Sm-EDTMP for bone pain palliation in skeletal metastases. *Eur J Nucl Med Mol Imaging,* 31, S171-S178.

Mazzaferri E. L. (1997). Thyroid Remnant 131I Ablation for Papillary and Follicular Thyroid Carcinoma. *Thyroid,* 7, 265271.

Minutoli, F. et al. (2006). 186Re-HEDP in the palliation of painful bone metastases from cancers other than prostate and breast. *Q J Nucl Med,* 50, 355-362.

Nilsson, S. et al. (2005). First clinical experience with alpha-emitting radium-223 in the treatment of skeletal metastases. *Clin Cancer Res,* 11, 4451-4459.

Nilsson, S. et al. (2007). Bone-targeted radium-223 in symptomatic, hormone-refractory prostate cancer: a randomised, multicentre, placebo-controlled phase II study. *Lancet Oncology,* 8, 587-594.

Regalbuto, C. et al. (2009). Radiometabolic treatment of hyperthyroidism with a calculated dose of 131-iodine: results of one-year follow-up. *J. Endocrinol. Invest,* 32, 134-138.

Roche, E. and Prentky, M. (1994). Calcium regulation of immediate early responce genes. *Cell Calcium*, 16, 331-338.

Sgouros, G. et al. (2004). Patient-Specific Dosimetry for 131I Thyroid Cancer Therapy Using 124I PET and 3-Dimensional-Internal Dosimetry (3D-ID) Software. *J. Nucl. Med*, 45, 1366-1372.

Silberstein, E. B. (2001). Painful osteoblastic metastases: the role of nuclear medicine. *Oncology*, 15, 157-163.

Snyder, W. et al. (1975). "S" absorbed dose per unit cumulated activity for selected radionuclides and organs MIRD Pamphlet No. 11. New York (NY): Society of Nuclear Medicine.

Srivastava, S. C. et al. (1998). Treatment of metastatic bone pain with tin-117m stannic diethylenetriaminepentaacetic acid: a phase I/II clinical study. *Clin Cancer Res*, 4, 61-68.

Strigari, L. et al. (2011). Dosimetry in nuclear medicine therapy: radiobiology application and results. *Quart. J. Nucl. Med. Mol. Imag*, 55(2), 205-221.

Tennvall, J. et al. (1988). Palliation of multiple bone metastases from prostatic carcinoma with strontium-89. *Acta oncologica*, 27, 365-369.

3

Medical Cyclotron

Reina A. Jimenez V
Policlínica Metropolitana, Venezuela

1. Introduction

In this chapter we intend to illustrate the reader about the use of Cyclotrons to produce easy handle radioisotopes, to be used for medical diagnostics or therapies in Nuclear Medicine. Firstofall, we will describe different activation processes to generate artificial radioisotopes, characteristics needed to be safely used in medicine, such as the relationship between fathers and daughters that can compromise patient or environment health. It also will be describe radioisotopes desire behavior inside human body in order to clarify which isotopes can be activated or not in a cyclotron facility to be used in human medical applications. Nuclear Medicine radioisotopes must fulfill four main characteristics in order to be easy handle by operators and be easily and quickly disposed by patients and not to represent environmental radioactive contamination harm, so they have to have:

1. Low activity
2. Low energy
3. Short half life
4. Decay to a stable daughter

In Nuclear Medicine, equipment also has to have a high sensitivity to small amounts of radiation and to different types of radioisotopes. The ideal radioisotopes must be easily eliminated by the patient just after the study has been done in a short period of time which is a function of the physical half life of the isotope and the patient excretion system. The total time elapse for patient elimination of any trace of radioisotope used for study is known as Effective Half Life Time $T_{1/2}^{eff}$ and is related to the time isotope population is reduced to its half due to the radioactive decay of father to daughter (Physical Half Life) $T_{1/2}^{phy}$ and the time patient systems needs to eliminated of isotope from it system (Biological Half Life) $T_{1/2}^{bio}$ in this way:

$$\frac{1}{T_{1/2}^{eff}} = \frac{1}{T_{1/2}^{phy}} + \frac{1}{T_{1/2}^{bio}}$$

So it is not easy to find natural occurrence radioisotopes to fulfill this equation in order to make $T_{1/2}^{eff}$ shorter than biological times of cellular repair. Fortunately in mid 20Th century, there was a huge development of activation processes when man learn how to manipulate atom and its nuclei, so now we have a big amount of radioisotopes for an equally big amount of pacific applications. There are two kinds of manmade machinery capable of modify stable nuclide: Nuclear reactors and particle accelerators. Accelerator can also be divided into two big groups: Linear accelerators and spiral path accelerators or Cyclotrons. The radioisotopes used in Medicine can be from natural ocurrences like ^{137}Cs (used in the last century in Teletherapy machines and in low dose rate brachytherapy) or ^{192}Ir (used nowadays in high dose rate brachytherapy), or can be produced in Reactors or Cyclotrons. Most common reactor products used in Medicine are:

For diagnostic purposes: ^{51}Cr, ^{125}I, ^{131}I, ^{59}Fe, ^{42}K, ^{177}Lu, ^{99}Mo (fission product), ^{75}Se, ^{24}Na, ^{99m}Tc, ^{133}Xe (fission product), ^{159}Yt.

For therapeutic purposes: ^{213}Bi, ^{60}Co, ^{165}Dy, ^{169}Er, ^{125}I, ^{131}I, ^{192}Ir, ^{212}Pb, ^{177}Lu, ^{103}Pd, ^{32}P, ^{188}Re, ^{186}Re, ^{153}Sm, ^{89}Sr (fission product), ^{90}Y (fission product).

For diagnostic and therapeutic or other purposes: ^{60}Co, ^{166}Ho, ^{125}I, ^{99}Mo (fission product), ^{177}Yt.

Most common radioisotopes produced in Cyclotrons used in Medicine are:

For diagnostic purposes: ^{11}C, ^{13}N, ^{15}O, ^{18}F, (PET studies), ^{64}Cu, ^{67}Ga, ^{68}Ga, ^{111}In, ^{123}I, ^{124}I, ^{81m}Kr, ^{99}Mo (activation product), 82Rb, 201Th.

For therapeutic purposes: ^{67}Cu.

For diagnostic, therapeutic or other purposes: ^{57}Co, ^{82}Sr, ^{68}Ge. All of them have to fulfill the four conditions mentioned above.

Knowing all this restrictions radioisotope has to accomplish, to be safely used in human, now we can talk about the characteristics of a cyclotron to produce such an isotope. Later in this chapter we will describe such an installation regarding shielding, environmental safety, radiopharmacy lab, etc.

In Venezuela, we start to install the first baby cyclotron for medical purposes on 2001, so our last section of this chapter is to illustrate how this installation works and how its programs has been accomplish to the present date.

2. Basic physics of particle activation

"Particle activation" means "artificial radioactivity" or "man made radioisotopes", far away from "natural radioactivity" which is a basic characteristic of our Universe, that has been present all over the universe history, and it contains only four natural decay series characterized by their numbers of nucleons as is shown in Table 1., artificial radioactivity is a very young phenomena born in 20th century.

Series	Parent	Nucleons	Stable end
THORIUM	$^{232}Th_{90}$	4n	$^{208}Pb_{82}$
NEPTUNIUM	$^{237}Np_{93}$	4n+1	$^{209}Bi_{83}$
URANIUM	$^{238}U_{92}$	4n+2	$^{206}Pb_{82}$
ACTINIUM	$^{235}U_{92}$	4n+3	$^{207}Pb_{82}$

Table 1. Natural decay series.

Firstofalll we have to define radioactivity: It is a property of nature in which atoms have such a big amount of energy so they need to discharge it to the surrounding media. The aim of it is to become stable, i.e. have the less amount of energy need to exist, because atom stability is the more cost/efficiency retail in matter. Atom then has design some method to discharge energy and diminish it energy level to become stable. Radioactive atoms can emit some energy packs splitting them in pieces of several dimensions and energy content to reach its stability:

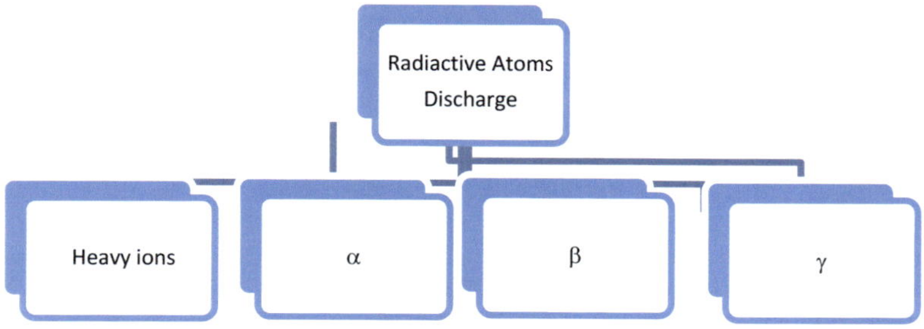

Fig. 1. Decay mode of radioactive atoms to reach stability.The action of atoms to split means mass and energy transfer to media. For example, in a ^{226}Ra atom energy excess push it to split out a $^{4}_{2}He$ nucleus (an alpha particle) and 1.4 MeV package of pure energy and another atom of ^{222}Rn, so where there was one atom now there are three different species born out it mass and energy

There are several methods for atoms to transfer energy to the media. Remember Einstein´s principle of $E = mc^2$, which means energy is matter and matter is energy. So in their attempt to become stable emits energy/matter to discharge it excess in several ways as in figure 1.
And scientist began to use this atom fraction to hit different nucleus of known atoms and to observe which was the results of the reverse experiment.
Back in 1929, Ernest Lawrence device a Cyclotron to fulfill his own need to generate high speed ions without needing high voltages he has not access to in Berkeley University. This history began 10 years before when Lord Rutherford used alpha particles coming from Madame Curie´s ^{226}Ra as projectiles to impact a Nitrogen nucleus to transform it into Oxygen.

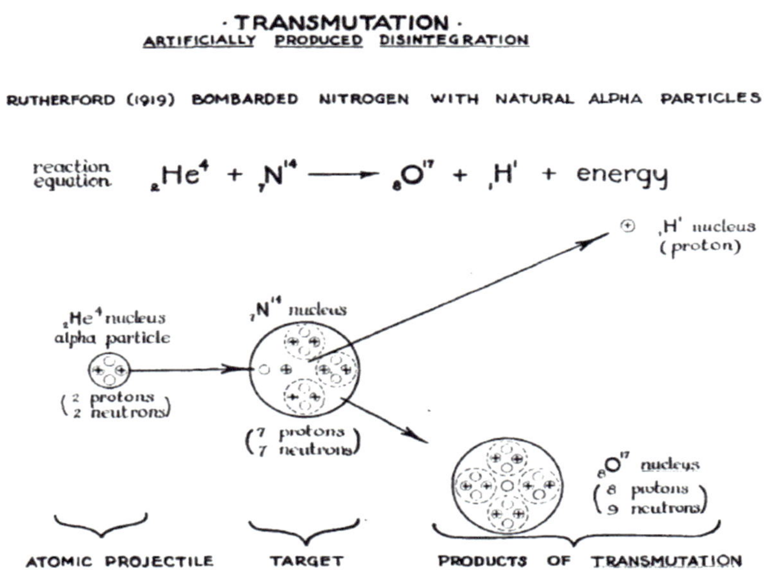

Fig. 2. Lawrence´s illustration about Rutherford Experiment.

In the same line of thoughts, Lawrence needs more projectiles to study this new phenomena. That 15th century dream of turning Lead into Gold was now though to be possible. Radioisotopes not always decay to a stable daughter but they continue trying, emitting different kinds of particles until they reach stability. In the sake for such stability they transform themselves into a partner they "believe" is more stable: The fifteen Century "Transmutation of Matter" occurs not for lead to become gold but something alike. Men made transmutation, which arise to be only the modification of the "positive electricity in the atomic nucleus", as Lawrence said.[1] He described his method of accelerating particles in Cyclotron as "resonance method" or "method of multiple acceleration:

The methods of multiple acceleration by resonance with an oscillating electric field have the advantage that they do not require high voltages. The general resonance principle is familiar even to the layman. A child in a swing knows that a high swinging velocity can be achieved by one big push, corresponding to the single acceleration of an ion by application of high voltage, or by a succession of small pushes properly timed with the swinging motion, corresponding to the resonance acceleration of ions. One type of apparatus that uses this resonance principle involves both a magnetic field and an oscillating electric field. We have in our laboratory two of this sort. The larger one of the two, which has been used in the nuclear investigations that I shall speak about, is shown on the next slide (Fig. 5). The most prominent feature of the apparatus is the giant electro-magnet, weighing something like 85 tons. Thus far we have accelerated deuterons to energies only slightly above five million, and the most energetic deuterons we have actually used in nuclear investigations had energies of about 4.5 million volts. The time, of course, will come when we will want to go up to higher voltages, and from our recent experience we are confident that, by using the full power of the magnet, we will be able to produce deuterons of energies above ten million volts, and possibly above fifteen million volts.

The ions are accelerated in the vacuum chamber between the poles of the magnet. The function of the magnetic field is to cause the ions to travel with constant angular velocity most of the time in circular paths. Within the chamber there are two semicircular hollow electrodes, between which is applied a high frequency potential difference. The ions circulate around from within one electrode to within another, and as they cross the diametrical region they gain increments of kinetic energy corresponding to the potential difference. Inasmuch as the angular velocity of the ions is determined by the magnetic field alone, they can be made to spiral around in synchronism with the oscillating electric field, with the result that they can be made to gain successive increments of velocity, and hence, going faster and faster on ever widening spirals, finally they emerge at the periphery of the apparatus where they are withdrawn by a deflecting electrostatic field through a thin aluminum window to the outside world. The swiftly moving deuterons travel a distance of about 17 cm before being stopped by their loss of energy in passing through air. The beam is visible as a bright blue glow; for the beam passing through the air excites the atoms and molecules to the emission of visible light. Experiments on the radioactivity induced by deuteron bombardment are carried out simply by placing the substance to be bombarded in the path of the deuteron beam just outside the aluminum window for any desired period of time, and then, taking the bombarded target away to an ionization chamber or a Wilson cloud expansion chamber, or any other apparatus used for studying the radiation given off from the activated target.

Fig. 3. Lawrence description of Cyclotron accelerating method.

Few time pass, until man used that newly produce radioactive material to treat and diagnoses different affections. John Lawrence, Ernest brother was the first to use his brother product ^{32}P to treat leukemia starting the medical applications of cyclotron products.

Method of particle activation then, need a Nuclear Reactor or an accelerator (Cyclotron, Syncrothron or Linac) to be produced: Nuclear Reactor is an installation in which big rod of natural occurring radioisotopes are set inside a pile with some stable, neutron absorbent, material. The radioisotopes (Th, U) initiates a chain reaction, the stable rod (such as carbon (graphite)) are used to absorb chain reaction debris, in order to moderate the amount of energy (heat) that is produce by nuclear reactions.

They are considered of two kinds: *Power Nuclear Reactors* which are dedicated to use the energy to produce electricity, for example, boiling water to move turbines with the steam and in this way produce electric power. *Nuclear Research Reactors* are used as a source of neutron of different energies to impact different atoms nuclei to become radioactive. In both cases they need the fission product from the original radioactive atom to undergo the chain reaction. For example, ^{235}U absorb a neutron, it become ^{236}U and this split into ^{92}Kr and ^{141}Ba with several neutron that can impact other ^{235}U and become ^{236}U to repeat the reactions.

[1] E.O.Lawrence:(1939) University of California: "Artificial Radiactivity" speech.

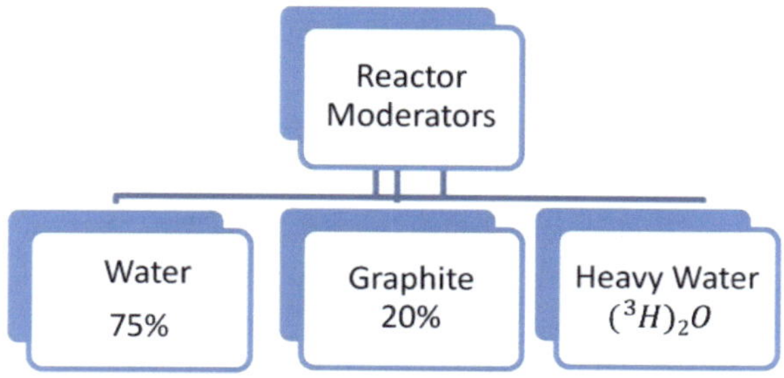

Fig. 4. Materials for particle absorption in a Reactor.

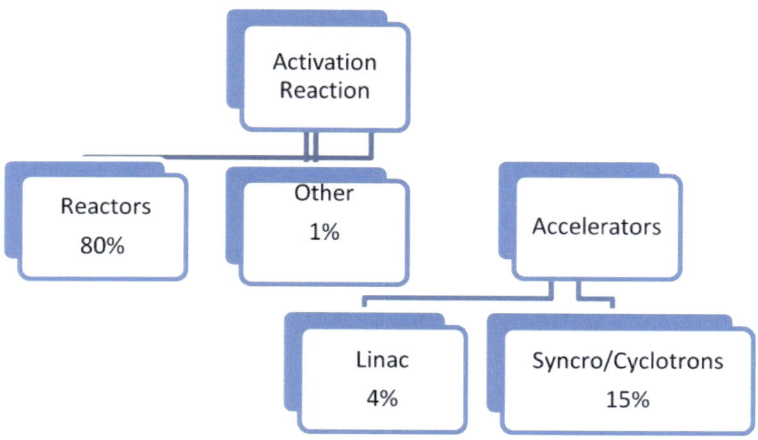

Fig. 5. Percentage of activation products worldwide coming from Reactors or Cyclotrons including medical, industry and research production.

In the other hand, cyclotron are electrical machines that generates particle acceleration thru helping them to undergo a circular or elliptical path in which particles gain energy by external manipulation of electric an magnetic fields.

Cyclotrons comes from a bigger family of electrical machines called Accelerators, because the make particles to gain energy letting them gain kinetic energy by applying electrical and magnetic fields to the particle trajectory so it can absorb energy from the media where it is travelling. Back to high school physics we can understand easily how cyclotrons accelerate particles: you must remember that force in an electrical field is:

$$F = qE \tag{1}$$

And also you remember that when you have and electrical and magnetic fields you can write

$$\vec{F} = q(\vec{v} \times \vec{B}) \tag{2}$$

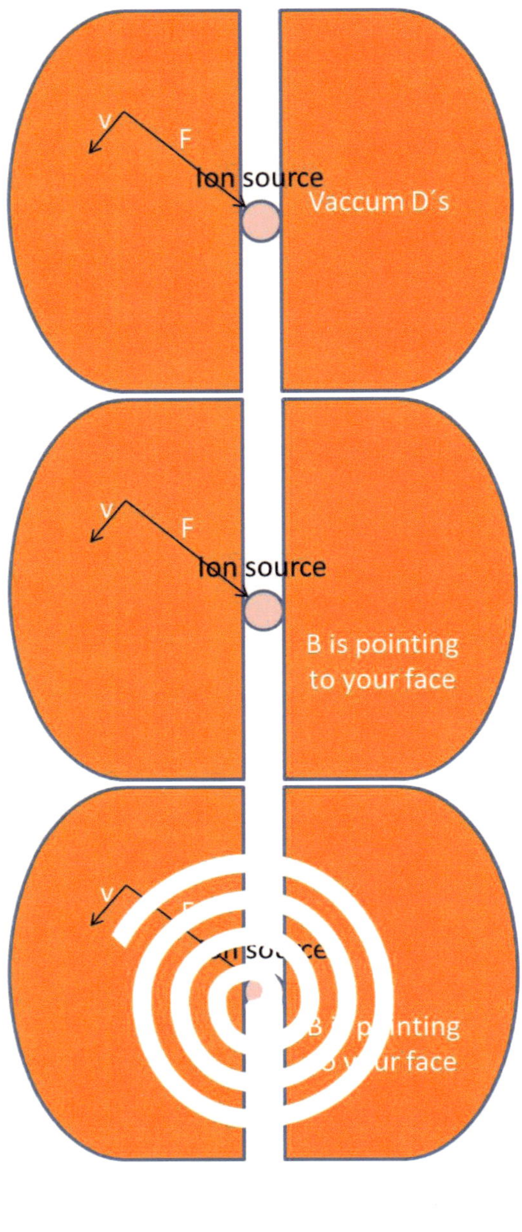

Fig. 6. Cyclotron schematics: a) ion input location, b) $\vec{B} = \vec{v}x\vec{F}$, c) Ion path.

Where q is the charge, v is the velocity and B is the magnetic field
Or in its escalar form

$$F = qvB \tag{3}$$

But you know that when you send a particle in a circular path also the centrifugal force yields:

$$F = \frac{mv^2}{r} \tag{4}$$

Where m is the mass of the particle to be accelerated and r is the radius of the circular path.
If you equal 3 with 4 you can obtain the radius you need for a particular energy you want

$$r = \frac{mv}{qB} \tag{5}$$

Velocity has two components, linear that is tangential to the spiral trajectory and angular that is about circular path cover by the particle, so

$$v = \omega r \tag{6}$$

Where ω is the angular velocity and

$$\omega = 2\pi f \tag{7}$$

Where f is the angular frequency of the movement, so using 3 and 4 we can know about cyclotron frequency

$$\frac{mv^2}{r} = qvB \tag{8}$$

Because potential energy has to become kinetic energy so,

$$qV = \frac{mv^2}{2} \tag{9}$$

Where V is the potential between the d´s where the particle gain energy

$$v^2 = \frac{2qV}{m} \tag{10}$$

$$where\ V = Er = vB \tag{11}$$

So $v = \frac{rqB}{m} = \omega r = 2\pi f r$ and finally

$$f = \frac{qB}{2\pi m} \tag{12}$$

And remembering Einstein, particles with this energies travels near speed of light

$$f = \frac{qB}{2\pi\gamma m_0} \tag{13}$$

With

$$\gamma = \frac{1}{\sqrt{1 - (v/c)^2}} \tag{14}$$

3. Methods of particle activation

Alpha particle Bombardment: Using natural produced alpha particles light elements can be activated, and as far as Pottasium. Such projectile induce the emission of a proton, the liberation of energy and a transmutation, not all the transmutation products are radioactive Neutron Capture: Firstly observed when matter is bombarded with deuteron, which also involve the emission of a proton, as we will illustrate forward.

4. Reaction of particle activation

1. Nuclear Activation in Reactors:

   (n,γ) Reaction: Radioactive capture: Undergo mostly by thermal neutron

$$^{59}_{29}Co + ^{1}_{0}n \longrightarrow ^{60}_{29}Co + \gamma \qquad \text{(s=36 b)}$$

$$^{98}_{42}Mo + ^{1}_{0}n \longrightarrow ^{99}_{42}Mo + \gamma \qquad \text{(s=0.12 b)}$$

In such a reaction father and daughter are of the same chemical species so they cannot be separated, reason why the target must have a very high enrichment rate.

   (n,α) Reaction followed by β- decay

$$^{130}_{52}Te + ^{1}_{0}n \longrightarrow ^{131}_{52}Te \xrightarrow{\beta^-} ^{131}_{53}I + \gamma$$

   Tellurium and iodine are easily chemical separated

   (n,p) Reaction: Neutron Capture

$$^{32}_{16}S + ^{1}_{0}n \longrightarrow ^{32}_{15}P + ^{1}_{1}H$$

$$^{58}_{28}Ni + ^{1}_{0}n \longrightarrow ^{59}_{28}Co + ^{1}_{1}H$$

This is similar to the first reaction produced in his cyclotron that be named "neutron capture" despite he was using deuterium as projectile, he observed that neutron stayed inside target nuclear and the remaining mass was expel as a proton.

   (n,α) Reaction: Light fission

$$^{6}_{3}Li + ^{1}_{0}n \longrightarrow ^{3}_{1}H + ^{4}_{2}He$$

2. Activation Equation:

$$\frac{dN_1}{dt} = \Phi \sigma_{act} N(t)$$

Where:

N_1 = Atoms of the target

Φ = Neutron flux

σ_{act} = Activation cross section

$N(t)$ = Number of atoms activated in a time period elapsed t

So, the number of activated atoms is:

$$N_1 = \Phi \frac{\sigma_{act} N(t)(1-e^{-\lambda t})}{\lambda}$$

And the activity of the sample is:

$$A = \lambda N_1 = \Phi \sigma_{act} N(t)(1-e^{-\lambda t})$$

t is the time of irradiation in seconds

A is the activity at the saturation value that is a function of reactor neutron flue at which target has been exposed.

3. Nuclear reaction in cyclotron production

(p,n) Reaction

$$^{18}_{8}O + ^{1}_{1}H \longrightarrow ^{18}_{9}F + ^{1}_{0}n$$

(d,α) Reaction:

$$^{20}_{10}Ne + \longrightarrow ^{18}_{9}F + ^{4}_{2}He$$

(p,α) Reaction

$$^{14}_{17}N + ^{1}_{1}H \longrightarrow ^{11}_{6}C + ^{4}_{2}He$$

$$^{16}_{8}O + ^{1}_{1}H \longrightarrow ^{13}_{7}N + ^{4}_{2}He$$

(d,n) Reaction

$$^{14}_{7}N + ^{2}_{1}H \longrightarrow ^{15}_{8}O + ^{1}_{0}n$$

$(d,2n)$ Reaction

$$^{68}_{30}Zn + ^{2}_{1}H \longrightarrow ^{65}_{31}Ga + 2^{0}_{1}n$$

$$^{124}_{52}Te + ^{1}_{1}H \longrightarrow ^{123}_{53}I + 2^{1}_{0}n$$

$(\alpha,2n)$ Reaction

$$^{65}_{29}Cu + ^{4}_{2}He \longrightarrow ^{67}_{31}Ga + 2^{1}_{0}n$$

5. Differences and similarities between reactors and cyclotrons

Cyclotron is not the only way of activating matter. Going through history, side by side cyclotron development in America, Europe was devoted to the natural radioactive material discovered by many scientists, from Madame Curie (1898), Pierre, Irene and also Joliot till Enrico Fermi, Otto Hahn, Lise Meitner and Fritz Strassman (1939). Neils Bohr and Jhon A. Wheeler published their explanation of the method for moderating, "modulating", chain reactions in a paper published only 2 days after WWII starts in 1939. The first reactor was then brought into criticality in Fermi´s Lab on December 2nd, 1942 in very controlled experiment including radiation safety and protection considerations. Proving that chain reaction can be controlled, it was matter of time to find uses for the products obtain from a nuclear reactor. The neutron from reactors are projectiles for many (n,p), (n,β), reactions to produce many radioisotopes. So time has come to begin talking about which of all this radioactive products can be used in medicine. The first radioactive material used in humans with medical purposes was 226Ra, (1898) used by Madame and Mousier Curie to treat skin lesion they called "benign". Their daughter Irene used 214Bi to measure blood flow, this two products come directly from the ^{238}U natural decay series. By the artificial radioisotopes side, the first one was that ^{32}P John Lawrence (1929) used to treat leukemia. After of it, a lot of radioisotopes and a lot of uses have been developed for diagnostic and therapy uses, so for this time, we can say that the radioisotopes used in Medicine distributions is as it is shown in Table 2:

	Reactors Produced		Cyclotrons Produced
	Fission Products	Neutron activation	
Diagnostic Purposes	^{133}Xe, ^{99}Mo	^{51}Cr, ^{125}I, ^{131}I, ^{89}Sr, ^{153}Sm, ^{59}Fe, ^{177}Lu, ^{42}K, ^{75}Se, ^{24}Na, ^{99m}Tc, ^{159}Yt	^{11}C, ^{13}N, ^{15}O, ^{18}F, ^{57}Co, ^{82}Sr, ^{68}Ge ^{64}Cu,^{67}Ga, ^{68}Ga, ^{111}In, ^{123}I, ^{124}I, ^{81m}Kr, ^{82}Rb, ^{201}Tl
Therapeutic Application	^{89}Sr, ^{90}Y	^{213}Bi, ^{60}Co, ^{165}Dy, ^{169}Er, ^{125}I, ^{131}I, ^{192}Ir, ^{212}Pb, ^{177}Lu, ^{103}Pd, ^{32}P, ^{186}Re, ^{188}Re, ^{153}Sm	^{67}Cu, ^{57}Co, ^{82}Sr, ^{68}Ge

Table 2. Distribution of the radioisotope production for medical applications.

Like the Curie's began using their newly discovered natural radioisotopes to treat cancer lesion in the skin, very short time after the construction of the cyclotron and the production of its radioisotopes, makes the medical applications to be easily spread.

But there is another mechanism for particle activation and it comes from the nuclear reactor where a bunch of natural radioisotopes "bars" are used to produced spontaneous fission products to aim the nucleus of stable atom or its electronic crown.

Nowadays reactors are the core of the nuclear power plants, but in their beginnings they were developed for research proposes to military applications only. Due to the natural "nuclear fuel" reactors were better in cost/efficiency fashion and in the late 30's and early 40's many budgets and efforts were driven to their construction to regulated nuclear chain reaction and its control, until the atomic bomb development to win WWII.

But passing thru that dark hour, all the money spend in its development seems to be not that important.

And cyclotron has to compete (and win) against reactors that were redeeming themselves by producing "atoms for the peace" trying to justify the large budget assign to them during WWII.

And for a long period of time the guilt drop the balance to reactors side until middle 70's when positron emission tomography arised based in a component containing ^{18}F: ^{18}FDG (Fluorodexoxy glucose).

This isotope was only produced in cyclotron and the compound could be synthetized in a straight forward relative easy way.

This made cyclotrons an Hospital equipment because, due to the short half-life of ^{18}F, it was necessary to stablish the supplier so near to the costumer as it can be, and being a hospital a places were pureness and asepsie is well know, and treat with reverential respect, which other place would be better to activated pure ^{18}F and synthetize the ^{18}FDG in a sterile form to be safe to apply in human.

And between 1929 and 1974 lot of things happened to cyclotron to develop its actual characteristic. From Lawrence Cyclotron to Hospital one, until CERN´s a lot of energy has pass through.

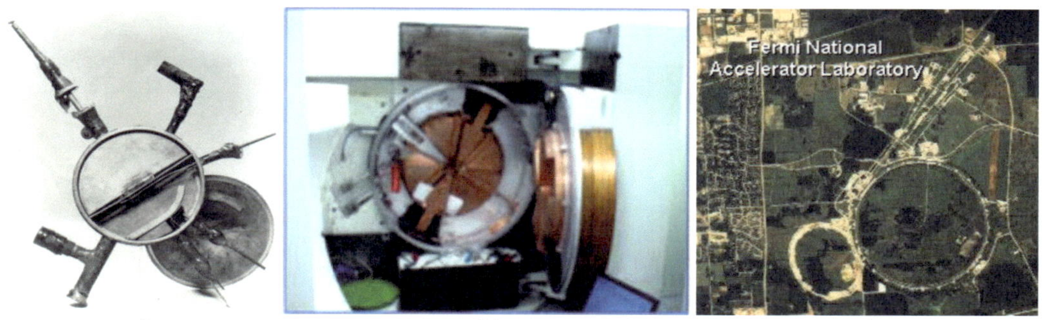

a) b) c)

Fig. 7. Different cyclotron size: a) Lawrence´s first one, b) Venezuela First one (courtesy of Dorly Coehlo), c) Fermi National Laboratory at CERN.

And size matters, and Cyclotrons win as best hospital candidates due to Reactors are bigger, harder and difficult to be set in a hospital installation. Can you imagine a nuclear reactor inside a health installation? Radiation Protection Program will consume all the budget available. Size, controlled reactions, electrical control, made cyclotrons easy to install, and baby cyclotrons come selfshielded so hospital don´t need to spend money in a extremely large bunker. Now on, we are going to talk about our first experience with the set up of a baby cyclotron for medical uses inside the first PET installation in Latin America. "Baby" means its acceleration "D" diameters are suitable to be set inside a standard hospital room dimensions, with all its needs to be safetly shielded for production transmision and synthetized for human uses for imaging in Nuclear Medicine PET routine. When we ask why Cyclotrons are better than reactors for radioisotopes production to be used in Medicine, we also have to have in mind that they has:

1. Less radioactive waste
2. Less harmful debris

3. They can be installed inside hospital decentralizing radioisotope production.
4. Almost zero risk of nuclear accidents (Because there is no chain reaction to control)
5. There is no risk of nuclear proliferation

Compare with a reactor.

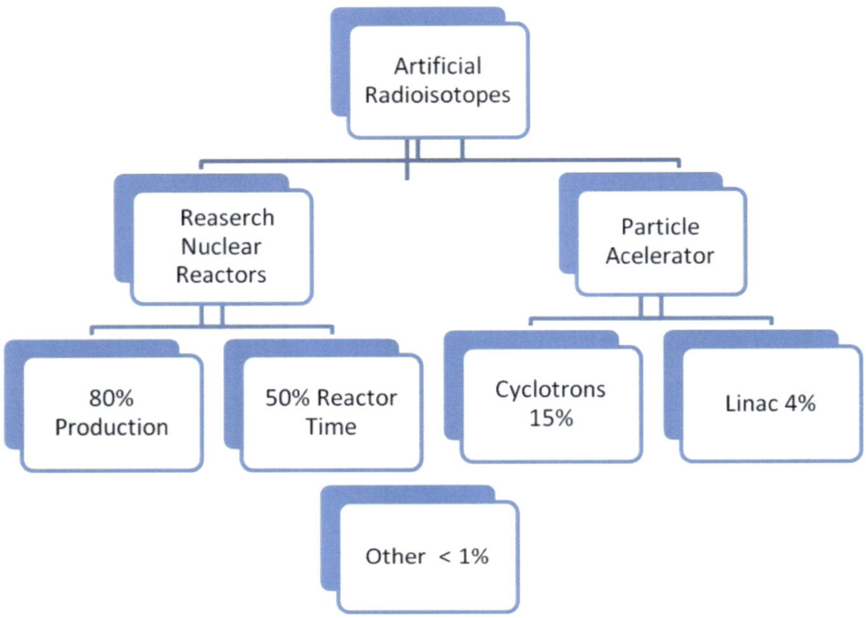

Fig. 8. Artificial radioisotopes.

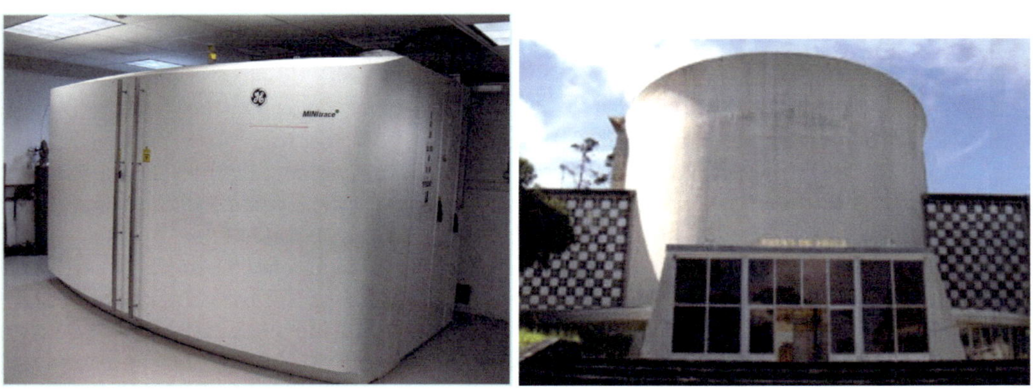

a) b)

Fig. 9. Difference in size between a) Venezuelan medical cyclotron (courtesy of Indira Lugo) and b)Venezuelan research reactor (in desuse).

Medical Cyclotrons generally often comes with 4 targets to activated: Fluor 18, Oxigen 15, Nitrogen 13 and Carbon 11. In Venezuela we have one with only one target to activated fluor 18 to sintethized ^{18}FDG, for PET studies.

6. Activation products medical uses

Remembering what we want for a radioisotopes to be safely used in medicine, Natural decay series has had a very bad performance. For example, ^{226}Ra was used in Medicine until users realized that its daughter was ^{222}Rn, a gas. Since ^{226}Ra was encapsulated in stainless steel tubes the accumulation of Radon from Radium decay inside the tube, cause the gaseous pressure to increase in a non controlled way, so more than 10 years after its encapsulation, the gas pressure was so high as to break the capsule and escape. So as ^{222}Rn is a radioactive gas and it half life is not short (almost 4 days), contamination was hard to contain, so Radium use was declined.

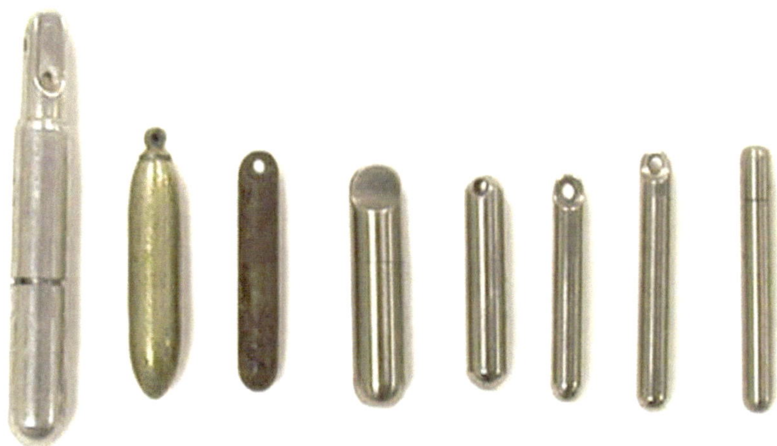

Fig. 10. Radium Tubes.

Activation products from Cyclotrons are in general of short half life, so the control can be focus in the energy users can handle. In such a way, we can say activation products can be tailored to our needs. But medical uses are little complicated. Nuclear Medicine consist in mix the radioisotope with a pharmaceutical product which is characterized by the organ they are going to address the isotope. What Nuclear Medicine really needs is to send the radioisotope to get inside the organ we want to study, and as the radioisotope is inside a molecule that can be metabolized by this organ, this metabolization function can be easily watch and measure with the appropriate radiation detectors. The name "radiopharmaceuticals" refers to the metabolically stable combination of a biochemical molecule to which radioisotope in bind that act as the vehicle through which, organ of interest can be reach. There are several mechanism for the radioisotope to join the address molecule such as:

1. Ionic compound: In which the radioisotopes determine the metabolic route to be follow as in ^{131}I to thyroid uses, because thyroid likes iodine and do not distinguish between different isotopes of the same element iodine.

2. Isotopic Exchange: In which the radioactive isotope goes to replace the stable isotope of it own species
3. Incorporation: In which radioisotope get inside the molecule but not interacting with the chemical compound, so it did not change its structure neither biochemical nor physical properties
4. Coprecipitation: In which radionuclide is precipitated in the same reaction with the chemical compound. Many are the radioisotopes that can be combined with different molecules to be address to different parts of human body with diagnostic or therapeutic purposes, so we can group them as in the table below:

Imaging:

Isotope	Symbol	Z	T1/2	Decay mode	Photons Energy	β energy	Uses
Fluorine-18	^{18}F	9	109.77m	β+	511 (193%)	0.664 (97%)	PET: Cancer detection and monitoring of treatment progress, in flurodexoxiglucose. (FDG) Tracer in flurothymidine (FLT) and fluromisonidazole (F-MISO), and ^{18}F-choline
Gallium-67	^{67}Ga	31	3.26d	EC	93 (39%)	185 (21%), 300 (17%)	SPECT: Tumor imaging, infections localization
Krypton-81m	^{81m}Kr	36	13.1s	IT	190 (68%)	-	Refrigerant
Rubidium-82	^{82}Rb	37	1.27m	β+	511 (191%)	3.379 (95%)	Tracer in positron emission tomography
Technetium-99m	^{99m}Tc	43	6.01h	IT	140 (89%)	-	Pulmonary ventilation studies.
Indium-111	^{111}In	49	2.80d	EC	171 (90%)	245 (94%)	Brain studies, infection and colon transit studies.
Iodine-123	^{123}I	53	13.3 h	EC	159 (83%)	-	Gamma emitter: diagnosis of thyroid function, without the beta radiation of I-131.
Xenon-133	^{133}Xe	54	5.24d	β-	81 (31%)	0.364 (99%)	Studies of pulmonary function and organic blood flow.
Thallium-201	^{201}Tl	81	3.04d	EC	69-83* (94%)	167 (10%)	Diagnostic aid in the form of thallous chloride TI 201
Carbon-11	^{11}C	6	20.39m	β+	--	0.96 (100%)	PET: Studies of brain physiology: epileptic focus, dementia, etc
Nitrogen-13	^{13}N	9	9.965m	β+	--	1.2 (100%)	PET: Cardiology
Oxygen-15	^{15}O	8	122.24s	β+	--	1.8 (100%)	PET: Cardiology and cancer detection
Cooper-64	^{64}Cu	29	13 h	β+	--	0.65 (61%) 0.58(39%)	genetic studies: copper metabolism: Wilson's and Menke's diseases. PET: tumours, and therapy.
Cooper-67	^{67}Cu	29	2.6 d	$β^-$	--	0.56 (100%)	Beta emitter therapy
Gallium-68	^{68}Ga	31	68 min	$β^+$	--	1.90 (100%)	PET: tumor detection, daughter in ^{68}Ge generator
Germanium-68	^{68}Ge	32	271 d	EC	--	0.1 (100%)	^{68}Ga generator parent

Therapy:

Isotope	Symbol	Z	T1/2	Decay mode	Photons energy	β energy
Yttrium-90	90Y	39	2.67d	β-	-	2.280 (100%)
Iodine-131	131I	53	8.02 d	γ, β-	364 (81%)	0.807 (100%)

Table 3. Common Isotopes Used in Nuclear Medicine for diagnostic studies or therapy procedure.

In the table above we can see some radioisotopes that say they are parent or daughter in a generator, but what is a generator?

7. Generators

In Nuclear Medicine environment, sometimes is useful to have a regular provision of radioisotopes for studies to be performed without the restrictions of providers time dependences, for example when studies has to be done anytime of the day in emergency conditions. If physician suspects an infection in a patient admitted in Emergency Room, it will be of utmost usefulness to have Nuclear Medicine images done with appropriate radiopharmaceuticals to solve the question about the most effective treatment to be offer to the patient. Either way, sometimes in Cardiology it is of high importance to know about percentage of isquemic muscle, but patient has not the luxury of time to undergo a catheterism, so it is more effective and quick to have Nuclear Medicine images and cine of the heart. In many cases like this, have a good availability of radiotracers make the differences between a correct and opportune answer or a misdiagnosis.

This is the reason why radioisotopes generators have become so popular beside the fact that in countries like Venezuela where there is no nuclear production, sometime become very hard to warranty a regular supply. A radioisotopes generator is a device in which you can contain a pair father/daughter in which the daughter is the product of interest for studies purposes and father only come to generate the full amount of daughter needed. Due to the short half life we need for the radioisotope to be safe handle in hospital conditions, it would be useful to find a pair father and daughter that warranty the in time provision of radioisotope needed. During the generator useful life father has to decay completely to the useful daughter so it can be easily recharged, disposed or returned to provider. Such pair must that accomplish some conditions like:

1. Father has to have long enough half life (physical) such as to overcome travel time from provider to user. In this way father will be generating enough amount of daughter that can be extract in site for studies and will continue generating daughter to fulfill the needs for its entire useful time.
2. Father must be shipped in pyrogen free condition
3. Daughter has to decay in a sufficient short life be secure for image acquisition and radiation protection of patient
4. Father and daughter have to have different chemical characteristics so the can be easily separate to be sure the daughter is so pure to be safe for human applications and there are no traces of the father in the injection solution.

5. This separation must be passive in terms of no violent chemical reaction must be involved in the process, to warranty the chemical safeness
6. The daughter must be eluted with a human compatible solution to warranty biological safeness
7. The human intervention would be minimum to warranty the minimum exposure to radiation
8. Radiation protection now is not the unique concern but chemical and biological protection is also very critical
9. The granddaughter must be of very long time as to be consider stable

After radiochemist discover some pairs of father/daughter that accomplish this characteristics, some were built in a shielded container to be send to hospital to extract the daughter. It makes radiosotopes clinically useful and commercially available.

Medicine is not the only client for radioisotopes generator, also we will talk about some other uses of them that are increasing its popularity thru years. So let´s have a few words about their relationship. As in any father/daughter relationship there are different kinds, in radioactive "family" we can talk about two kind of equilibrium that this families reach, they are called transient and secular equilibrium. Equilibrium meaning when father and daughter exist in significant proportion to one another. Secular equilibrium is a condition that they can reach when father physical half life is 2 or 3 magnitude orders greater that daughter´s (100 to 1000 times greater). It means when daughter decay many times father seems no to be affected. While transient equilibrium is a condition that is reach when father physical half life is about 10 times daughter´s. It is, when daughter decay few times father can decay to its 50%, i.e a full half life. Note that if physical half life of the daughter is larger that the father equilibrium can never be reach because father will be ever alone.

Secular Equilibrium Generators

$$^{68}Ge \xrightarrow{\varepsilon,275d} {}^{68}Ga \xrightarrow{\beta^+,\varepsilon,\gamma,1.14\,h} {}^{68}Zn$$

$$^{81}Rb \xrightarrow{\beta^+,\varepsilon,4.7h} {}^{81m}Kr \xrightarrow{\gamma,13s} {}^{81}Kr$$

$$^{82}Sr \xrightarrow{\varepsilon,25d} {}^{82}Rb \xrightarrow{\beta^+,\varepsilon,\gamma,75s} {}^{82}Kr$$

$$^{113}Sn \xrightarrow{\varepsilon,118d} {}^{113m}In \xrightarrow{\gamma,1.7\,h} {}^{113}In$$

Transient Equilibrium Generators

$$^{99}Mo \xrightarrow{\beta^-,\gamma,67h} {}^{99m}Tc \xrightarrow{\gamma,6\,h} {}^{99}Tc$$

$$^{188}W \xrightarrow{\varepsilon,275d} {}^{188}Rh \xrightarrow{\beta^-,17\,h} {}^{188}Os$$

Although this last one has a promising future in metastatic disease pain reliever and as a monoclonal antibody marker, the most popular generator in Nuclear Medicine is the Mo/Tc one. It is Techenetium is highly biocompatible in the Nuclear Medicine fashion so it can be used in a large number of studies.

This Mo/Tc generators can be produced in cyclotrons or reactors and as in many radioisotope produced, the advantages of using that from cyclotron in front of that of reactors is that in cyclotron you can use ^{98}Mo enriched target to be activated by neutron irradiation in a (n,γ) reaction, while ^{99}Mo coming from fission include very expensive production beside the complex regulations due to the highly enriched Uranium targets.

TARGET ORGAN	^{99m}Tc RADIOPHARMACEUTICALS
Brain	DTPA (DiethylTriaminoPentacetic Acid) ($CaNa_3{}^{99m}Tc$)
Brain Perfusion	ECD (EthylCysteinate Dimer)
Kidneys	DTPA (DiethylTriaminoPentacetic Acid) Calcium Gluconate Lactobionate Calcium Glucoheptonate Manitol Dextrose Penicilamine 2,4 dimercaptosuccinic acid
Liver	^{99m}Tc Sulphur Sn Hidroxide Sodium Phytate Sodium Calcium Phytate
Lungs	Inorganic Macroagregate Albumin Macroagregates Microspheres (50μ)
Bone	Poliphosphate Monofluorphosphate Diphosphonate Pirophospate (MDP) Metilendiphosphonate
Dynamic Studies	Albumina Microspheres (0.5-4 μ)
Tumors	Bleomicine Tetracycline Citrate
Spleen	Red Blood Cell Markers
Spleen and Bile	Vitamine B6 glutamic HIDA (Hepatobiliary IminoDiacetic Acid)
Blood Pool	^{99m}Tc Albumina
White Blood Cell or platelets (infection or inflammation)	^{99m}Tc HMPAO (HexaMethylPropileneAmineOxime)

Table 4. Radiuopharmaceuticals used with ^{99m}Tc for diagnostic studies.

8. Baby cyclotron characteristics

Baby cyclotrons are known as a hospital equipment be cause they are build to fulfill the medical proposes, in general, they can afford until 4 targets to activated most of radioisotopes needs to do PET studies

In Venezuelan experience the first installed cyclotron has the following characteristics:

- Generated beam for activation: H +
- Energy required for the activation: 9.6 MeV
- Output Beam minimal current: 50 μ A
- Material to Activate: $H_2{}^{18}O$
- Activation Product: $^{18}F^-$ (fluorine ion).
- Running average activity: 800 mCi
- Activation efficiency: Greater than 60%

Also the device dimensions where 3.6 x 2 x 2 m^3 for the acceleration d´s and inner shielding. And the room has to have at least 7 x 5 m^2 only for the cyclotron and another 6 x 5 m^2 for the synthesis lab. But the very concerning issue is the weight of the entire system, only in inner shielding it has 37 tons and the magnet alone has a weight of 11 tons the full system is over 50 tons

This cyclotron produce protons of 9.6 millions of electron volts (MeV) of energy with a maximum current of 50 μA, the target is made of oxigen to transmute to fluor. In this activation process there are some particles going out the path of the main beam so they have to be stopped by the inner shielding as to warranty 10 μSv/h at 1 m from shleding and 1 m from floor. Also the magnetic regulation permit 1 G at 6 m from the center of the D´s

8.1 Venezuelan medical cyclotron

In our experiences, the utmost importance matter in a Cyclotron is the Quality Assurance Program in which must be include:

1. Electrical Aspects
2. Mechanical and performance aspects and
3. Radiation Safety Aspects

In a broad approximation, we can say that:

8.1.1 Electrical aspects that have to be under control are:

- On/off switches
  - For operation
  - For Emergency
- Failure Interlocks
  - Safety Interlocks
    - Audible alarm
    - Luminous alarm
- Processing unit connection
- Selfdiagnostic

8.1.2 Mechanical and performance aspects to be under control are:

- Radiofrequency
  - Driver

    - Stability
- Mechanical movements of inner and outer doors
- Beam Energy
- Output flux
- Output dose and exposition
- Target effectiveness
- Activation effectiveness

8.1.3 Radiation Safety aspects to be under control are:

- Area classification and signs
- Area monitorization
- Personal dosimetry
- Activation control
- Airborne debris
- Chimney
- Personnel Medical Check up:
    - Previous to begin working in the facility
    - Annual (prevocational) check up
    - Posterior to end laboral relationship with the facility
- Shielding
- Radiation Safety Committee

8.1.4 Daily journey: Also three aspects need to be controlled step by step, accounting to:

- Radioisotope Production
- Handling radioactive material for studies
- Possible emergency

8.1.4.1 In radioisotope production it must be carefully checked:

- Pre-start conditions
- Area and ventilation ducts monitoring during cyclotron is on
- Activation and contamination control after cyclotron is turn off
- Pre and post Hot Cell monitoring
- Radioactive waste disposal entry and release record
- Fractionation residues and contamination
- Radioactive waste disposal
    - Place design
    - Waste classification
    - Decay rate
    - Free release dates

8.1.4.2 Radioactive material handling for diagnostic studies

- Total activity produced in a cyclotron run
- Fractionation doses
- Patient injection site and procedure

- Patient waiting room= Controlled area
- Adverse reaction, contraindication, diabetic patients

8.1.4.3 Possible emergencies

- Coolling system failure
- Door interlocks during cyclotron is on
- In use production line rupture
- Vial rupture
    - Inside hot cell
    - Inside fractionation hood
    - Outside

8.1.4.4 Radioactive material spills

- Inside hot cell
- Inside fractionation hood
- During transportation

This a resume of our general procedure manual, reproduced for physicians to know about all procedures that will be under their responsibility because they are legally, the responsible for the facility and its practices, as is establish in BSS and many other documents regarding medical practice. Here we only intent to introduce a general framework about medical cyclotrons so we will only mention some useful concepts and its application in a new facility.

8.1.5

Regarding to electrical aspects we must emphasize that failure interlock never must be deactivated, before the in charge expert check it out and solve the situation, only after he/she sign the log describing the solution, operation can continue. It is important to remember that ignoring this interlocks and alarms has conducted, many times, to major accidents injuring personnel and patients.

Before turning on cyclotron for a production run, the following operation parameters must be checked:

STEP ONE: MORNING CHECK OUT BEFORE TURNING CYCLOTRON ON: (EXAMPLE)

Water leakage	***NO***	
Normal operative ventilation	***OK***	
Electrical power on, stable and normal	*Control cabinet*	***OK***
	Rf cabinet	***OK***
Vacumm	7×10^{-7} mbar (7×10^{-5} Pa)	
Water conductivity	5 μSiemens	
Water cooling temperature	**20±2 °C**	
Gas valves	*Production*	Máx 0.5 MPa (73 psi)
	Operation	3 ±0.1 MPa (435 ± 14 psi)
	Transport	0.5 ±0.2 MPa (73 ±29 psi)
Shielding closed	***OK***	
Nobody in	***OK***	

Cyclotron door closed	***OK***
Room door closed	***OK***
Safety system on (green)	***OK***

8.1.6

On mechanical and performance settings it is important to become religious with the daily log for parameters to be safely establish before start working, to be sure of, what we want to obtain is what we really will obtain after cyclotron runs in the desire conditions

STEP TWO: TUNNING ON CYCLOTRON (EXAMPLE)

Turn on all the computers		
Run autocheck		
Define in the console	Current	
	Irradiation time	
	Charge	
	Activity	
	Target water level	

8.1.7

For personnel safety there exist three types of emergency interlocks:

- Radiological emergency: as described
- Ergonomical emergency: as feet trapped under the cyclotron doors
- Nature emergency: earthquake, flood, etc

8.1.8

In radiation safety aspects it is important to notice that radiation protection is not a solely part body but a team work . Everybody in the facility must be involved in Radiation Protection (RP) tasks and in the Radiation Safety (RS) Program and must be accomplish this minimal recommendations:

RADIATION PROTECTION BASIC RECOMMENDATIONS: (EXAMPLE)

1.	Use your badge all the time you are in the facility (body, ring, alarm dosimeters)
2.	Use also the handy personal monitor that has been assign to you anytime you access the supervised and controlled areas
3.	Inside cyclotron room, hot lab and fractionation lab, use cloak, glove and glasses
4.	Do not use decorative rings (jewelry), scarf, bracelet or any other accessory that could transport contamination outward
5.	Never get in cyclotron room during production
6. 7.	Never use mouth pipettes Never handle radioactive material outside cells or hoods
8.	Use long forceps or tweezers
9.	Never use controlled fridge for food or beverage
10.	Radioactive waste must be dispose by its nature and classification in the selected area for them

11.	Monitor your working area before and after each assignation and whenever a contamination is suspected
12.	Wash your hands before living controlled area
13.	Monitor your hands before living controlled area and return to 12 until background is reached. In any case contact RSO
14.	Record every activity (cyclotron, Hot Lab, Synthsys lab, Fractionation Lab) in corresponding log
15.	Any unusual event must be report in corresponding log
16.	In any radiological event communication chain must be follow
17.	In case of inhalation or ingestion follew corresponding emergency procedure as it is written

8.1.8.1

In such a large facility it is mandatory to exist an ad hoc committee known s "Radiation Safety Committee" (RSC) as it is establish in Venezuelan safety standard NVC3299. In our case, this comitte must ever be conformed by:

1. Radiation Safety Officer
2. One delegate from maintenance and engineering department
3. One delegate from directive or administrative board
4. One delegated of security department
5. One delegate from technician staff
6. One delegate from nursing staff
7. One delegated from physician (at least)

Many other specialist, physician, physicist, chemist can be include

8.1.8.2

For radiation area classification, national standard recommendation will be follow as in NVC 2257: Any area must be classified as "Controlled" if in any moment of daily operation the exposition rate is above 0.5 mR/h. In this sense , cyclotron room, synthesis lab, hot lab, injection room pet/ct room are controlled areas by default. Classification of different areas will be consult to RSC and RSO and will be solve only after 24 h continuous measurements, and any other consideration in standard classification may be voted and solved by more that 75% of delegates

This is the figure that will take all the decisions regarding al RS concerns and its decisions must be voted to win with more of the 75% of the committee delegates.

In radioisotope uses (for diagnostic or therapies) any patient application can be supervised by committee and logs must be all time up to date. All the details for all the task mentioned above must be clearly describe in each procedure manual and clearly understand by any of the participant of each task

Notification chain must also be clearly establish and accomplish from personnel who needs to report, thru RSO, until the National Regulatory Authority

8.1.8.3 Cyclotron Cycle

- In cyclotron room protons hits water target transmuting ^{16}O into ^{18}F.
- In Hot Lab ^{18}F ions are measured in activity, pureness, pyrogenicity, volume, etc
- Synthesis Lab FDG is produced by substitution of oxygen ion by the activated fluorine ion inside the molecular chain yielding to labeled ^{18}FDG

8.1.8.4 Parasite Activation

One of the most relevant issues in Cyclotron facility is the activation of the materials inside the cyclotron room during daily operation. As cyclotron room is a close and hardly shielded facility all activation products will ever be contained inside its room and the activation levels will only be monitored and measured during providers maintenances, in this opportunity, frotis are taken of the most suitable materials to be activated and they are measure in spectrometer. On the other hand, gaseous activation is continuously monitored with proper devices set inside the chimney. As first defense line, the facility has a 200 m circuit through which gaseous particles travel during 24 hours before getting into the chimney to be release to the atmosphere. As our cyclotron do not have gaseous target all the airborne particles come from the air inside the room, so they are characterized by their extremely short half lives, around nano or micro seconds. Periodcally, frotis are taken from the chimney to be measure in spectrometer.

For any maintenance that need the "backdoor" of the cyclotron to be removed, exposition rate must be below 0.5 mR/h as it is establish in NVC2259. If it is not, maintenance personnel must wait until this level is reached.

Finally, it must be said that in operation conditions Cyclotron is fully shielded allowing a maximum of 10 mSv at 1 m in the axial direction of the magnet, and such a value is only reached one or twice a day in the production time that is less than 2 hours accounting all the running.

8.2 Synthesis laboratory

In Pet studies a cyclotron is nothing without radiochemical laboratory , because cyclotron only produce the ion, in our case, ^{18}F and it has to be joined to the glucose analogue molecule (fluordexoxiglucose) to be driven to the body. In it fluor is send into molecule via electrophilic fluorination or nucleophilic fluorination reaction in which stable fluor is substitute by the activated ^{18}F.

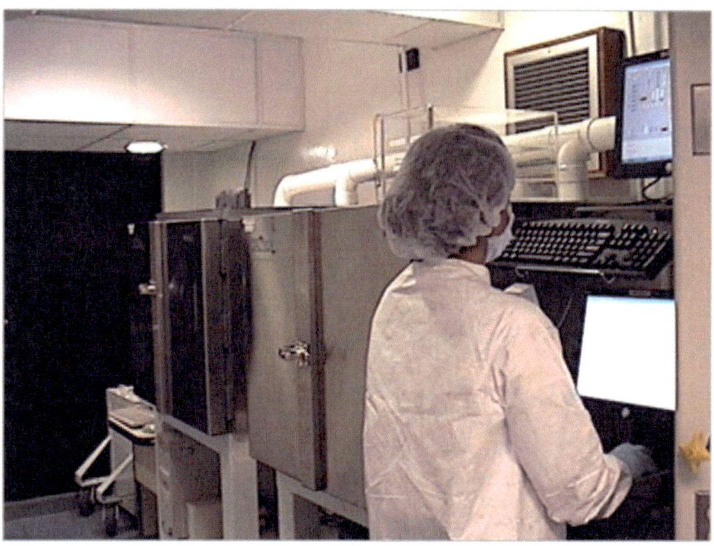

Fig. 11. Synthesis Lab in Venezuelan Cyclotron facility (courtesy Dorly Coehlo)

8.3 Patient radiation protection

Before finishing let´s have few words about the protection of patients. In patient protection we have to had in mind not only the physical half life because sometimes biological half life is longer and radiation protection must to be concern to the excretion system of patient so Nuclear Medicine define an effective half life to take into account the two contributions to patient doses coming from physical and biological behavior of radioisotope. Biological half live is the time living organism needs to excrete any radioisotope trace of radioactive material. It depends no only of physical time but on effectiveness of excretion system of the body. So effective life is :

$$\frac{1}{T_{1/2}^{eff}} = \frac{1}{T_{1/2}^{phy}} + \frac{1}{T_{1/2}^{bio}}$$

ISOTOPES	HALF LIVES (days)		
	$T_{Physical}$	$T_{Biological}$	$T_{Effective}$
^{3}H	4.5×10^{3}	12	12
^{14}C	2.1×10^{6}	40	40
^{22}Na	850	11	11
^{32}P	14.3	1155	14.1
^{35}S	87.4	90	44.3
^{36}Cl	1.1×10^{8}	29	29
^{45}Ca	165	1.8×10^{4}	164
^{59}Fe	45	600	42
^{60}Co	1.93×10^{3}	10	10
^{65}Zn	244	933	193
^{86}Rb	18.8	45	13
^{90}Sr	1.1×10^{4}	1.8×10^{4}	6.8×10^{4}
^{99m}Tc	0.25	1	0.20
^{123}I	0.54	138	0.54
^{131}I	8	138	7.6
^{137}Cs	1.1×10^{4}	70	70
^{140}Ba	12.8	65	10.7
^{198}Au	2.7	280	2.7
^{210}Po	138	60	42
^{226}Ra	5.8×10^{5}	1.6×10^{4}	1.5×10^{4}
^{235}U	2.6×10^{11}	15	15
^{239}Pu	8.8×10	7.3×10^{4}	7.2×10^{4}

Table 4. Physical and Biological half lives

Radioisotopes like P and Sr like to stay in bone, so as far as they can be used to treat bone lesions the maximize its doses due to the combination of physical and biological exposure. Phosphorous decay faster so Sr is better to treat bone metastasis due to it relatively long physical and biological half life. For diagnostic studies Tc has proven to be the best due to its short physical and biological lives, so it is excrete from the body just after images has be taken.

9. References

Books

International Atomic Energy Agency. Technical Document 1340: Manual for Reactor Produced Radioisotopes. January 2003.1-257.

RUTH, T. World View of Radioisotope Production. 2008. 1-60.

International Atomic Energy Agency. Technical Report Series No 471: Cycotron Produced Radionuclides: Guidelines for setting up a Facility. January 2003.1-257.

Publications

NVC2257: Norma Venezolana Covenin 2257: Radiaciones Ionizantes: Clasificación, señalización y demarcación de zonas de trabajo. ISBN: 980-06-1559-8

NVC2259: Norma Venezolana Covenin 2259: Radiaciones Ionizantes: Límites anuales de dosis. ISBN: 980-06-1560-1

NVC3299: Norma Venezolana Covenin 3299: Programa de Proteccion Radiologica . Requisitos ISBN: 980-06-1854-6

Massila, K., Stein, R. & Suhizan, S. & Azlianor, A. World Academy of Science, Engineering and Technology: Theoretical Isotopes Generator: An Alternative Towards Isotope Pattern Calculator. 2007. 146-149.

McGoron, A. Radioisotopes in Nuclear Medicine. 1-8.

Medical Radioisotopes Production without a Nuclear Reactor. May 2011. 1-38.

Nichols, A., Evaluation of Decay Data: Relevant IAEA Coordinated Research Projects. March 2008. 1-82.

Palige, J., Majkowska, A. & Herdzik, I. & Ptaszek, S. Nukleonika: $^{69}Ge\backslash^{68}Ga$ Radioisotopes Generator as a Source of Radiotracers for Water Flow Investigations. 2077. 77-80.

Sahoo, S., Sahoo, S. Production and Application Of Radioisotopes. 2006. Physics Education. 5-11.

World Nuclear Medicine. Radioisotopes in Nuclear Medicine. January 2011. 1-13

Moreira, R: XIV Seminari de Ingenieria biomedica: Principios y Elementos de un Cyclotron.uruguay 2005

Santos , A: X Congreso Brasileiro de FIsica Medica: Implementaçaode un PET/CT num Servicio de Medicina Nuclear. Brazil, 2005

Gorospe, L et al: PET/CT: Aspectos de Protocolo y Controversias Legales. Radiologia 2008: 50:207-214

Finley,D: Particle Accelerator for High Energy Physics. FERMIlAB. July 2002

Ruth, T. World View of Radioisotope Production. 2008. 1-60.

Fišer, M et al: Cyclotron targets and production technologies used for radiopharmaceuticals in NPI Czechoslovak Journal of Physics, Volume 53, Supplement 1, January 2003 , pp. A737-A743

Electronic References

http://en.wikibooks.org/wiki/Basic_Physics_of_Nuclear_Medicine/Production_of_Radioisotopes

http://hyperphysics.phy-astr.gsu.edu/hbase/Nuclear/biohalf.html#c2

http://medical-dictionary.thefreedictionary.com/rubidium+82

http://www.docstoc.com/docs/28954013/Medical-Isotope-Production-and-Use

http://www.nucmedtutorials.com/dwradiopharm/rad7.html

http://www.ornl.gov/sci/isotopes/r_w188g.html
http://www.telatomic.com/nuclear/isotope_generator.html
http://www.wolframalpha.com/input/?i=germanium+68
http://www.world-nuclear.org/info/inf55.html

1 E.O.Lawrence:(1939) University of California:"Artificial Radiactivity" speech

4

Radionuclide Infection Imaging: Conventional to Hybrid

Muhammad Umar Khan and Muhammad Sharjeel Usmani
Departments of Nuclear Medicine/PET Al-Jahra Hospital & Kuwait Cancer Control Centre, Kuwait

1. Introduction

Radionuclide imaging has been frequently used for detection and localization of infectious and inflammatory diseases for over five decades. Although there are many infection seeking agents available and currently being used but there is a general consensus that none of them is ideal. No clear cut guidelines exist to recommend a particular radionuclide imaging procedure for a particular clinical indication, however, in some instances the literature does provide us with ample evidence for the choice of the infection specific agent whereas one may have to depend upon the routine management protocols to decide which radionuclide imaging procedure to perform in a particular situation. In fact, presently, the clinical utility of radionuclide infection imaging varies under different circumstances and clinical scenarios; but with the incorporation of hybrid imaging systems, the fusion of functional and anatomical data in form of SPECT-CT and PET-CT has certainly improved the sensitivity and specificity of detecting and localizing an infectious process. Ga-67 citrate, bone seeking radiotracers, radiolabelled leukocytes, antibody and antibody fragments labelled white cells are used in different clinical situations such as osteomyelitis, diabetic foot, infected vascular grafts, infected hip or knee prostheses, intra-abdominal infections including acute appendicitis, cardiovascular, pulmonary infections, malignant otitis externa with variable sensitivity and specificity. Similarly, the ability of F-18 FDG PET to detect infection, inflammation and granulomatous diseases due to their increased glycolytic activity has provided us with another effective agent especially in cases of fever of unknown origin, vasculitis, chronic osteomyelitis, sarcoidosis, inflammatory bowel disease and assessing response to therapy. New advances in the form of SPECT-CT have now also incremented the diagnostic capability of conventional scintigraphic procedures to localize infection. Finally, many investigational new infection seeking agents are in the process of being developed in search of an ideal. These include Tc-99m ubiquicidin, Tc-99m labelled Interleukin-8, N-formyl products, chemotactic cytokines etc. Therefore, with on going research in development of infection specific agents and the advent of hybrid imaging the future offers definite hope for better infection detection and localization in our patients.

2. Gallium scintigraphy

2.1 Gallium-67 citrate: Pharmacological and physiochemical characteristics

Ga-67 citrate has been used since 1971 to detect and localize infectious and inflammatory process. The exact mechanism of uptake has been studied extensively and various factors are thought to govern the tracer accumulation at the infection site. Most of the circulating Ga-67 is in the plasma and nearly all of it complexes with transferrin. Due to the increased blood flow and vascular membrane permeability the Ga-67/transferrin complex is delivered to the inflammatory sites or foci. Ga-67 is also thought to bind to lactoferrin which is present in high concentrations in the inflammatory foci. Direct bacterial uptake and accumulation as well as Ga-67 transportation bound to the leukocytes is also another factor studied. Bacteria and some fungi produce low molecular weight chelates called siderophores present on their cell surfaces and these have a high affinity for Ga-67. The Ga-67/siderophore complex facilitates the transport of Ga-67 within the cell itself. This mechanism of Ga-67 uptake may be attributable to the accumulation of Ga-67 within an abscess in neutropenic patients.

Ga-67 is a cyclotron produced radioisotope and emits principle gamma rays (93, 184, 296, 394 KeV). These are suitable for imaging. The dosage of Ga-67 typically used is 185-370 MBq for infection imaging, however, in our personal experience even a lesser dose did produce adequate images worth interpretation. Around 15-25% of the injected dose is excreted via the kidneys by 24 hours. After 24 hours the principle route of excretion is the colon. At 48 hours 75% of the injected dose remains in the body and is equally distributed among the liver, bone, bone marrow and soft tissues. The physical half-life of Ga-67 is 78 hours while the biological half-life of around 25 days gives ample opportunity to take delayed images even after days post injection.

2.2 Gallium-67: Imaging protocols and pre-requisites

Ga-67 imaging is usually performed 18-72 hours post injection, however, we also routinely image the patients at 6 hours post injection particularly if the suspected focus of infection is in the abdomen. This we have found to be helpful in a number of cases. Limited spot views or whole body imaging can be done depending upon the clinical indication and the use of a medium energy collimator is a standard. Patients' preparation with laxatives and enemas has been considered by some but the effectiveness of such preparation seems limited. Recent Gadolinium exposure as in an MR contrast study or multiple blood transfusions resulting in excess ferric ion may alter the Ga-67 biodistribution by saturation of the protein-binding sites. This needs to be sorted out in history while preparing the patient for injection and imaging.

2.3 Gallium-67: Clinical utilities and applications

Ga-67 citrate has been extensively used in the past four decades in clinical practice for several pathological conditions particularly whenever infection or inflammation has been in question. Ga-67 has demonstrated high sensitivity for both acute and chronic infectious process as well as non-infectious inflammation. Moreover, the Ga-67 tracer activity parallels acute inflammation, returning to normal as the disease process resolves.

The most common of the clinical scenarios where Ga-67 has been and is still utilized include fever of unknown origin (FUO), sarcoidosis, pulmonary infections like pneumocystis carnii pneumonia (PCP), drug-induced pulmonary toxicity as is seen with bleomycin or amiodarone, and in cases of malignant otitis externa. Further Ga-67 has been successfully utilized in spinal discitis and vertebral osteomyelitis. Mediastinal infections in immunocompromised patients have been detected by Ga-67.

In patients with the clinical diagnosis of FUO, anatomical imaging is less helpful as functional changes occur prior to anatomical alteration at a suspected site resulting in normal anatomical imaging. FUO has numerous causes and neoplasms including lymphoma account for up to 25% of these cases. Although PET/CT and labelled leukocytes are more frequently employed for FUO but Ga-67 can still be helpful with good detection rates where these formal are not available (Figure 1).

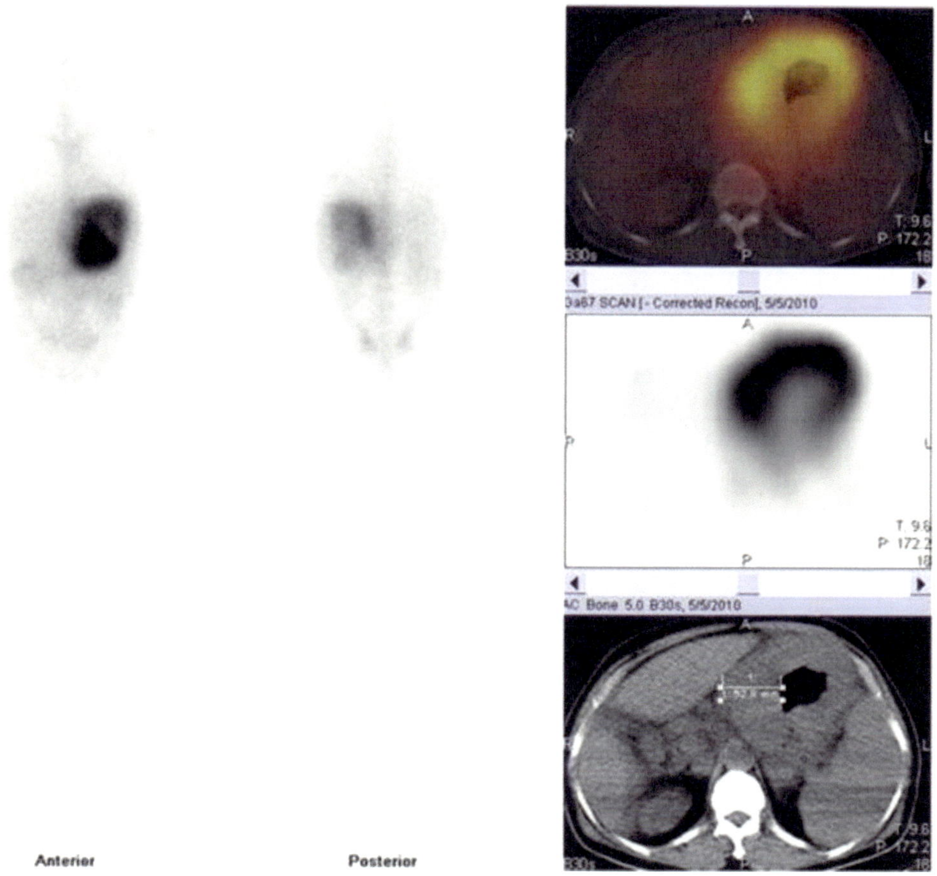

Fig. 1. A 40-year-old male with FUO. Ga-67 scintigraphy shows intense tracer accumulation in the left side of abdomen. SPECT/CT images localize the abnormal uptake to the thickened gastric wall measuring over 50mm. SPECT/CT report raised the suspicion of lymphoma and suggested subsequent endoscopic biopsy; the report of which showed findings consistent with gastric lymphoma.

Sarcoidosis is a systemic disorder that involves the lungs in up to 90% of the cases. Hilar lymph nodal involvement is evident in over 80% of the cases. Pulmonary accumulation of Ga-67 in these patients parallels active disease and there exists a good concordance between the Ga-67 intensity of uptake and the disease severity. Ga-67 scintigraphy has a sensitivity of 70% for detecting pulmonary parenchymal disease and a 95% for hilar adenopathy. The overall sensitivity is about 90%. If these patients are further subjected to a Thallium scintigraphic exam, it is usually negative. A characteristic Ga-67 scintigraphic pattern seen in patients with sarcoidosis is termed as the "Panda sign" (due to typically increased and more prominent lacrimal, parotid and nasopharyngeal activity). This can be seen in up to 80% of patients with stage I disease. Moreover the pre-tracheal and bilateral hilar adenopathy gives rise to an inverted "Y" which is termed as a "Lambda sign" (Figure 2). It is important, however, to remember that the panda sign can be seen in cases of Mikulicz syndrome (uveoparotid fever), lymphoma, Sjogren's syndrome and HIV. Some Pulmonologist believe that a panda sign on Ga-67 scintigraphy even without a lambda sign, but with hilar adenopathy on CXR or CT is still suggestive of sarcoidosis and do not opt for a biopsy.

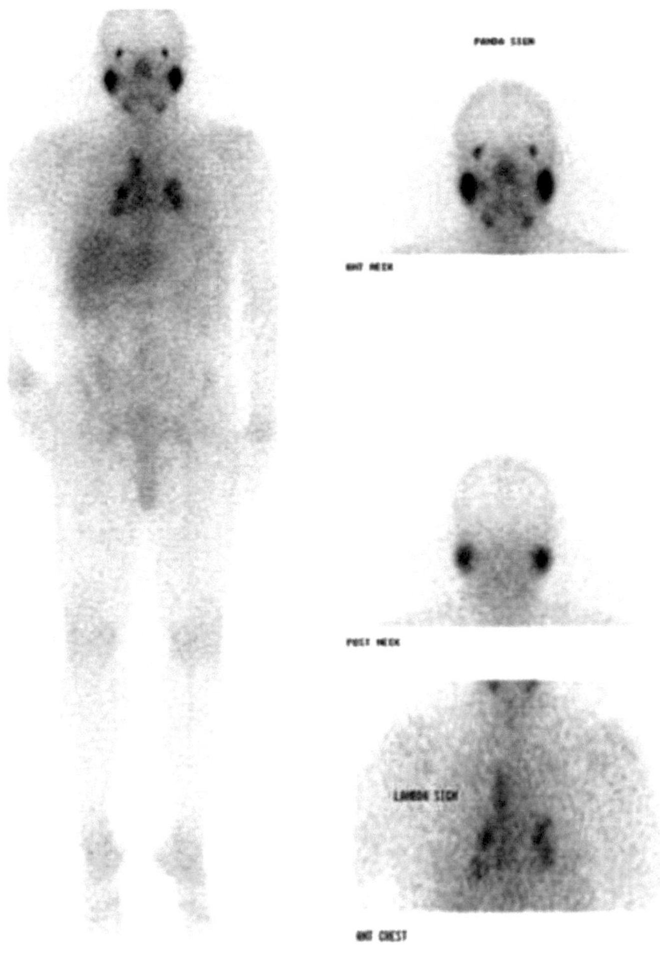

Fig. 2. A 28-year-old male with suspicion of sarcoidosis. Ga-67 scintigraphy shows typical "Panda" and "Lambda" signs.

The sensitivity of Ga-67 scintigraphy for PCP in HIV patients has been reported to be as high as 90-95%. The scintigraphic pattern is that of diffuse increased pulmonary uptake which is disproportionate to the clinical and radiological findings. However, due to a long list of differentials that can give rise to a similar scintigraphic picture the specificity can be increased by considering the intensity and distribution of the tracer as well as the comparison of activity either with the liver uptake or the sternum. Diffuse heterogeneous pulmonary activity which is more intense than the liver has specificity for PCP between 95-100%.

In cases of drug-induced pulmonary toxicity (Bleomycin, Cyclophosphamide, Methotrexate, Nitrofurantoin, Amiodarone) radiologically the abnormalities are not evident at early stages of the toxicity. In such a scenario, Ga-67 provides early detection with usually moderate increased uptake seen in the lungs on the scan. More recently, Ga-67 scintigraphy (Figure 3) as well as PET/CT has been used to evaluate malignant otitis externa. These modalities are also used to evaluate the response to therapy in such cases. Vertebral osteomyelitis has been detected and evaluated by Ga-67, however, the specificity can be increased if the interpretation is done in conjunction with the bone scan. An accepted criterion in such a clinical scenario is to have Ga-67 uptake greater than uptake seen on the bone scan with incongruent tracer distribution. Labelled leukocytes, however, are more accurate for the evaluation of vertebral osteomyelitis.

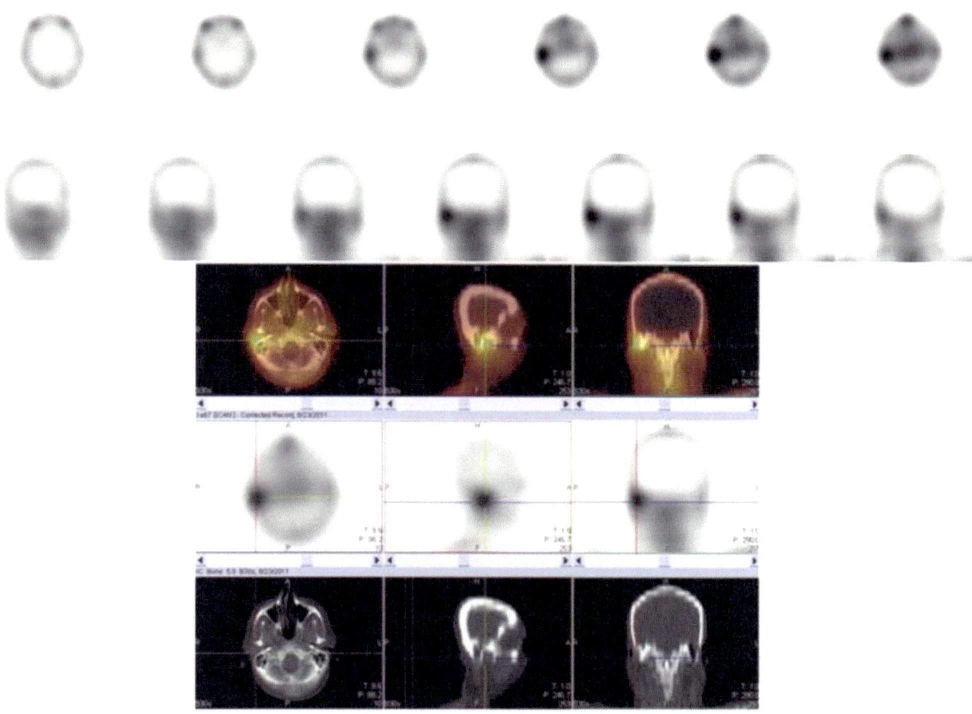

Fig. 3. A 46-year-old female with clinical diagnosis of right malignant otitis externa referred for Ga-67 scintigraphy. Transverse and coronal SPECT images show intense tracer uptake in the right auricular region. SPECT/CT images localize the abnormal uptake to right external auditory meatus without evidence of any underlying bony cortical breech.

2.4 Gallium-67: Hybrid SPECT/CT imaging

Ga-67 scintigraphy is primarily characterized by poor spatial resolution and low specificity due to paucity of anatomical and morphological information. (Bar-Shalom et al., 2006) studied patients with multiple infectious conditions including FUO and concluded that SPECT/CT was found to be beneficial in determining the precise anatomical sites of infection in 85% of discordant studies. In particular, substantial benefits were observed in scans of the chest and abdomen. In our own experience the addition of SPECT/CT to Ga-67 scintigraphy has a definite incremental value that helps resolve many difficult clinical scenarios (Figure 4).

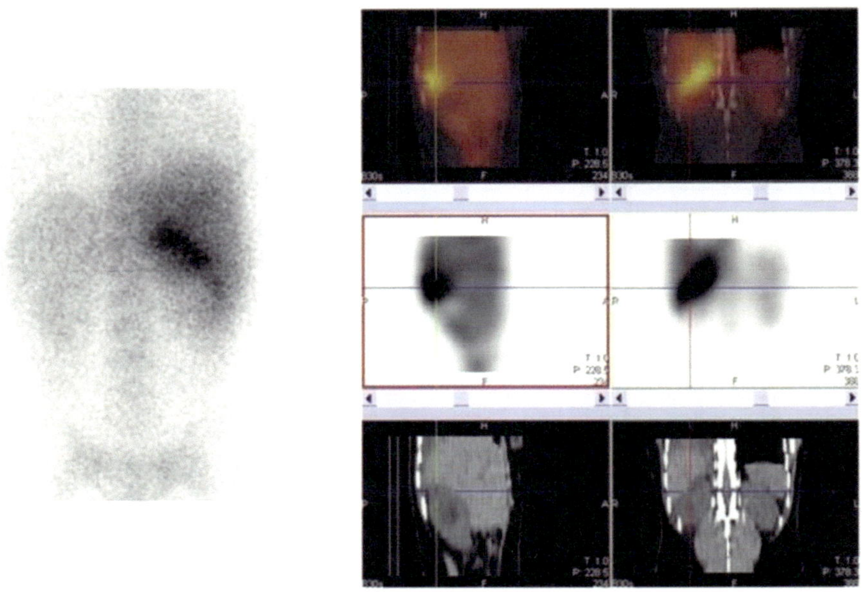

Fig. 4. A 21-year-old female with history of polycystic kidney disease referred for Ga-67 scintigraphy to evaluate suspected infected right renal cyst. Ga-67 scintigraphy shows linear intense tracer accumulation in the infra-hepatic region. SPECT/CT images localize the abnormal uptake to an area in the upper pole of right kidney just above a hypodensity (renal cyst) that shows photopenia on SPECT images. Subsequent guided biopsy drained abscess just beneath the renal capsule.

3. Bone scintigraphy

3.1 Tc-99m MDP: Pharmacological and physiochemical characteristics

Tc-99m Methylene-Diphosphonate (MDP) has been extensively used in the work up of osteomyelitis. The mechanism of uptake of diphosphonates has not been completely elucidated but the general presumption is that they are adsorbed to the mineral phase of bone with relatively lesser binding to the organic phase. Some also have postulated chemo-adsorption to the hydroxyl-apatite mineral component of the osseous matrix itself. Tc-99m (Technetium 99m) is a generator produced radioisotope with the principle gamma photon of 140 KeV optimal for imaging with low energy high resolution parallel-hole collimator. The physical half-life of Tc-99m is 6 hours making possible delayed imaging with good target to background ratio. Approximately 50% of the injected dose is localized to the bone. The tracer uptake is dependent upon the blood flow and the rate of new bone formation.

3.2 Tc-99m MDP: Imaging protocols and pre-requisites

When bone scintigraphy is performed for the evaluation of osteomyelitis, the study is done in three phases. These include a dynamic sequence termed as the flow or perfusion phase, followed by immediate static image of the area of interest termed as the blood-pool phase or soft tissue phase. The third phase is the static delayed imaging of the area of interest usually acquired 2-4 hours post injection. Some also perform a fourth phase at 24 hours which is usually a static spot view of the region of interest. The usual adult dosage is 740-925 MBq. Patients are instructed to be well hydrated and void frequently after the injection.

3.3 Tc-99m MDP: Clinical utilities and applications

Three-phase bone scintigraphy is the radionuclide procedure of choice for diagnosing osteomyelitis in non-violated bone i.e. bone that is not affected by underlying conditions. It is highly sensitive for diagnosing osteomyelitis and can detect the process 7-14 days before the manifestation of radiological changes. The reported sensitivity of 90-100% and specificity of 70-95% for identification of osteomyelitis is in non-violated bone. In adults a negative bone scan essentially rules out infection. Focal hyperperfusion, focal hyperemia, and focally increased bony uptake on delayed images are the characteristic scintigraphic findings for osteomyelitis. Many times due to some underlying bone conditions the specificity of the bone scan for osteomyelitis is further compromised. In such situations, the additional images at 24 hours (4th - phase) may improve specificity. This is due to the fact that uptake in woven or immature bone present in osteomyelitis continues for several more hours than normal bone. The accuracy of 4-phase bone scan that is more specific but less sensitive than a 3-phase bone scan is approximately 85%. Further the specificity of bone scan can also be improved by addition of Ga-67 scintigraphy. The overall accuracy of bone scan/Ga-67 scintigraphy is approximately 65-80%.

3.4 Tc-99m MDP: Hybrid SPECT/CT imaging

Three-phase bone scintigraphy and MRI are considered the modalities of choice for diagnosing osteomyelitis. Moreover, MRI can assess the associated soft tissue complications. MRI has its limitations as well. The replacement of marrow fat with edema and exudate results in a decreased signal on T1 and an increased signal on T2-weighted images. Such findings are not specific for osteomyelitis and can be seen with acute infarction, fracture or even tumour. Therefore the overall sensitivity and specificity of MRI for detection of acute osteomyelitis ranges from 92-100% and 89-100% respectively. CT is more sensitive to detect cortical destruction. On site-based analysis by (Bar-Shalom et al., 2006) scintigraphy (planar & SPECT) and SPECT/CT showed concordant results for diagnosis and localization of 50% of infection sites. SPECT/CT defined the precise anatomical localization of 44% of infectious sites that were erroneous or equivocal on scintigraphy in this study. In another preliminary report, (Horger et al., 2003) found that SPECT/CT improved the diagnostic performance of three-phase bone scan for osteomyelitis avoiding false-positive or equivocal results. In our own experience SPECT/CT has always had an incremental value to routine planar imaging and in many clinical situations in particular further characterizing the abnormalities to reach definitive imaging diagnosis (Figure 5).

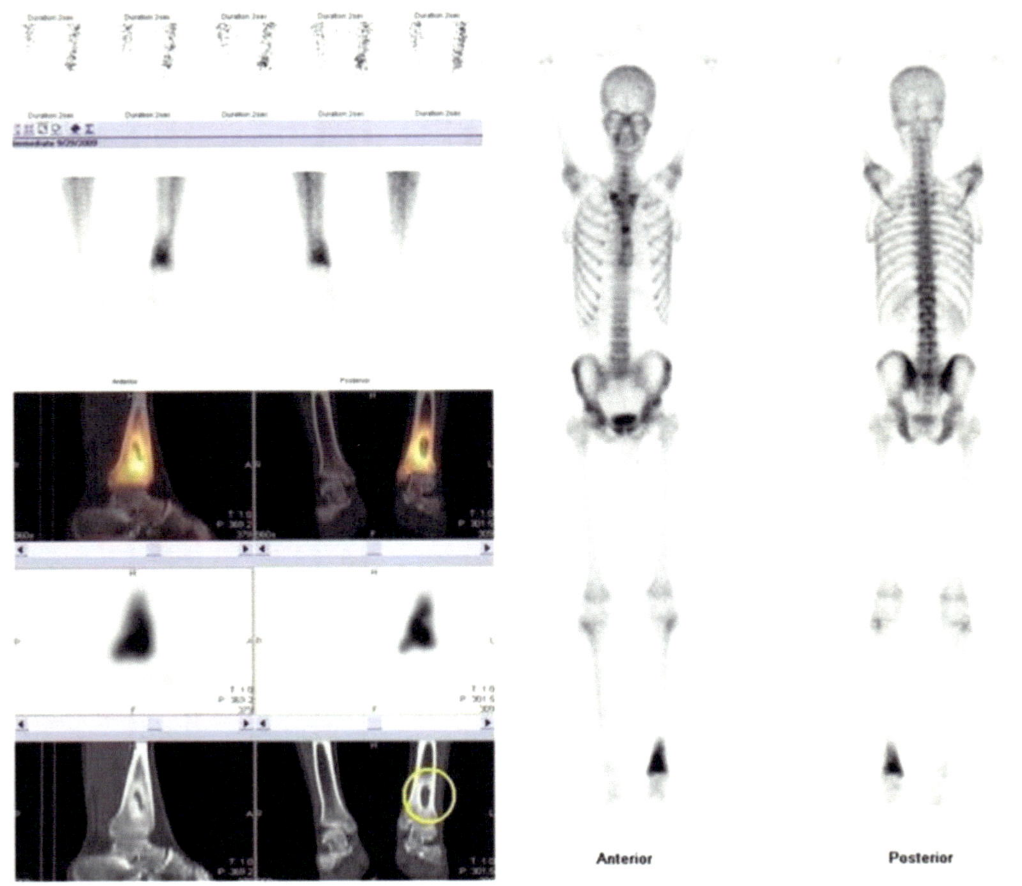

Fig. 5. A 19-year old male referred for evaluation of pain left lower limb. Tc-99m MDP images show hyperaemia, increased pool activity and intense increase tracer uptake in the distal end of left tibia. SPECT/CT images show a well-defined low attenuation metaphyseal lesion with central radiolucent area surrounded by peripheral bone sclerosis clearly confined to within the bone itself sparing the joint cavity. Findings consistent with diagnosis of osteomyelitis with features typical of a Brodie's Abscess.

4. Radiolabelled leukocytes scintigraphy

4.1 Radiolabelled leukocytes: Pharmacological and physiochemical characteristics

These days radiolabelled leukocytes are the most commonly used method to detect and localize infection. The leukocytes can be labelled using either Indium-111 (In-111) oxyquinoline or Tc-99m hexamethylpropylene amine oxime (HMPAO). In-111 oxine is a highly lipophilic ligand which diffuses across leukocyte membranes. Once inside the cell, it dissociates into oxine (8-hydroxyquinoline, which diffuses out of the cell) while In-111 is retained within the cytoplasm as a result of binding with intracellular proteins. In-111 labelled leukocytes localize at sites of infection through diapedesis, chemotaxis, and enhanced vascular permeability. In-111 has a physical half-life of 67 hours. It decays by electron capture with gamma emissions of 173 and 247 KeV. In-111 labelled leukocytes are normally distributed to the liver, spleen, and bone marrow. Intense pulmonary activity is seen soon after injection, which clears rapidly, and it is probably due to leukocyte activation during labelling, which impedes their movement through the pulmonary vascular bed, prolonging their passage through the lungs.

Tc-99m HMPAO is a lipophilic agent that readily crosses the cell membrane of leukocytes. Once inside the cell the compound becomes hydrophilic and remains trapped. It is subsequently bound to intracellular organelles, primarily the nucleus and mitochondria. The bond to granulocytes is more stable than to monocytes and the tag elutes from these cells five times more rapidly. The normal biodistribution of Tc-99m HMPAO labeled leukocytes is more variable. In addition to the reticuloendothelial system, activity is also normally present in the genitourinary tract, large bowel, blood pool, and occasionally the gallbladder. Physiologic bowel excretion limits the usefulness of this agent for imaging abdominal infections.

4.2 Radiolabelled leukocytes: Labeling technique

There are a number of methods for labelling leukocytes, however, the basic principles and technique remains uniform. Approximately 40 ml of blood is withdrawn from the patient into a syringe that contains anticoagulant. This syringe containing blood is then kept in an upright position for about 1–2 hours to promote gravity erythrocyte sedimentation, a process that is facilitated by the addition of hydroxyethyl starch. The process can be accelerated by using hypotonic lysis of the red cells instead of gravity sedimentation as well. After the erythrocytes have been separated, the leukocytes must be separated from platelets. The leukocyte-rich plasma is centrifuged, and the leukocyte "pellet" that forms at the bottom of the tube is removed, incubated with the radiolabel, washed, and re-injected into the patient. The usual dose of In-111 labelled leukocytes is 10–18.5 MBq; while the routine dose of Tc-99m HMPAO labelled leukocytes is 185–370 MBq. The majority of leukocytes labelled are neutrophils, and hence the procedure is most useful for identifying neutrophil-mediated inflammatory processes, such as bacterial infections. The procedure is less useful in conditions where the predominant cellular response is other than neutrophilic such as tuberculosis.

A total white count of at least 2000/mm^3 is needed to obtain satisfactory images. ABO compatible donor WBC's may be used in neutropenic patients (i.e. White cell count less than 2000/mm^3). Radiolabelled leukocytes should be administered within 1–2 hours of cell labelling. Labelled cells stored longer than 3 hours have a significant loss of cell viability. Temperatures higher than 70°F tend to increase cell damage and should be avoided. Cell labelling should be performed by trained laboratory personnel in a laminar flow hood using sterile procedures. Care must be taken to ensure correct identification of patients and blood products. All patients and laboratory procedures should have an appropriate quality control program.

4.3 Radiolabelled leukocytes: Imaging protocols and pre-requisites

In-111 labelled leukocyte is usually performed 18-24 hours post injection because early imaging at 4 hours usually misses out on two-thirds of the lesions detected on later images. However, it is critical to obtain early (1-4 hour) images when evaluating patients for inflammatory bowel disease or those suspected of possible ischemic bowel disease.

Occasionally, 48 hour delayed images may be necessary due to prolonged circulation of labelled cells in about 10% of cases. Limited spot views or whole body imaging can be acquired depending upon the clinical indication. Images should be acquired with a medium-energy parallel-hole collimator. Energy discrimination is accomplished by using a 15% window centered on the 173 KeV photopeak and a 20% window centered on the 247 KeV photopeak. Simultaneous In-111 leukocyte/Tc-99m MDP bone images can be obtained using a gamma camera that can acquire and discriminate the 140 KeV Tc-99m photons from the In-111 photons. Each In-111 leukocyte/Tc-99m bone image is acquired using a medium energy collimator for 50K counts in the In-111 window or for 15 minutes, 4 hours and/or 16–30 hours post injection of In-111 leukocytes. Tc-99m Sulphur colloid imaging can also performed after or simultaneously with In-111 leukocyte imaging if bone marrow distribution is in question.

The interval between injection of Tc-99m HMPAO labeled leukocytes and imaging varies with the indication; in general, imaging is usually performed 3-4 hours post injection. Some centers perform only 2 hours post injection images and occasionally 24 hour delayed images may be necessary due to prolonged circulation of labelled cells.

4.4 Radiolabelled leukocytes: Clinical utilities and applications

Labelled leukocytes have been used for the diagnosis of complicated osteomyelitis after fractures and surgery i.e. violated bone, vascular graft infections, and various soft-tissue insults. In-111 labelled leukocytes are probably the preferable agent for imaging suspected sites of infection in the abdomen, while Ga-67 is preferable for detecting pulmonary pathology in the setting of FUO. There are advantages as well as certain disadvantages associated with both In-111 and Tc-99m labelled leukocytes. Advantages of the In-111 label are those of virtually constant normal distribution of activity that is limited to the liver, spleen, and bone marrow and its more stable in-vivo characteristics. Further In-111 labelled leukocytes can be used in simultaneous dual-isotope acquisitions. On the contrary, the drawbacks of the In-111 label include a low photon flux due to less than ideal photon energies. When compared to the Tc-99m label, the latter has a high photon flux and somewhat ideal photon energies; with relatively more radioactivity injected, the ability to detect abnormalities within a few hours post injection is a plus for Tc-99m label. Disadvantages of Tc-99m labelled leukocytes include genitourinary tract activity, which appears shortly after injection, and colonic activity, that appears by 4 hours post injection thereby obscuring potential foci of infections at these sites.

Labelled leukocytes have been studied by many to be an accurate technique for the diagnosis of osteomyelitis in the setting of violated bones as well as in diabetic foot infection. The overall sensitivity and specificity of Tc-99m HMPAO labelled leukocytes is 88% and 91%, respectively, for osteomyelitis in previously violated bones. However, Tc99m HMPAO labelled leukocytes imaging is performed only after a positive finding on a three phase bone imaging, because the latter is highly sensitive but significantly less expensive, making it more appropriate as a first-line screening procedure. (Devillers et al., 2000) reported an overall sensitivity, specificity, and accuracy of 93%, 100%, and 96%, respectively, for Tc-99m HMPAO labelled leukocytes and 100%, 17%, and 53.3%, respectively, for Tc-99m MDP bone imaging. In our own experience combined Tc-99m HMPAO/Tc-99m MDP imaging proved useful in diagnosing osteomyelitis. The specificity of Tc-99m MDP bone scanning improved from 30% to 78% with the addition of Tc-99m HMPAO labelled leukocytes (Figure 6).

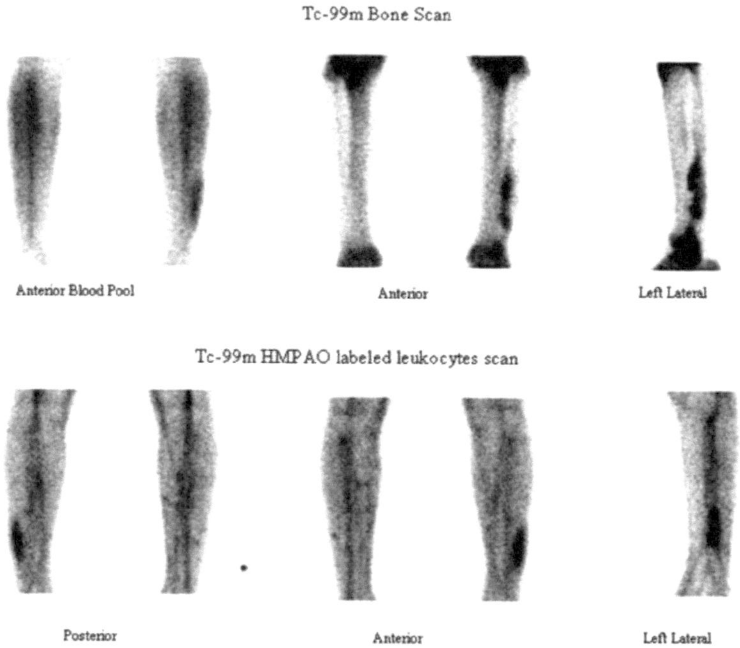

Fig. 6. A 30-year old female with chronic left leg pain, presented with tenderness and swelling at left lower leg. Tc-99m MDP bone scan show increased pool activity and increase tracer accumulation at the distal ½ of left fibula on delayed images. Tc-99m HMPAO labelled leukocytes scan showed increase tracer uptake in the distal left fibula corresponding to the site seen on bone scan, findings consistent with scintigraphic evidence of osteomyelitis.

Labelled leukocytes imaging have been used in the diagnosis of orthopaedic implant infection after positive findings on three phase bone scanning. False positive scans can occur due to dystrophic ossification, peri-prosthetic granulomas, altered distribution of red marrow, and damage to the polyethelene surface of the prosthesis and metallosis. Combined leukocyte-marrow imaging can overcome many of the problems created by variable marrow distribution post-operatively. (Palestro et al., 1990) reported good results with combined In-111 labelled leukocytes/bone marrow imaging, with 86–100% sensitivity and 97–100% specificity in hip and knee prosthesis infections. (Joseph et al., 2001) also noted the ability of added sulphur colloid scanning to eliminate the false positive results. Our own experience suggest Tc-99m HMPAO labelled leukocytes scan appears significantly valuable in detecting osteomyelitis in patients with prosthetic implants (Figure 7).

Labelled leukocyte imaging is the procedure of choice for the evaluation of patients with diabetic foot. Sensitivity and specificity of In-111 labelled leukocytes for diabetic foot osteomyelitis is between 72%-100% and between 67%-100%, respectively. Sensitivity of Tc-99m HMPAO labelled leukocytes has been reported to be 90% and 93% while the specificity has been observed to be 86% and 100% by various groups. Interestingly, the combination of Tc-99m HMPAO labelled leukocytes scan with Tc-99m three phase bone scan has yielded both high sensitivity and high specificity (92.6% and 97.6%, respectively), moreover this combination is of benefit in patients with Charcot osteoarthropathy. The reported sensitivity

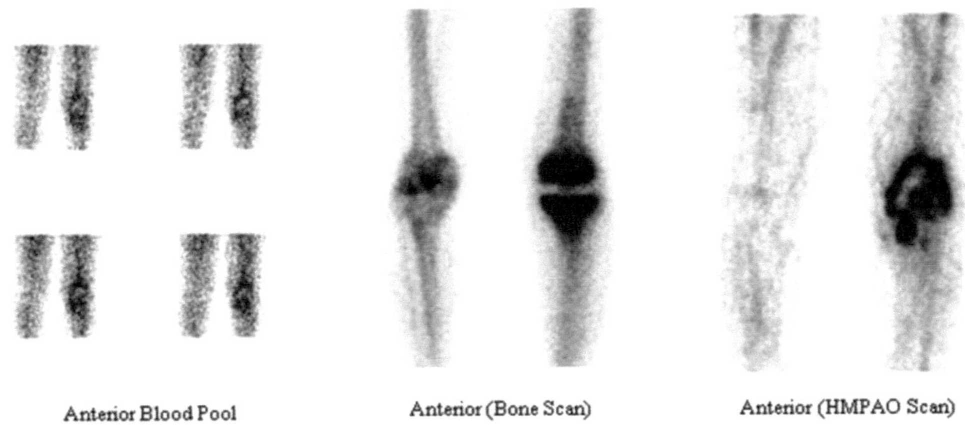

Fig. 7. A 70-year old female with history of left total knee replacement three years ago, presented with pain and swelling in the left knee prosthesis. Tc99m MDP bone scan show increased pool activity and intense increase tracer accumulation around left knee prosthesis. Tc-99m HMPAO labelled leukocytes scan showed increase tracer localization with rinds of tracer uptake at the femoral component of left knee prosthesis suggesting prosthetic infection.

of 92.6% and a specificity of 97.6% by (Poirier et al., 2002) for Tc-99m HMPAO/Tc-99m MDP bone imaging for the diagnosis of osteomyelitis in diabetic foot ulcers appear promising and it is believed that neuroarthropathy does not affect the performance of this scan. In our own institutional experience this combination for diabetic foot ulcers proved to be useful in diagnosing underlying osteomyelitis (Figure 8).

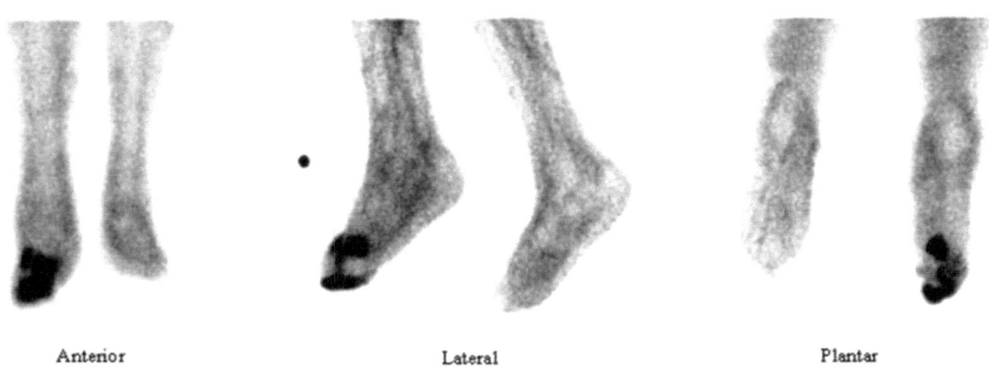

Fig. 8. A 50-year old male with history of diabetic right big toe amputation done 3 years ago, now presented with discharge from the right foot. Tc-99m HMPAO labelled leukocytes scan showed features consistent with osteomyelitis at right 3rd metatarsal bone with overlying soft tissue infection in the right distal foot.

Leukocyte labelled imaging is not as sensitive for infection of the spine as it is for other musculoskeletal infections and may be falsely negative in up to 80% of cases. The difficulty in interpretation may be related to the large percentage of spinal osteomyelitis which produces a cold, rather than a hot lesion (marrow uptake in the spine may be higher than in the adjacent inflammatory site which may mask the abnormality or cause the appearance of a cold defect). MRI is presumably the modality of choice when evaluating patients for suspected vertebral osteomyelitis.

In-111 labelled leukocytes scans are superior to Ga-67 for evaluation of suspected abscess in abdomen and pelvis due to the lack of a normal bowel excretory pathway. Some abscesses accumulate In-111 labelled leukocytes very slowly, and 48 hour delayed imaging may be necessary to identify these lesions. In appendicitis a focal area of increased activity in the right lower quadrant may be identified. Labelled leukocyte can be used to assess for disease activity and distribution of inflammatory bowel disease and excellent correlation is found between endoscopy, histology, and scintigraphic findings for disease extent and activity. (Annovazzi et al., 2005) reported in a meta-analysis that leukocytes labelled with In-111 oxine or Tc-99m HMPAO should be considered as the procedures of choice in acute phases of disease, since endoscopic and barium studies are contraindicated.

Labelled leukocyte imaging has been successfully utilized to detect both cardiovascular and central nervous system infections with limited clinical consequences. Leukocyte scintigraphy provides valuable information about contrast-enhancing brain lesions seen on radiological imaging. Positive findings indicate that the origin of the brain lesion is almost assuredly infectious; a negative result rules out infection with a high degree of certainty. However, false positive results can be seen in brain tumours, and false-negative results in patients receiving high-dose steroids. Labelled leukocyte imaging is the radionuclide procedure of choice for diagnosis of graft infection, with a sensitivity of more than 90%; neither duration of symptoms nor pre-treatment with antibiotics adversely affects the study. The specificity of labelled leukocyte imaging is more variable, ranging from 53% to 100%. Causes of false-positive results include peri-graft hematomas, bleeding, graft thrombosis, pseudoaneurysms, and graft endothelialisation, which occur within the first 1–2 weeks after placement.

4.5 Radiolabelled leukocytes: Hybrid SPECT/CT imaging

SPECT/CT has incremental value for interpretation of labelled leukocytes imaging for an array of clinical indications in different regions of the body, by distinguishing normal physiologic distribution from accumulation due to underlying infectious process. Benefit has been observed when characterizing foci of labelled leukocytes accumulation near the major vessels. The hybrid technology helps in discriminating blood-pool activity from infectious sites, particularly in evaluation of suspected vascular graft infection and fever of unknown origin. Moreover, SPECT/CT with Tc-99m HMPAO labelled leukocytes is useful to image bone and joint infections, providing accurate localization especially some cases where planar images alone are not able to distinguish soft tissue from bone and to precisely define the extent of infection, thus modifying clinical patient management and therapeutic approaches in several cases. In particular those with diabetic foot infection, it helps support treatment planning and avoiding more invasive procedures. (Filippi & Schillaci, 2006) more recently reported that SPECT/CT avoided unnecessary bone amputation in significant numbers of patients.

(Filippi & Schillaci, 2006) have evaluated the usefulness of SPECT/CT for interpreting Tc-99m HMPAO labelled leukocytes in bone and joint infection. SPECT/CT fusion correctly characterized and localized the site of abnormal uptakes in all patients with osteomyelitis, having a substantial impact on the clinical management. Moreover, those patients with a suspicion of infection post orthopaedic implants, SPECT/CT offered a more accurate anatomic localization of the site of infection than SPECT alone allowing differentiation between prosthesis and soft-tissue uptake. Similarly, (Bar-Shalom et al., 2006) observed that using In-111 labelled leukocyte SPECT/CT contributed to accurate identification of infection in 55% of patients suspected to have osteomyelitis and 67% of those suspected to have a vascular graft infection.

5. Tc-99m labelled Anti-granulocyte antibody scintigraphy

5.1 Tc-99m labelled Anti-granulocyte antibody: Pharmacological and physiochemical characteristics

Three anti-granulocyte antibodies have been used including anti-NCA-95 immunoglobulin IgG, fanelosomab (a monoclonal murine M class immunoglobulin), sulesomab (a murine monoclonal antibody fragment anti-NCA-90 Fab) and anti-CD15. Presently most routinely sulesomab (Leukoscan ®) is used in clinical practice.

Leukoscan consists of a small murine monoclonal antibody fragment, sulesomab, labelled with Tc-99m. The radiolabelled antibody fragment (Fab) reacts with the normal cross reacting antigen (NCA-90) present on the surface of virtually all neutrophils. Therefore areas where neutrophils have accumulated can be detected and this proves useful in determining the location and extent of infection and inflammation. Uptake at sites of infection is therefore related to migration of antibody labelled circulating granulocytes and non-specific non-antigen related uptake of free antibody. The use of radiolabelled monoclonal antibodies against surface antigens as present on granulocytes has the advantage that labelling procedures are easier and do not require handling of potentially contaminated blood. Since the leukocytes are not removed from the patient, it is considered as in-vivo labelling process. Mounting of an immune response and production of human anti-mouse antibodies (HAMA) may pose a concern; however, in our experience and available published data the level of adverse events and probability of HAMA response are both low.

5.2 Tc-99m labelled Anti-granulocyte antibody: Imaging protocols and pre-requisites

Tc-99m Sulesomab is presented as a lyophilised powder (0.31 mg per vial) to be reconstituted with sodium chloride. Approximately 555-925 MBq is injected intravenously. Imaging should be performed 1–8 hours post injection. We usually perform imaging at 10 minutes and 2-4 hours post injection with occasional 24 hour delayed imaging in certain situations to have better target to background ratio for better delineation of lesions.

5.3 Tc-99m labelled Anti-granulocyte antibody: Clinical utilities and applications

Tc-99m Sulesomab is commonly indicated as an adjunctive diagnostic imaging of infection/inflammation in patients with suspected osteomyelitis, including patients with diabetic foot ulcers. As Tc-99m MDP bone scan has a low specificity, Tc-99m Sulesomab imaging as a follow-up test reduces the false-positive rate of Tc-99m MDP imaging. The overall sensitivity and specificity for the diagnosis of infections is 86% and 72%, respectively.

In patients with diabetic foot ulcers, the diagnostic accuracy of Tc-99m Sulesomab compared with In-111 and Tc-99m HMPAO labelled leukocytes scanning was observed not to be significantly different (81 and 75%, respectively). However, Tc-99m Sulesomab imaging has a significantly higher sensitivity. In our own experience Tc-99m Sulesomab imaging has an incremental diagnostic value in the detection and ruling out osteomyelitis especially when used subsequent to Tc-99m MDP imaging (Figure 9).

Tc-99m fanolesomab has been used for diagnosis of acute appendicitis. It has a good overall accuracy with a positive predictive value (PPV) of 74-87% and a negative predictive value (NPV) between 95-100%. A high NPV is helpful for the patients to avoid unnecessary surgery, however, a number of false positives have been an issue with this radiopharmaceutical.

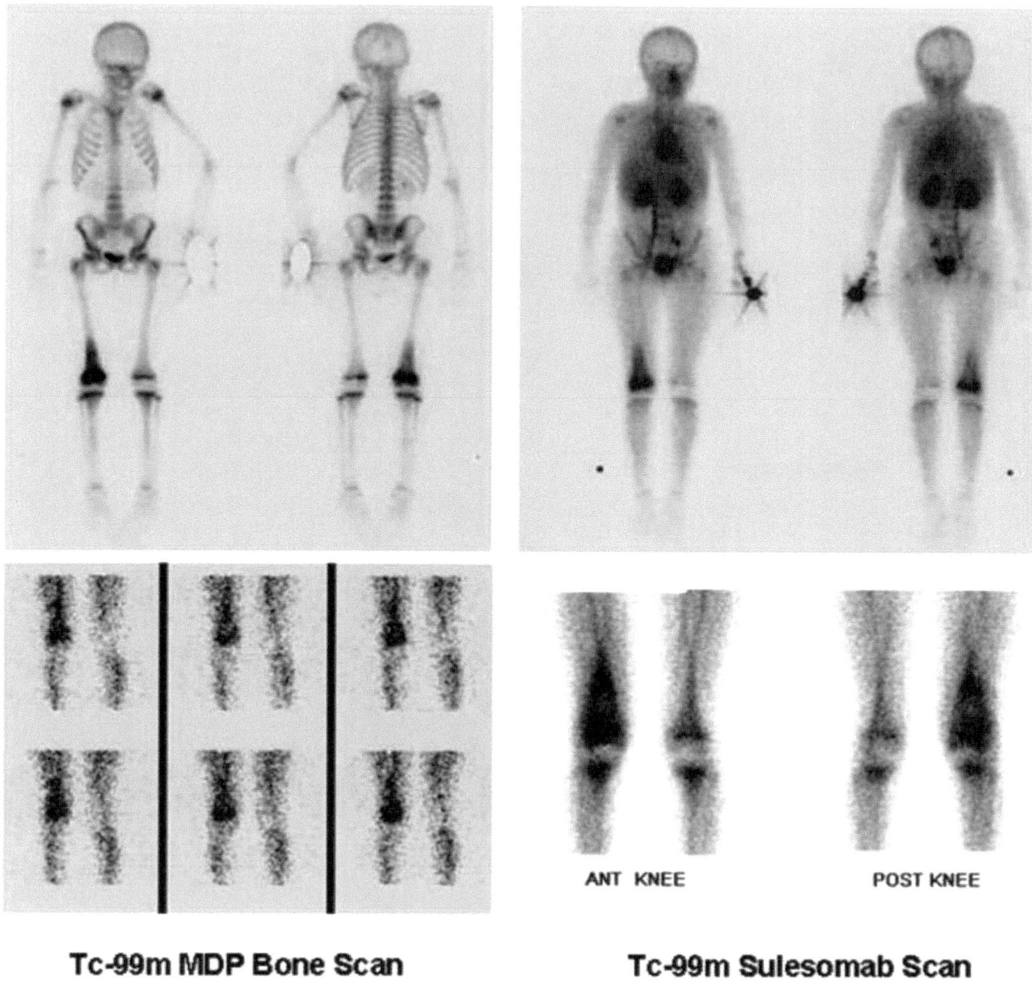

Fig. 9. A 10-year old girl, presented with tenderness and swelling at right distal femur. Tc-99m MDP bone scan show hyperperfusion and increases tracer accumulation at the distal 1/3rd of right femur. Tc-99m Sulesomab imaging show increased tracer uptake at distal right femur corresponding to the site seen on bone scan, confirming osteomyelitis.

5.4 Tc-99m labelled Anti-granulocyte antibody: Hybrid SPECT/CT imaging

(Horger et al., 2003) showed that SPECT/CT changed the interpretation of radioimmunoscintigraphy with Tc-99m labelled anti-granulocyte antibodies in 28% of suggestive foci evaluated in 27 patients in whom relapsing post-traumatic osteomyelitis was suspected. In another recent study (Graute V et al., 2010) concluded that SPECT/CT substantially improves the utility of imaging with Tc-99m labelled anti-granulocyte antibodies for diagnosis and localization of suspected joint infections and provide information on the extent of the infection. We have found that SPECT/CT imaging not only helps anatomical localization of the infectious site but also provides lesion characterization and extent of involvement of the infectious process (Figure 10).

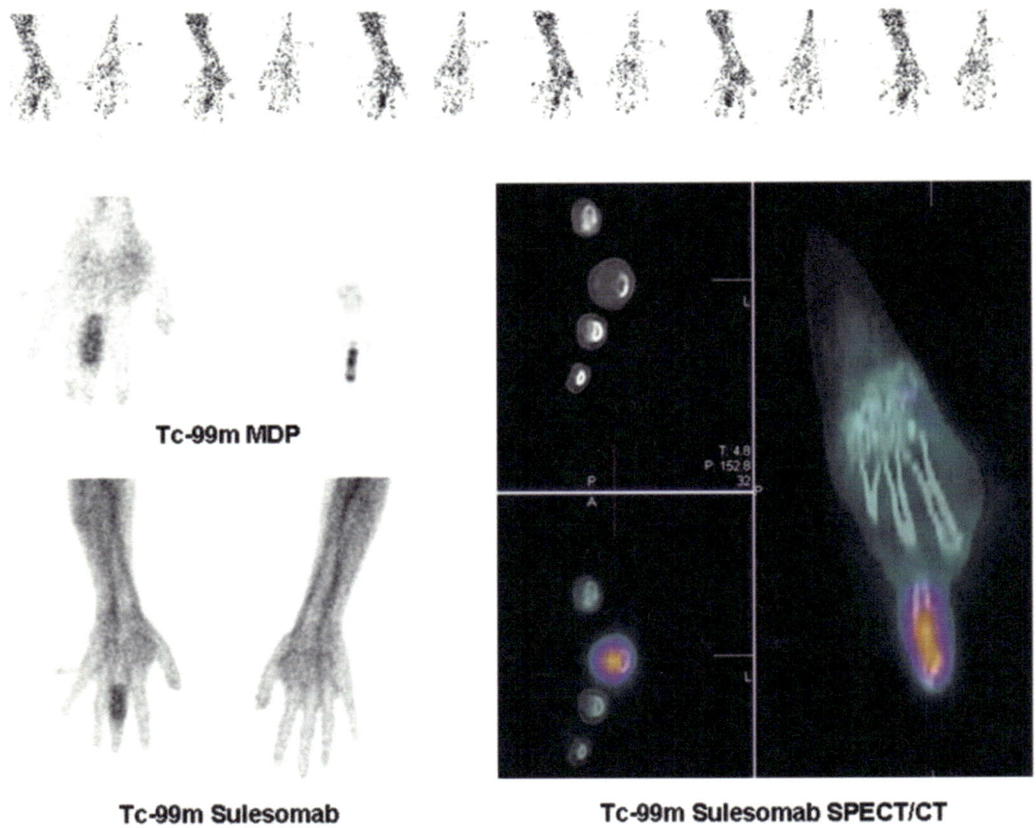

Fig. 10. A 25-year old female referred for evaluation of osteomyelitis in the left middle finger. Tc-99m MDP bone scan show hyperaemia, increased pool activity and intense linear increased tracer uptake in the left 3rd proximal phalanx extending up to the mid of middle phalanx. Tc-99m Sulesomab images show increased uptake at the same site confirming osteomyelitis. Further correlative SPECT/CT images show evident cortical distortion with low attenuation changes.

6. F-18 fluorodeoxyglucose positron emission tomography

6.1 F-18 FDG: Pharmacological and physiochemical characteristics

Fluorine 18 (F-18) Fluorodeoxyglucose (FDG) Positron Emission Tomography (PET) has been extensively used for imaging malignant processes, however, it is also now an established agent for imaging benign processes such as infection, inflammation and granulomatous disease. Increased F-18 FDG uptake in these tissues is attributed to the increased glucose consumption through the hexose monophosphate shunt, which is the main energy source in chemotaxis and phagocytosis. The respiratory burst or the phagocytes activation results in increased F-18 FDG uptake. Marked F-18 FDG uptake is seen in neutrophils during acute phase of inflammation while during the chronic phase it is the macrophages and polymorphonuclear leukocytes that take up the tracer. Therefore, in cases of sterile inflammation it is mainly the neutrophils and macrophages that take up F-18 FDG. The mechanism of F-18 FDG uptake in infectious and inflammatory process is the same as in malignancy with metabolic trapping of the F-18 FDG-6-phosphate that cannot be further metabolised as it is not a substrate for the glucose 6-phosphatase isomerase enzyme. However, as the level of glucose 6-phosphatase remains the same in inflammatory cells as opposed to tumour cells where they are decreased, the F-18 FDG washes out from the inflammatory cells in due course. Further the numbers of GLUT (glucose transporter receptors) are less in inflammatory cells when compared with tumour cells.

The normal distribution of F-18 FDG includes the brain, myocardium, and the genitourinary system with variable uptake seen in the stomach, bowel and the bone marrow. Increase F-18 FDG activity can be seen in the spleen in patients with infection and presumably reflects the increased glucose usage by spleen in the setting of an infectious process.

6.2 F-18 FDG PET: Imaging protocols and pre-requisites

The patients are advised to fast for several hours before imaging. This reduces the F-18 FDG uptake in normal tissues. Moreover, it reduces the competition for glucose transporters. The physical activity of the patient is limited prior to injection and this reduces the F-18 FDG uptake in the striated muscles. Some centers also administer benzodiazepines 30-60 minutes prior to injection to reduce the brown fat and muscle uptake. Patient is routinely injected 370-550 MBq of F-18 FDG intravenously and laid to rest in a comfortable bed. Imaging is usually done at 60 minutes post injection, however, some centers may extend the uptake period to 90 minutes or may acquire images twice at different times (dual point) particularly in cases of granulomatous processes such as tuberculosis. Whole body imaging is preferred in cases where a focus of infection is to be investigated. F-18 is cyclotron produced radioisotope. The physical half-life of F-18 is 110 minutes. The principal gamma photons produced are of 511 KeV energy generated by positron emission.

6.3 F-18 FDG PET: Clinical utilities and applications

The indications for F-18 FDG PET for imaging infection are not different from those discussed previously, however, in particular investigation for the site of infection or ascertaining the cause in FUO, vasculitis, HIV-AIDS, infected prostheses, as well as osteomyelitis, diabetic foot infections, sarcoidosis and tuberculosis have been studied.

In case of FUO, the sensitivity and specificity of F-18 FDG PET has been observed to be 84-93% and 86-90% respectively. In most studies, it has helped in the management of about 35-37% cases. The reported PPV is 87% and the NPV 95%. Negative F-18 FDG PET makes it very unlikely that a morphologic origin of the fever will be identified. Infective endocarditis that can be a source of FUO has also been studied with F-18 FDG PET.

F-18 FDG accumulation has been observed in certain conditions resulting in vasculitis. These include giant cell arteritis, Takayasu arteritis, polymyalgia rheumatica, aortitis/peri-aortitis, infectious vasculitis and unspecified large vessel vasculitis. Inflammation of the vessel walls cannot be detected in the early phase on conventional anatomical imaging. F-18 FDG assists in early diagnosis, assessing the extent of the disease and has also been found superior to MRI in depicting disease activity and treatment response. High brain uptake, relatively high skin background and the smaller diameter of the vessels lower the sensitivity of F-18 FDG PET in temporal arteritis. Giant cell arteritis in arteries greater than 4mm in diameter is nicely demonstrated by F-18 FDG PET. It is important to remember that vasculitis can be one of the causes of FUO as we have observed in some of our referred patients (Figure 11). Assessment for this is done by observing both non-attenuation corrected and attenuation corrected PET images.

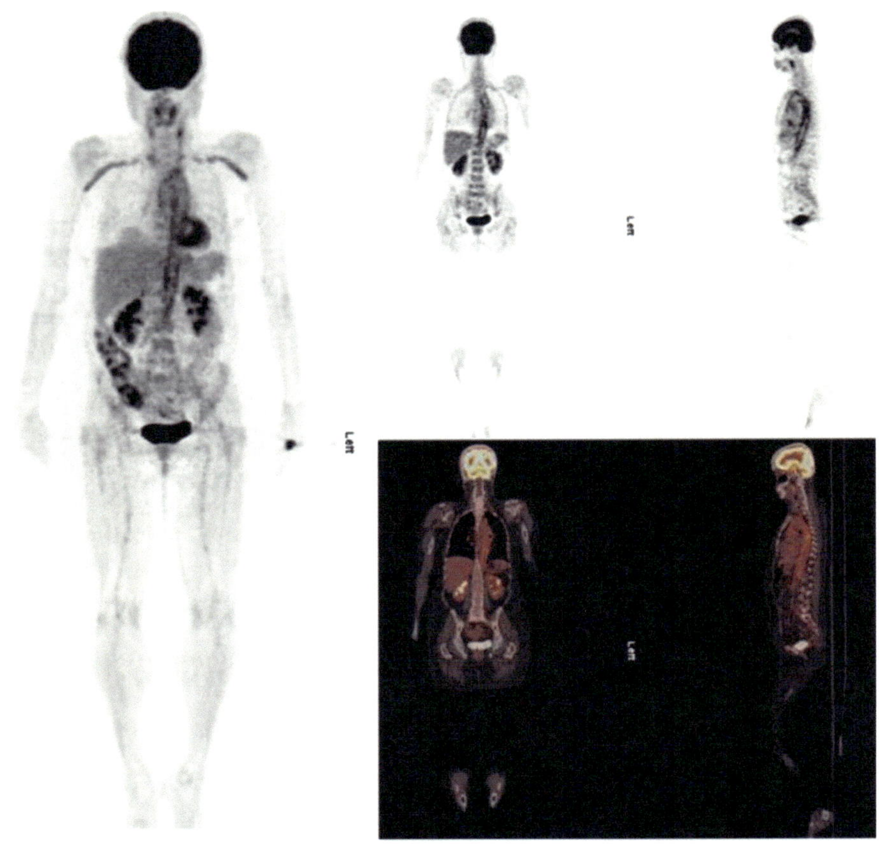

Fig. 11. A 56-year old female with FUO referred for detecting potential site(s) of infection. F-18 FDG PET/CT scan show diffuse increased FDG uptake evident in major blood vessels including the carotids, brachiocephalics, aortic arch, descending thoracic aorta extending up to the renal level. Findings consistent with the inflammatory etiology of vasculitis.

In patients with HIV-AIDS, there is increased likelihood of opportunistic infections as well as malignancy. (O'Doherty et al., 1997) reported that F-18 FDG PET has a sensitivity of 92% and specificity of 94% in localizing abnormalities that required treatment in these patients; however, they also concluded that it is not possible to clearly distinguish infectious from a malignant process in these patients. Toxoplasmosis is the commonest of the opportunistic infections in AIDS patients. Most commonly the central nervous system is affected. F-18 FDG has been reported to be superior and more accurate than MRI in differentiating CNS lymphoma from conditions such as toxoplasmosis, progressive multi-focal leukoencephalopathy and syphilis. Further on quantitative assessment it has been shown that the standardized uptake values of toxoplasmosis are significantly lower than lymphoma with virtually no overlap.

F-18 FDG PET has been used extensively to evaluate painful lower limb joint prostheses. It has a limited significance especially when distinguishing infected joint prosthesis from aseptic prosthetic loosening. As inflammation is part of both the conditions, there is increased F-18 FDG peri-prosthetic accumulation observed in both. F-18 FDG PET is considered highly sensitive for evaluation of chronic osteomyelitis. Unlike bone scintigraphy F-18 FDG uptake normalizes in less than 2-3 months following treatment, thereby, reducing the false positive scans seen when osteomyelitis is suspected in complicated fractures. F-18 FDG PET has also been used with variable utility in diabetic foot infections, sarcoidosis, tuberculosis, organ transplantation and inflammatory bowel disease. In case of sarcoidosis the imaging findings are similar to those seen and discussed with Ga-67 scintigraphy. Further F-18 FDG PET can detect metastatic infectious foci with high sensitivity even if other imaging is negative.

6.4 F-18 FDG PET: Hybrid PET/CT imaging

Hybrid PET/CT systems in fact gained more popularity than the SPECT/CT systems and PET imaging is synonymously used for PET/CT imaging. The incorporation of anatomical data fused with the functional PET images results in accurate localization of the abnormalities and moreover detailed characterization of the lesions can be ascertained. In our experience PET/CT imaging for infectious process has limited utility, primarily in cases of FUO, vasculitis, malignant otitis externa and assessment of chronic osteomyelitis. However, as more evidence based data surface, this modality may prove to be an important method in detection and management of a number of infective conditions.

7. Brief considerations and limitations regarding anatomic imaging modalities

Radiograph or plain films are almost always the initial imaging study for diagnosing and assessing osteomyelitis. Finding on plain films to suggest or support infectious process include periosteal elevation or thickening, cortical thickening, irregularity with loss of trabecular architecture, sclerosis, osteolysis, and new bone formation. It is however important to note that these changes may not be evident at least until 5-7 days in children and 10-14 days in adults. Plain films show lytic changes only after at least 50%-75% of the bone matrix is destroyed.

Ultra-sonography is mostly utilized in evaluation and diagnosing of fluid collections, involvement of the periosteum, along with assessing surrounding soft tissue abnormalities. It may provide guidance for diagnostic or therapeutic aspirations, subsequent drainage and/or tissue biopsy.

Anatomic imaging modalities including CT and MR imaging provide excellent structural resolution for the detection and characterization of infectious or inflammatory conditions. These provide a high-quality assessment of infection related structural abnormalities. However, the limitation is that these techniques rely solely on structural changes and, therefore, differentiation between active and structural but indolent alterations following surgery or other interventions is difficult to differentiate and these modalities are generally of limited value in detecting early disease regardless of the cause. In evaluation of infectious process CT scans may assist in the assessment of disruption of the bony cortex and soft-tissue involvement. Furthermore, CT may also reveal edema, intra-osseous fistula and cortical defects that lead to soft tissue sinus tracts.

CT is better suited for an evaluation of cortical bone, whereas MR imaging is more useful for the evaluation of internal architecture of structures such as the bone marrow, muscles, tendons, ligaments, cartilage etc. MR imaging has high accuracy in the acute osteomyelitis evaluation and detection primarily delineating adjacent soft tissue infection; particularly when no prior alterations in osseous or soft structure are present. However, in patients who have undergone previous surgical intervention, MR imaging may not be able to clearly distinguish signal abnormality secondary to bone marrow edema or enhancement related to a reactive phenomenon and that related to infection. Similarly, the diagnostic accuracies of both CT and MR imaging to evaluate osteomyelitis generally decrease in the presence of metallic implants due to streak and susceptibility artefacts.

MR imaging has a higher sensitivity and specificity than plain films and CT. Further findings become positive earlier in the disease process with MR than with plain films. MR imaging is particularly better at depicting bone marrow abnormalities with sensitivity of 82%-100% and specificity of 75%-95%. Vertebral osteomyelitis is one condition where MR has a characteristic pattern of confluent vertebral body and disk involvement; the diagnostic accuracy in such cases amount to 90%. MR imaging findings in osteomyelitis usually are related to the replacement of marrow fat with water secondary to edema, exudate, hyperemia, and bone ischemia. Findings include the following: decreased signal intensity in the involved bone on T1-weighted images, increased signal intensity in the involved bone on T2-weighted image, and increased signal intensity in the involved bone on short-tau inversion recovery (STIR) images. A decreased intensity on T1-weighted images with no change on T2-weighted images may indicate surgical or post-traumatic scarring of bone marrow. The MR imaging limitations are primarily due to the reason that findings of osteomyelitis are nonspecific, and similar changes may occur as a result of fractures, tumours, and a number of various intramedullary or juxtamedullary processes that result in bone marrow edema.

8. Future prospects and novel agents

The future for infection imaging looks promising with the search for an ideal agent still on. There has been a progression in the development of leukocytes labelled in-vitro by F-18 FDG. Moreover, leukocytes labelled with Copper-64 (Cu-64) are being studied. Radiolabelled antibiotics are also in vogue. The theoretical reasoning for radiolabelled antibiotics would be that such would incorporate into and metabolized by bacteria, thereby, making it possible to localize the site of infection. Tc-99m Ciprofloxacin has been studied, some results published with regards to its use in post-operative infections, however, this did not go into routine clinical practice due to conflicting data. Tc-99m labelled anti-microbial peptides are also being studied including Tc-99m labelled recombinant human beta-defensin-3 that exerts bactericidal effects on gram positive and gram negative bacteria as well as some yeasts, and Tc-99m ubiquicidin whose uptake is related to number of viable bacteria. Most recently (Lupetti et al., 2011) in a review have mentioned radiolabelled antimicrobial peptides, fluconazole and chitin targeting agents that have been studied to image fungal infection in mice. There is a limitation of difficulty in differentiating bacterial and fungal infections. However, radiolabelled fluconazole has the ability to distinguish Candida albicans infection from bacterial infections/sterile inflammation.

Tc-99m ubiquicidin (Tc-99m UBI29-41), Tc-99m labelled lactoferrin (hLF1-11), Tc-99m fluconazole and I-123 labelled chitinase are being further studied at the moment. Tc-99m UBI29-41 was clinically tested in trial setting as human infection imaging agent (Akhtar et al., 2005) with promising results. They suggested an optimal imaging time of 30 minutes post injection for this agent. Another team (Salber et al., 2008) assessed and compared Tc-99m ubiquicidin and F-18 ubiquicidin autoradiography to anti-Staphylococcus aureus immunofluorescence in rat muscles abscesses. However, most recently, (Assadi et al., 2011) assessed the diagnostic accuracy of Tc-99m UBI29-41 scintigraphy for osteomyelitis making a comparison to Tc-99m MDP Bone scan and MR imaging. The authors concluded that for fast imaging with high accuracy, Tc-99m UBI29-41 is suitable for detection of osteomyelitis. In this most recent study the accuracy for Tc-99m UBI29-41 for detection of infection was observed to be 100% as compared to 90% for Tc-99m MDP bone scan. MR imaging was done in more than half of these cases and showed an accuracy of 75% for detecting osteomyelitis. Further in another most recent preliminary study by (Nazari et al., 2011) evaluated the role and ability of Tc-99m UBI29-41 to assess response to antibiotic therapy in orthopedic infections with quantitative analysis. With these recent encouraging reports, Tc-99m UBI29-41 seems a novel agent of the future for infection imaging.

N-formyl products (fMLF or fMLP) labelled with Tc-99m are also being studied in rabbits for localization of infection. Tc-99m labelled Interleukin-8 (IL-8) seems another promising agent for the future as after initial animal model experiments it has been tried in humans with promising initial results.

9. Conclusion

Radionuclide imaging plays a significant role in infection detection and localization. Currently the selection of infection imaging agent depends upon the availability and local expertise especially in cases of labelling leukocytes which require time consuming labelling procedures. SPECT-CT provides essential anatomical localization especially in cases of vertebral osteomyelitis, diabetic foot, and infected prosthesis, cardiovascular, abdominal and pulmonary infections. Gallium scintigraphy can be replaced with FDG PET where available. FDG PET is a preferred procedure of choice for pyrexia of unknown origin, vasculitis, sarcoidosis, infected grafts and inflammatory bowel disease, moreover quantitative FDG PET analysis appears another promising further advance. Finally, with the progress in hybrid imaging the diagnostic power of conventional scintigraphy in detection and localization of infection has greatly augmented and the development of newer infection seeking agents pave the way for improved patient management in future.

10. Acknowledgment

The authors would like to acknowledge and thank Dr AbdulRedha A. Esmail and Dr Fahad Marafi for their contribution of the PET/CT images. We would also like to extend our thanks to our colleagues and staff of Departments of Nuclear Medicine and PET Unit, Al-Jahra Hospital and Kuwait Cancer Control Centre for their help and contribution.

11. References

Akhtar, MS.; Qaisar, A. Irfanullah, J. et al (2005). Antimicrobial peptide 99mTc-ubiquicidin 29-41 as human infection-imaging agent: clinical trial. *Journal of Nuclear Medicine*, Vol.46, No.4, (April 2005), pp.567-573, ISSN 0161-5505

Annovazzi, A.; Bagni, B. Burroni, L. et al (2005). Nuclear medicine imaging of inflammatory/infective disorders of the abdomen. *Nuclear Medicine Communication*, Vol.26, No.7, (July 2005), pp. 657–664, ISSN 0143-3636

Assadi, M.; Vahdat, K. Nabipour, I. et al (2011). Diagnostic value of 99mTc-ubiquicidin scintigraphy for osteomyelitis and comparisons with 99mTc-methylene diphosphonate scintigraphy and magnetic resonance imaging. *Nuclear Medicine Communication*, Vol.32, No.8, (August 2011), pp. 716-723, ISSN 0143-3636

Bar-Shalom, R B.; Yefremov, N. Guralnik, L. et al (2006). SPECT/CT Using 67Ga and 111In-Labeled Leukocyte Scintigraphy for Diagnosis of Infection. *Journal of Nuclear Medicine*, Vol.47, No.4, (April 2006), pp. 587–594, ISSN 0161-5505

Bleeker-Rovers, CP.; de Kleijn, EM. Corstens, FH. et al (2004). Clinical value of FDG PET in patients with fever of unknown origin and patients suspected of focal infection or inflammation. *European Journal of Nuclear Medicine and Molecular Imaging*. Vol.31, No.1, (January 2004), pp. 29-37, ISSN 1619-7070

Bleeker-Rovers, CP.; Bredie, SJ. van der Meer, JW. et al (2004). Fluorine 18 fluorodeoxyglucose positron emission tomography in the diagnosis and follow-up of three patients with vasculitis. *American Journal of Medicine*. Vol.116, No.1, (January 2004), pp. 50-53, ISSN 0002-9343

Bleeker-Rovers, CP.; Rennen, HJ. & Boerman, OC. (2007). 99mTc-labeled interleukin 8 for scintigraphic detection of infection and inflammation: First clinical evaluation. *Journal of Nuclear Medicine*, Vol. 48, No. 3, (March 2007), pp. 337-343, ISSN 0161-5505

Calder, JD.; Gajraj, H. (1995). Recent advances in the diagnosis and treatment of acute appendicitis. *British Journal of Hospital Medicine*, Vol.54, No.4, (August 1995), pp. 129-133, ISSN 1462-3935

Datz, FL. (1996). Abdominal abscess detection: Gallium, 111In-, and 99mTc-labeled leukocytes, and polyclonal and monoclonal antibodies. *Seminars in Nuclear Medicine*, Vol.26, No.1, (January 1996) pp. 51-64, ISSN 0001-2998

Devillers, A.; Garin, E. Polard, JL. et al (2000). Comparison of Tc-99m-labelled antileukocyte fragment Fab' and Tc99m-HMPAO leukocyte scintigraphy in the diagnosis of bone and joint infections: a prospective study. *Nuclear Medicine Communication*, Vol. 21, No.8, (August 2000), pp. 747–753, ISSN 0143-3636

Filippi, L.; Schillaci, O. (2006). Usefulness of hybrid SPECT/CT in 99mTc- HMPAO-labeled leukocyte scintigraphy for bone and joint infections. *Journal of Nuclear Medicine*, Vol.47, No.12, (December 2006), pp. 1908–1913. ISSN 0161-5505

Filippi, L.; Uccioli, L. Giurato, L. & Schillaci, O. (2009). Diabetic Foot Infection: Usefulness of SPECT/CT for 99mTc-HMPAO-Labeled Leukocyte Imaging. *Journal of Nuclear Medicine*, Vol.50, No.7, (July 2009) pp. 1042–1046, ISSN 0161-5505

Gnanasegaran, G.; Barwick, T. Adamson, K. et al (2009). Multislice SPECT/CT in benign and malignant bone disease: when the ordinary turns into the extraordinary. *Seminars in Nuclear Medicine*, Vol.39, No.6, (November 2009), pp. 431-442, ISSN 0001-2998

Gotthardt, M.; Bleeker-Rovers, CP. & Boerman, OC. (2010). Imaging of inflammation by PET, conventional scintigraphy, and other imaging techniques. *Journal of Nuclear Medicine*, Vol.51, No.12, (December 2010), pp. 1937-1949, ISSN 0161-5505

Graute, V.; Feist, M. Lehner, S. et al (2010). Detection of low-grade prosthetic joint infections using 99mTc-antigranulocyte SPECT/CT: initial clinical results. *European Journal of Nuclear Medicine and Molecular Imaging*, Vol. 37, No.9, (August 2010), pp. 1751-1759, ISSN 1619-7070

Harwood, SJ.; Valdivia, S. Hung, GL. et al (1999), Use of Sulesomab, a radiolabeled antibody fragment, to detect osteomyelitis in diabetic patients with foot ulcers by leukoscintigraphy, *Clinical Infectious Diseases*, Vol.28, No.6, (June 1999) pp. 1200-1205, ISSN 1058-4838

Horger, M.; Eschmann, SM. & Pfannenberg, C. (2003). The value of SPET/CT in chronic osteomyelitis. *European Journal of Nuclear Medicine and Molecular Imaging*, Vol.30, No.12, (December 2003), pp. 1665–1673, ISSN 1619-7070

Ingui, CJ.; Shah, NP. & Oates, ME. (2007). Infection Scintigraphy: Added value of single-photon emission computed tomography/computed tomography fusion compared with traditional analysis. *Journal of Computer Assisted Tomography*, Vol.31, No.3, (May 2007), pp. 375-380, ISSN 0363-8715

Joseph, TN.; Mujtaba, M. Chen, AL. et al (2001). Efficacy of combined technetium-99m sulfur colloid/indium-111 leukocyte scans to detect infected total hip and knee arthroplasties. *Journal of Arthroplasty*, Vol.16, No.6, (September 2001), pp. 753-758, ISSN 1532-8406

Kumar, R.; Nadig, MR. Balakrishnan, V. et al (2006). FDG-PET imaging in infection and inflammation. *Indian Journal of Nuclear Medicine*, Vol.21, No.4, (April 2006) pp104-113, ISSN 0970-8499

Kurdziel, KA. (2000). The panda sign. *Radiology*, Vol.215, No.3, (June 2000), pp. 884-885, ISSN 0033-8419

Love, C.; Palestro, CJ. (2004). Radionuclide imaging of infection. *Journal of Nuclear Medicine Technology*, Vol.32, No.2, (June 2004), pp. 47-57, ISSN 0091-4916

Love, C.; Tomas, MB. Tronco, GG. et al (2005). FDG PET of infection and inflammation. *Radiographics*, Vol.25, No.5, (September 2005), pp. 1357-68, ISSN 0091-4916

Lupetti, A.; de Boer, MG. Erba, P. et al (2011). Radiotracers for fungal infection imaging. *Medical Mycology*. Vol.49, No. Suppl 1 (April 2011), S62-69, ISSN 1460-2709

Mariani, G.; Bruselli, L. Kuwert, T. et al (2010). A review on the clinical uses of SPECT/CT. *European Journal of Nuclear Medicine and Molecular Imaging*, Vol.37, No.10, (October 2010), pp. 1959-1985, ISSN 1619-7070

McAfee, JG.; Subramanian, G. & Gagne, G. (1984). Technique of leukocyte harvesting and labeling: Problems and perspectives. *Seminars in Nuclear Medicine*, Vol.14, No.2, (April 1984), pp. 83-106, ISSN 0001-2998

Nazari, B.; Azizmohammadi, Z. Rajaei, M. et al (2011). Role of 99mTc-ubiquicidin 29-41 scintigraphy to monitor antibiotic therapy in patients with orthopedic infection: a preliminary study. *Nuclear Medicine Communication*, Vol.32, No.8, (August 2011), pp. 745-751, ISSN 0143-3636

O'Doherty, MJ.; Barrington, SF. Campbell, M. et al (1997). PET scanning and the human immunodeficiency virus-positive patient. *Journal of Nuclear Medicine*, Vol.38, No.10, (October 1997), pp. 1575-83, ISSN 0161-5505

Pakos, EE.; Trikalinos, TA. Fotopoulos, AD. et al (2007). Prosthesis infection: diagnosis after total joint arthroplasty with antigranulocyte scintigraphy with 99mTc-labeled monoclonal antibodies-a meta-analysis. *Radiology*. Vol. 242, No. 1, (January 2007), pp. 101-108, ISSN 0033-8419

Palestro, CJ.; Kim, CK. Swyer, AJ. et al (1990). Total-hip arthroplasty: periprosthetic indium-111-labeled leukocyte activity and complementary technetium-99m-sulfur colloid imaging in suspected infection. *Journal of Nuclear Medicine*, Vol.31, No.12, (December 1990), pp. 1950-1955, ISSN 0161-5505

Palestro, CJ. (1994). The current role of gallium imaging in infection. *Seminars in Nuclear Medicine*, Vol.24, No.2, (April 1994), pp. 128-141, ISSN 0001-2998

Palestro, CJ. & Torres, MA. (1997) Radionuclide imaging in orthopedic infections. *Seminars in Nuclear Medicine*, Vol.27, No.4, (October 1997), pp. 334–345, ISSN 0001-2998

Palestro, CJ. (2009). Radionuclide imaging of infection: in search of the grail. *Journal of Nuclear Medicine*, Vol.50, No.5, (May 2009) pp. 671-673, ISSN 0161-5505

Petruzzi, N.; Shanthly, N. & Thakur, M. (2009). Recent trends in soft tissue infection imaging. *Seminars in Nuclear Medicine*, Vol.39, No.2, (March 2009), pp. 115-123, ISSN 0001-2998

Poirier, JY.; Garin, E. Derrien, C. et al (2002). Diagnosis of osteomyelitis in the diabetic foot with a 99mTc-HMPAO leucocyte scintigraphy combined with a 99mTc-MDP bone scintigraphy. *Diabetes Metabolism*, Vol.28, No.6, (December 2002), pp. 485–490, ISSN 1262-3636

Salber, D.; Gunawan, J. Langen, KJ. et al (2008). Comparison of 99mTc- and 18F- ubiquicidin autoradiography to anti-Staphylococcus aureus immunofluorescene in rat muscle abscesses. *Journal of Nuclear Medicine*, Vol.49, No.6, (June 2005), pp.995-999, ISSN 0161-5505

Santiago, CR.; Giménez, CR. & McCarthy K. (2003). Imaging of osteomyelitis and musculoskeletal soft tissue infections: current concepts. *Rheumatic diseases clinics of North America*, Vol.29, No.1, (February 2003), pp. 89-109, ISSN 0889-8573

Scher, DM.; Pak, K. Lonner, JH. et al (2000). The predictive value of Indium-111 leukocyte scans in the diagnosis of infected total hip, knee, or resection arthroplasties. *Journal of. Arthroplasty*, Vol.15, No.3, (April 2000), pp. 295-300, ISSN 1532-8406

Tsan, MF. (1985). Mechanism of gallium-67 accumulation in inflammatory lesions. *Journal of Nuclear Medicine*, Vol.26, No.1, (January 1985), pp. 88-92, ISSN 0161-5505

van Eerd, JE.; Boerman, OC. & Corstens, FH. (2003). Radiolabeled chemotactic cytokines: New agents for scintigraphic imaging of infection and inflammation. *Quarterly Journal of Nuclear Medicine*, Vol.47, No.4, (December 2003), pp. 246-255, ISSN 1824-4785

Wegener, WA. & Alavi, A. (1991). Diagnostic imaging of musculoskeletal infection. Roentgenography; gallium, indium-labeled white blood cell, gammaglobulin, bone scintigraphy; and MRI. *Orthopaedics Clinics of North America*. Vol.22, No.3, (July 1991), pp. 401-418, ISSN 0030-5898

Zhuang, H. & Alavi, A. (2002). 18-fluorodeoxyglucose positron emission tomographic imaging in the detection and monitoring of infection and inflammation. *Seminars in Nuclear Medicine*, Vol.32, No.1, (January 2002), pp. 47-59, ISSN 0001-2998

Nuclear Medicine in Musculoskeletal Disorders: Clinical Approach

Noelia Medina-Gálvez[1] and Teresa Pedraz[2]
[1]*Hospital Universitario de San de Juan de Alicante, Department of Physical Medicine and Rehabilitation, Miguel Hernández University*
[2]*Hospital General Universitario de Alicante, Department of Rheumatology*
Spain

1. Introduction

Nuclear medicine supplies with functional perspective in the diagnosis of different pathologies of the musculoskeletal system. Bone scintigraphy is one of the most used nuclear medicine techniques in our clinical practice for location, evaluation and diagnosis of these pathologies because of its high sensitivity. This technique identifies functional changes before structural lesions have been established. For the study of musculoskeletal disorders, the usage of three-phase bone scintigraphy is applied more often than conventional bone scintigraphy. However, due to its low specificity, it has been replaced by other techniques such as magnetic resonance imaging (MRI) in the evaluation of localized lesions. New techniques in nuclear medicine which provide precision with high sensitivity are currently available, such as single-photon emission computed tomography (SPECT), useful in the evaluation of lumbar and hip pathology, or the presence of inflammation in small joints (hands and feet), and positron emission tomography (PET), which provides a metabolic imaging. Several radionuclides can be used in the scintigraphic evaluation, although the most commonly used for bone scintigraphy are labelled with technetium 99-m (99mTc), standing out diphosphonate compounds such as methylene diphosphonate (MDP). This radiopharmaceutical (Tc-99m-MDP) is used for studying metabolic bone diseases like Paget´s disease, transient osteoporosis and reflex sympathetic dystrophy. And it is also useful in the location of polytopic forms of avascular osteonecrosis, in the study of hidden painful radiologic bone lesions such as osteoid osteoma or others bone tumours, in the evaluation of soft-tissue lesions, and in the assessment of spread pattern of bone metastases. Furthermore, this radionuclide may locate bone fractures, identify the cause of pain in patients with chronic pain after arthroplasty, show the evolution of heterotopic ossification and provide information about musculoskeletal system infections (in combination with other radionuclides) and paediatric diseases. Other radionuclides commonly used in the evaluation of infectious or inflammatory processes in the musculoskeletal system are gallium citrate and indium 111-labelled leukocytes, since the latter increases the specificity of technetium radiotracer. Local treatments can be applied by radio isotopic techniques. One of these is radiosynoviorthesis, used in the treatment of patients with persistent monoarthritis in different stages (from inflammatory poliarthritis to pigmentary villonodular sinovitis).

The objective of this chapter is to make a simple but detailed review of the main nuclear medicine clinical applications in the appraisal and management of musculoskeletal problems.

2. Normal bone scintigraphy

Bone scan is a diagnostic technique used to assess the presence of anomalies in the distribution pattern of bone formation. It has high sensitivity, but specificity is frequently variable or limited. Three-phase bone scintigraphy is currently the most used technique because it allows evaluating the degree of hyperemia (flow phase), increased of articular permeability (blood pool phase) and the presence of alterations in bone remodeling (bone tissue phase). Traditional technique is based on the biological properties of bisphosphonates marked with 99mTc, usually MDP, when they are integrated into the bone metabolism after intravenous administration. Typically, 30% of the injected dose of Tc-99m-MDP remains in the skeleton, and most of bone uptake occurs in the first hour. The remainder is eliminated from the tissues and blood by the kidneys and imaging is obtained 3 - 4 hours later. In general, uptake of the tracer depends on local blood flow, osteoblastic activity and extraction efficiency. Normal scintigraphy imaging depends on technical equipment and employees, but it is also significantly influenced by other factors such as age and constitution of the patient, intake of drugs, degree of hydration, renal function and/or the presence of impaired circulation. Therefore a whole body study is recommended, with anterior and posterior screenings that allows assessing the symmetry or asymmetry in the distribution of the drug. However, a located study may be sufficient in some cases, since provides greater image quality and requires less time and is less expensive. In other patients, especially when a spine study is necessary or avascular osteonecrosis located in the hip or knee is suspected, it will require a SPECT, that is more sensitive for detecting abnormalities and provides, combined with tomography, three-dimensional images.

It is necessary to have knowledge of normal variants and patterns of abnormality to minimize misinterpretation. Whole body bone scan shows normal variations in the uptake of the radiotracer, as this is higher in areas with high bone remodeling. The age of the patient has a fundamental role in the appearance of the scan, especially during the growth period and in the elderly. In children, as they have a growing skeleton, there is a diffuse bone uptake and a striking uptake at the growth plates of bones, especially in metaphyseal-epiphyseal areas of long bones and cranial sutures. This decreases over the years until complete fusion of the epiphyses takes place. On the other hand, bone scan images are often of poor quality in old people. Aging may be reflected in scintigraphic images by a diffuse reduction of bone uptake of the radioisotope, although diffuse uptake at the dome or symmetrical uptake in the peripheral joints (secondary to osteoarthritis) may be present. Associated degenerative processes may lead to increased uptake in the involved joints. Obese people also get lower quality images. In addition, insufficient hydration and/or renal failure hamper the radiopharmaceutical removal of soft tissues and modify the end result.

The sternum and the sacroiliacs joints are normal uptake areas in scintigraphic studies (**Fig. 1**). Other areas that may appear as normal increased uptake (**table 1**) are forewings of the iliac bone, coracoid process, tip of the scapula and, sometimes, costochondral junction, lower portion of the cervical spine, kneecaps and some muscle attachments. Thoracic kyphosis and lumbar lordosis may cause the parts of the column that are farther away, appear as less warm. In patients with scoliosis, concave side usually appears hotter than the convex. There is also a physiological uptake located at renal pelvis and the bladder, since radiotracers are eliminated by the kidneys (Murray, 1998; Schneider, 2006).

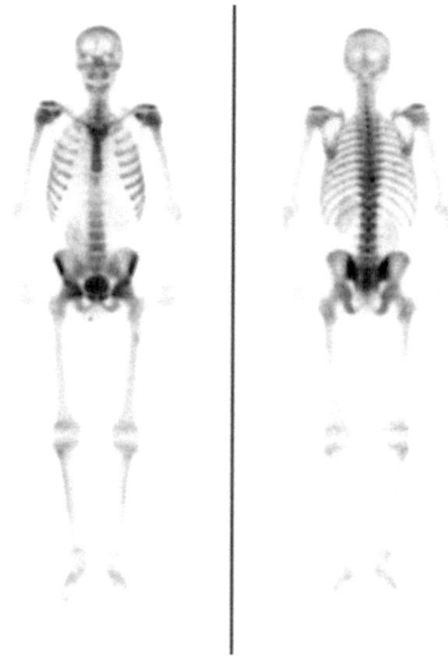

Fig. 1. Normal bone scintigraphy.

Head and neck:	Skull sutures, pterion, occipital protuberance, angle of mandible, hyperostosis frontalis, sinuses (ethmoidal and maxillary), dental disease and microcalcification of thyroid cartilage
Thorax:	Sternoclavicular joint, acromioclavicular joint, sternal foramina, costochondral uptake, manubrium sternum/xiphisternum, tip of scapulae, symmetrical muscle insertion in the posterior ribs of paraspinal muscles (stippled appearance)
Abdomen and pelvis:	Kidney, bladder, bladder diverticulae, pelvic diastasis (post partum women)
Long bones:	Deltoid tuberosity/deltoid insertion, trochanteric bursitis

Table 1. Normal Variants of uptake on 99mTc-MDP Bone Scan.

Many causes may lead to false pathologic imaging or pitfalls (Naddaf et al., 2004). Bladder diverticula or bladder image over pubic bones, urine leakage or urinary retention and patient rotation are some common examples. Artifacts on bone scintigraphy can be technical or patient-related (**Table 2**). The technical artifacts include equipment, radiopharmaceutical, and image processing-related problems. Equipment-related artifacts may be due to inadequate quality-control procedures and calibration. Faulty radiopharmaceutical preparation alters biodistribution and can compromise the diagnostic quality of the images. Increased tracer uptake in the stomach, thyroid, and salivary glands can be seen if there is free pertechnetate, in the radiopharmaceutical. A number of factors, for example, presence of reduced aluminum ions, if the radiopharmaceutical is left unused for a long time, inappropriately high pH and addition of dextrose solutions, may affect uptake of radioactivity in bone.

Finally, the most common artifact on the bone scan is due to extravasation at the site of injection, that may occasionally cause confusion with a bone abnormality, and it is therefore important to document the site of injection in all patients. Further, ipsilateral lymph node(s) may be seen due to extravasation of radiotracer and can on occasion cause confusion,

Radiopharmaceutical:	Free pertechnetate (stomach, thyroid, salivary glands)
Technical:	Injection site, lymph node (radiotracer extravasations), injection into central venous catheter, arterial injection
Patient:	Urine contamination, patient motion, breast prosthesis, metallic prosthesis (elbow, shoulder, knee and hip)
Metallic:	Belt buckle, medallion, jewellery, pace maker
Instrumentation:	Photomultiplier tube, cobalt peak, image contrast
Treatment:	Postradiotherapy

Table 2. Common Artifacts in Bone Scintigraphy.

particularly if overlying the scapula or a rib (Gnanasegaran et al., 2009). Photon-deficient areas commonly seen on the bone scan are due to metallic objects. Patients should be asked to remove metallic objects wherever possible before performing the scan. Urinary contamination is a common problem, which may simulate focal lesions, especially if close to or overlying the bone. It is useful to remove the clothing or to wash the skin and reimage the patient around the region of interest to avoid any confusion. The patient should void before the study and rarely delayed imaging or bladder catheterization may be required. Further, radioactive urine in the bladder is a frequent cause of artifact in patients evaluated with SPECT for pelvic metastases (prostate cancer) or low-back pain. Increased radioactive urine in the bladder can cause streak artifacts on the reconstructed images and overlap bony structures. Further, intense tracer retention in the bladder is reported to cause pixel overload, resulting in a relatively cold area close to the region of interest of the femoral heads, which hinders its interpretation.

3. Rheumatoid arthritis

Rheumatoid arthritis (RA) is a chronic autoimmune systemic disease of unknown origin, with an overall prevalence of 1%. It mainly affects joints with symmetrical and polyarticular pattern and may lead up to progressive structural damage, functional disability and extra-articular complications. It can affect many organ systems and it is also associated with a higher prevalence of other diseases such as infections, neoplasms and cardiovascular disease. It has been shown that 50% of patients with RA are disabled within 10 years of onset of disease and survival is reduced (Malviya et al., 2010; as cited in Solomon et al., 2003, Wolfe et al., 1994, 2002, 2003).

Conventional radiology is the most wide-spread technique for the appraisal of RA, since it allows the evaluation of the presence or absence of erosions, joint space narrowing or articular osteopenia, but only when symptoms have been present for several months or years. The importance of early diagnosis in patients with RA, based on the possibility of modifying the prognosis with an early treatment, has led to the introduction of new techniques that identify the characteristic changes in an accurate and reliable way. MRI and High-Frequency Ultrasonography (US) have shown their reliability for detecting early bony, vascular and soft tissue changes in patients with RA and are the techniques most commonly used with this aim. Nuclear medicine techniques, such as imaging with nanocolloids, PET or three-phase bone scintigraphy may also be useful in this field. Three-phase bone scintigraphy is still used in clinical practice in patients with RA because it allows the detection of changes (hyperemia, increased permeability, altered bone metabolism) before the structural lesions appear, and may display the pattern of joint involvement and even predict the development of erosions (Colamussi et al., 2004; as cited in Mottonen et al.,

1988). The intensity of uptake on scintigraphy is correlated to some clinical and laboratory indexes of disease activity (De Leonardis et al., 2008; as cited in Park et al., 1977) and the monitoring during treatment can evaluate the effectiveness of it (De Leonardis et al., 2008; as cited in Palmer et al., 1993; Elzinga et al., 2010). It is also a useful technique when an additional pathology (eg, osteonecrosis, stress fractures or metastatis) is suspected. Furthermore, in patients with nonspecific polyarthralgia, normal bone scan excludes the presence of active arthritis (Colamussi et al., 2004; as cited in Shearman et al., 1982). It is a sensitive tool but not highly specific, and may be altered in other diseases such as osteoarthritis. Nevertheless, planar bone scintigraphy is clearly less sensitive than SPECT in the evaluation of early stages of this disease or mild abnormalities. Multipinhole SPECT of the hands has been used to identify patients with minimal changes in bone metabolism (Gotthardt et al., 2010). This technique proven to equal MRI in sensitivity and also detected increased bone metabolism in two patients in whom MRI had negative results, demonstrating that multipinhole SPECT may be even more sensitive than MRI in some cases (Gotthardt et al., 2010; as cited in Ostendorf et al., 2010). PET may also be used for imaging of synovial inflammation. The most commonly used radiotracer in clinical PET scanning is fluorodeoxyglucose (18F-FDG), and since inflammation is a glucose-avid oxidative process, 18F-FDG-PET allows a quantitative measurement of the uptake of tracer concentration with a positive correlation with the degree of joint inflammation in patients with RA. Recently, it has been demonstrated its correlation with parameters of disease activity (swelling, tenderness, serum markers) and findings from gold standard techniques such as US and MRI. This quantitative assessment could be useful for evaluating the therapeutic effectiveness. Besides 18F-FDG, tracers such as 11C-choline may be used for measurement of cell proliferation and evaluation of synovitis with high accuracy (Gotthardt et al., 2010; as cited in Roivainen, 2003). Other techniques, including the imaging of sinovitis with 99mTc-nanocolloids, have shown high sensitivity and specificity in this field. Thus, nuclear medicine techniques, especially PET and multipinhole SPECT of small joints, may play a role in identifying RA at an early stage, but the usefulness of these techniques compared with MRI and US needs to be proven in RA imaging. Currently, US and MRI are the techniques of choice for serial assessments of patients with RA due to practical reasons and the required exposure of the patient to radiation in the nuclear medicine studies. Large systematic prospective studies on the efficient use of imaging modalities to assess the efficacy of treatment in early RA are lacking. Nevertheless, new imaging modalities are assuming an important role in the investigation and management of RA. Tagging important cellular and protein mediator may allow us improving the knowledge of RA pathophysiology. In recent years, the use of labelled immunoglobulins (Igs) that head for areas of inflammation and where they stay accumulated (aspecific polyclonal IgG-type antibodies labelled in most cases with Tc-99m), has been developed (**Table 3**).

mAbs	Type	Class	Isotope	Target
Infliximab (Remicade)	Chimeric	IgG1	99mTc	TNF-α
Adalimumab (Humira)	Fully human	IgG1	99mTc	TNF-α
Rituximab (Rituxan/Mabthera)	Chimeric	IgG1	99mTc	CD20
MAX.16H5	Murine	IgG1	99mTc	CD4
1.2B6	Murine	IgG1	111In	E-selectin
OKT-3 (Muromonab)	Murine	IgG2	99mTc	CD3

Table 3. Molecular imaging of RA by radiolabelled monoclonal antibody (mAbs).

The immunoscintigraphy has proven to be more sensitive than clinical examination for identifying synovitis and have a high positive predictive value for the onset of RA in patients with nonspecific arthropathy, and its usefulness for monitoring and assessing treatment response (Colamussi et al., 2004; as cited in De Bois et al., 1995a, 1995b, 1996). It can also be used to detect infection, although the preferred technique in these cases is labelled leukocyte scintigraphy, in which two tracers are often used: 99mTc-HMPAO or 111In-oxine (De Gersem & Jamar, 2010). Labelled leukocyte scintigraphy is also useful in assessing therapeutic response in RA patients and it has been correlated with other indices of activity in this disease (Collamussi et al., 2004; as cited in Al-Janabi et al., 1988). However, immunoscintigraphy seems to be more accurate than labelled leukocyte scintigraphy for the identification of synovitis in RA (Collamussi et al., 2004; as cited in Liberatore et al., 1992).

Other molecules and receptors (e.g. 64Cu-labelled anti-GPI, 68Ga-labelled annexin V or 123I-antileukoproteinase) are being identified as therapeutic targets and used to develop new radiopharmaceuticals which accumulate in areas of inflammation where they can be located and quantified. Their study and description will allow improving the understanding of the complex pathophysiology of RA and detecting changes in very early stages of this disease and will give us the possibility of a pre-therapy scintigraphic approach with radiolabelled monoclonal antibodies that will let us evaluate the presence of target molecules in the inflammatory lesion, thus helping in the selection of the most efficient therapy and predicting therapy response (Glaudemans et al., 2010; Malviya et al., 2010). But currently, these techniques are not used in clinical practice and remain like a research tool inside selected laboratories. Bioluminescence and fluorescence reflectance imaging are other approaches that allow imaging, and potentially the delivery of therapeutic agents at a molecular level (McQueen & Ostergaard, 2007).

4. Sacroilitis

Sacroiliac joint involvement is a common finding in the spondyloarthropathies (SpA) group and it is an important parameter included in the diagnostic criteria. Conventional radiology is essential in the evaluation of the sacroiliac joints, but it does not detect early abnormalities and, therefore, the use of other complementary techniques currently available, such as CT, MRI, US, and bone scintigraphy, is necessary to avoid delaying the diagnosis.

Until only a few years ago, bone scintigraphy was the gold standard technique for early diagnosis of inflammatory processes at this joint. The assessment of sacroilitis by scintigraphy is based on the quantification of radiotracer uptake in the sacrum and sacroiliac joints. This technique can help to differentiate between degenerative and inflammatory disorders in patients with nonspecific radiological changes. Both conventional bone scintigraphy and SPECT mode are sensitive techniques for early detection of SpA in patients with low back pain and who still do not have typical radiological changes, because the uptake of radiopharmaceutical at sacroiliac joints is produced before structural damage happens. However, in the sclerotic phase of evolved SpA, scintigraphy frequently does not detect any abnormalities. MRI, more sensitive in detecting early changes and more specific, has shifted to the bone scan. In this regard, a published review (Schneider, 2006; Song et al., 2008) realized with the aim to assess the diagnostic value of scintigraphy for detecting sacroilitis in patients with established and/or probable ankylosing spondylitis, has proven limited value of scintigraphy both in the early detection of sacroilitis and in patients with established ankylosing spondylitis. In patients with SpA and gastrointestinal symptoms but negative endoscopic or radiological test results, abdominal scintigraphy with labelled leukocytes can be used to assess the abdominal involvement (Colamussi et al., 2004; as cited in Elkayam et al., 2002).

5. Infection

In the setting of infection four entities can be established: osteomyelitis, septic arthritis, soft tissues infections and joint replacement infection.

5.1 Osteomyelitis

Osteomyelitis is defined by infection localized to bone. It can occur as a result of hematogenous seeding, contiguous spread of infection to bone from adjacent soft tissues and joints, or direct inoculation of infection into the bone as a result of trauma or surgery (Lalani, 2011). Three-phase bone scan with 99mTc-hydroxymethylene diphosphonate or Tc-99m-MDP has long been used as the standard method for the detection of osteomyelitis (Gotthard et al., 2010), and positive focally increased uptake on all three phases (**Fig. 2**) is usually seen (Love et al., 2003).

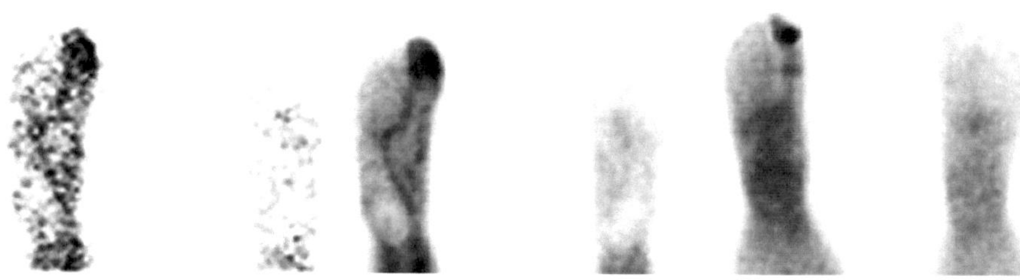

Fig. 2. Three-phase bone scan: Focally increased uptake on all three phases in a patient with osteomyelitis of the right great toe.

In contrast, in the setting of cellulitis there is increased activity only in the first two phases and normal or mild diffuse increased activity in the third phase (Brown et al., 1993; Horwich, 2011). Radiographic studies do not show any change for at least 1- 2 weeks after initial infection, contrary to the three-phase bone scan where imaging of the infection can be seen in the first 24 - 48 hours of the infection (Díaz & De haro, 2005). Bone scintigraphy has a high sensitivity exceeding 80% and a limited specificity reaching up to 50% (Gotthard et al., 2010, as cited in Hakim et al., 2006; Palestro et al., 2002). The limited specificity can be explained by uptake of the radiopharmaceutical at all sites of increased bone metabolism irrespective of the underlying cause. Other conditions such as tumors, fractures, joint neuropathy may mimic osteomyelitis at three-phase bone scintigraphy. To improve specificity, complementary imaging with gallium-67 (67Ga) citrate (for spinal infection) or indium-111-labelled autologous leukocytes (for the appendicular skeleton) is often performed (Love et al., 2003).
Gallium scans utilize the affinity of gallium-67 to acute phase reactants (lactoferrin, transferrin, and others) to demonstrate areas of inflammation that may be related to infection (Horwich, 2011). Intense uptake on 67Ga bone scintigraphy in two adjacent vertebrae with loss of the disc space is highly suggestive of spinal osteomyelitis (Palestro & Torres, 1997). This method is quite sensitive and more specific than three-phase bone scan (Horwich, 2011; as cited in Palestro, 1991; Tumeh, 1986). It is typically performed 24 hours following inyection and therefore should be reserved for patients who are clinically stable and do not require prompt

imaging results for urgent management decisions. Gallium not only enhances the specificity of the diagnosis but provides information about surrounding soft tissue infection (Palestro & Torres, 1997). If gallium scan is negative, it effectively excludes the diagnosis of osteomyelitis (Horwich, 2011; as cited in Pineda, 2006). A gallium scan can be performed concurrently with a technetium labelled three-phase bone scan, and the information gathered may be more useful than that of either examination alone (Horwich, 2011; as cited in Tumed, 1986). Both radionuclides can be injected at the same time and the scintigraphic images can be obtained three to four hours after injection, while gallium images will be obtained up to 24 hours later (Horwich, 2011). This combination is probably the best nuclear medicine tool for the evaluation of vertebral osteomyelitis (Palestro & Torres, 1997).

Labelled leukocyte imaging is a good alternative in the evaluation of osteomyleitis, but is of little value in vertebral osteomyelitis because this entity often presents as a non specific photopenic defect (Gotthard et al., 2010; as cited in Van Der Bruggen et al., 2010). But, in the diabetic foot diagnosis, labelled leukocyte imaging alone is sufficient to determine the presence of osteomyelitis in the forefoot. In the midfoot and hindfoot it may be necessary to combine leukocyte scintigraphy with others radiotracers to precisely localize the infection (Palestro & Torres, 1997). The combined imaging approach of 99mTc-colloid bone marrow/labelled-leukocyte scanning enhances the sensitivity and specificity above 90%, avoiding the problem of physiologic uptake into bone marrow. Because in osteomyelitis bone marrow is replaced by the infectious process, bone marrow imaging will be negative whereas leukocyte scanning in the same location will be positive (Gotthardt et al., 2010, as cited in Palestro et al., 2006).

In chronic osteomyelitis the specificity of Tc-99m-MDP bone scans is very low even with active exacerbation because positive uptake also occurs with the healing process (El-Maghraby et al., 2006). Other false negative results are possible in areas of relative ischemia, since radiotracer may not be adequately delivered to the target site (Horwich, 2011). 67Ga combined with Tc-99m-MDP allows identification of active chronic osteomyelitis. Discordance between 67Ga and Tc-99m-MDP with more intense 67Ga or different distribution is highly specific at 80-100% (El-Maghraby et al., 2006). 18F-FDG-PET is a promising modality for imaging musculoskeletal infection and might play an important role in the evaluation of chronic osteomyelitis and spinal infection (Strobel & Stumpe, 2007). The specificity for spinal infection drops only if patients underwent surgery less than 6 months before PET and if osteosynthetic material is present (Gotthardt et al., 2010; as cited in De Winter et al., 2003). However, because MRI may not be an option in patients with metallic implants in situ, PET currently is the most sensitive imaging modality in the evaluation of such patients (Gotthardt et al., 2010; as cited in De Winter et al., 2003). Furthermore, in cases of severe defenerative disk disease with oedema-like changes in the endplates and the adjacent discs, MRI can give false-positive results (Gotthardt et al., 2010; as cited in Palestro et al., 2006). Other tracers for diagnosing spinal osteomyelitis are also under investigation, including radiolabelled antibiotics and antifungical tracers (Gemmel et al., 2006).

5.2 Septic arthritis

Septic arthritis is the infection of the synovial tissues. It often occurs as a result of hematogenous seeding and less often by direct inoculation as a result of trauma or surgery (Díaz & De haro, 2005). Although it may occur at any age, it is most common in children under 3 years. Over 90% of cases are mono-articular (El-Maghraby et al., 2006). The most commonly involved joints are the hips and the knees (Díaz & De haro, 2005). Despite MRI and nuclear medicine methods are used for the diagnosis or a preliminary investigation of infectious arthritis, the definitive diagnostic test is the identification of bacteria in the synovial fluid aspiration (Díaz & De haro 2005). Though, some joints are difficult to examine. As in the osteomyelitis, there is an increased uptake on all three phases of three-phase bone scan (El-Maghraby et al., 2006). The hallmark of septic arthritis is symmetrical uptake in both sides of the joint (Díaz & De haro, 2005). However, a positive scintigraphy has a low specificity. The differential diagnosis is made more accurate when the osteoarticular scintigraphy is combined with gallium citrate or more commonly radiolabelled leukocyte or immunoglobulins. In the presence of septic arthritis, these agents demonstrate activity patterns of diffuse nature in the soft tissue in and around the joint with no focal abnormality in bone. However, this can be difficult to ascertain without demonstration of exactly where bone lies in relation to the soft tissue infection and may need combined imaging. Rosenthall et al have shown that a combined study does raise the sensitivity for the detection of septic arthritis from 54% with TC-99m-MDP alone to 84% for combined 67Ga/Tc-99m-MDP scanning (El-Maghraby et al., 2006; as cited in Rosenthall et al., 1982). Another combination is the labelled leukocytes/Tc-99m-MDP combined study, which is reported to be more specific than a 67Ga/Tc-99m-MDP study and produces fewer equivocal results (El-Maghraby et al., 2006; as cited in Tehranzadeh et al., 2001; Chengazi & O'Mara, 2003). For disc space infections, although the bone scan is often positive, gallium scintigraphy is the preferred method. Indium-111(111In)-leukocytes have been shown to be of limited value in the diagnosis of disc space infection; although some authors feel that the labelled white cell scan can be of benefit especially if the cold (photon deficient) lesions are considered diagnostic of disc space infection (Brown et al., 1993).

5.3 Cellulitis

Cellulitis is a soft tissue infection. The scan shows intense uptake in the first two phases of the study with diffuse extra-osseous activity, while the final image is normal after 2-4 hours. The presence of other processes that stimulate osteoblastic reaction, as in cases of suspected osteomyelitis in areas with trauma, surgery or arthritis, complicates the interpretation of the scintigraphic image which is completely non specific. Combined studies with different radiotracers such as 67Ga, 111In-leukocytes or 99mTc-HM-PAO improve the sensitivity and specificity, although MRI remains as gold standard technique (Díaz & De Haro, 2005).

5.4 Painful joint replacement

Prosthetic joint replacement is a common procedure and most patients have excellent results, but 20% of them develop pain during the follow-up. It may be secondary to infection, aseptic loosening or heterotopic bone formation (El-Maghraby et al., 2006). Differentiate betweeen loosening and infection is often a difficult problem, especially because clinical signs and symptoms, laboratory tests and radiographies are insensitive, nonspecific, or both. Cross-sectional imaging modalities are hampered by artifacts produced by the prosthetic devices. Radionuclide imaging is not affected by the presence of metallic hardware and is therefore useful for evaluating the painful prosthesis (Love et al., 2001). Negative scintigraphic study rules out septic or aseptic loosening. Both conditions, however, may show increased tracer uptake in bone scans, but the pattern and site of uptake may help to differentiate each other. In aseptic loosening, focal localized uptake at the tips is seen, whereas in the infection diffuse intense uptake will be seen in the three phases of bone scan. The sensitivity for bone scan in infection is relatively high, ranging from 70% to 100% but the specificity is variable ranging from 20% to 90% and the reported accuracy is around 50-70% (El-Maghraby et al., 2006; as cited in Rosenthall et al., 1982, Turpin & Lambert, 2001, Wilson, 2004). The combination of 67Ga-citrate and Tc-99m-MDP bone scans has better results, with accuracy around 70-80% (El-Maghraby et al., 2006). But lower results for this combination has also been reported because the uptake of both tracers can be found not only in infection, but also in the postoperative patient, in heterotopic bone formation, and loosening or inflammatory reaction to cement fixators (El-Maghraby et al., 2006; as cited in Turpin & Lambert, 2001).

Labelled leukocyte imaging is, at least theoretically, the ideal technique for diagnosing the infected prosthesis because in general, white cells do not accumulate at sites of increased bone mineral turnover in the absence of infection (Palestro, 1998). However, labelled-leukocytes yield false positive results due to reactive or displaced bone marrow as a result of surgery are present up to more than 24 months after implantation (El-Maghraby et al., 2006; as cited in Oswald et al., 1990). Labelled leukocytes accumulate not only in infection but in the bone marrow as well. This problem has been overcome by the addition of complementary bone marrow imaging, which is usually performed with Tc-99m sulfur colloid. Both, labelled leukocytes and sulfur colloid accumulate in the bone marrow, but only labelled leukocytes accumulate in infection. In contrast to the results reported for labelled leukocyte imaging alone, the results of combined leukocyte-marrow imaging of prosthetic joints have been uniformly excellent, with an accuracy of 90% or greater (Love et al., 2001; as cited in Palestro 1990, 1991) and has become the method of choice to evaluate surgical prostheses (El-Maghraby et al., 2006; as cited in Love et al., 2001; Turpin & Lambert, 2001). Although extremely accurate, leukocyte-marrow scintigraphy is hampered by significant limitations. The in vitro labelling process is labor intensive, is not always available, and requires direct contact with blood products. The need for marrow imaging adds to the complexity and cost of the study and is an additional inconvenience to patients, many of whom are elderly and debilitated (Love et al., 2001). In an effort to maintain the accuracy of the study while reducing or eliminating the disadvantages, several methods of labelling leukocytes in vivo have been investigated, but their role in prosthetic joint infection has not been established.

FDG-PET has been extensively investigated, the high-resolution tomographic images, availability of the agent, and rapid completion of the procedure are all desirable traits. Published results to date, however, are inconclusive in this setting (Love et al., 2009; as cited in Chacko et al., 2002; Joseph et al., 2001; Love et al., 2004; Manthey et al., 2002; Pill et al., 2006; Reinartz et al., 2005; Stumpe et al., 2004; Zhuang et al, 2001).

6. Avascular osteonecrosis

Osteonecrosis, also known as aseptic necrosis, avascular necrosis, ischemic necrosis, and osteochondritis dissecans, is a pathological process that has been associated with numerous conditions and therapeutic interventions. The exact prevalence of osteonecrosis is unknown. In the United States, there are an estimated 10,000 to 20,000 new patients diagnosed per year, and osteonecrosis is the underlying diagnosis in approximately 10 percent of all total hip replacements. The male-to-female ratio of this disorder is 8:1, but varies with different comorbidities (Jones, 2011). The mechanisms by which this disorder develops are not fully understood. Compromise of the bone vasculature leading to the death of bone and marrow cells (bone marrow infarction) appear to be common to most proposed etiologies. The process is most often progressive, resulting in joint destruction within three to five years if left untreated. A variety of traumatic and nontraumatic factors contribute to the etiology of osteonecrosis. Glucocorticoid use and excessive alcohol intake are reported to be associated with more than 90% of the cases. Osteonecrosis usually occurs in the anterolateral femoral head, although it may also affect the femoral condyles, humeral heads, proximal tibia, vertebrae, and small bones of the hand and foot. Many patients have bilateral involvement at the time of diagnosis, including disease of the hips, knees, and shoulders. The most common presenting symptom of osteonecrosis is pain and patients may have eventually limitation on range of motion. A limp may be present late in the course of lower extremity disease. A small proportion of patients are asymptomatic. In these cases the diagnosis is usually incidental. Asymptomatic involvement contralateral to a symptomatic site is frequently noted.

There is no pathognomonic feature of osteonecrosis. A clinical diagnosis is appropriately made in a symptomatic patient when imaging findings are compatible with this disease and other causes of pain and bony abnormalities are either unlikely or have been excluded by appropriate testing. The evaluation for suspected osteonecrosis should begin with plain film radiography, althought it can remain normal for months after symptoms of osteonecrosis begin. Features of osteonecrosis on plain film radiographs, radionuclide scans (**Fig. 3**), and MRI are helpful diagnostically and provide the basis for classification and staging systems. Early diagnosis of osteonecrosis is crucial: the earlier the stage of the lesion at the time of diagnosis, the better the prognosis. Clinically, early diagnosis and treatment of osteonecrosis might prevent unnecessary surgery (Pape et al., 2004). Therefore, early diagnosis and location of osteonecrosis have prognostic value and determine the therapeutic alternatives.

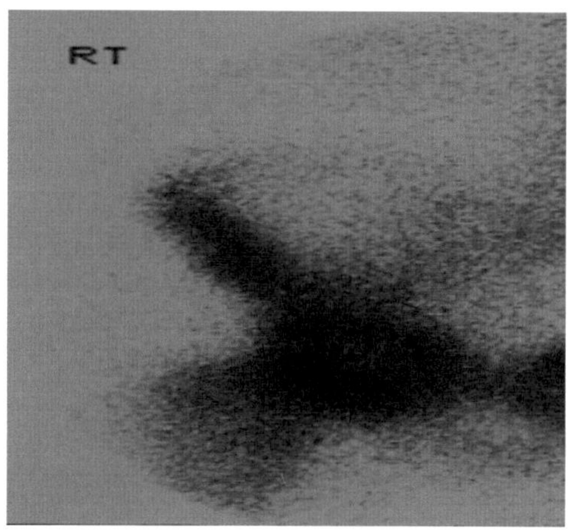

Fig. 3. Radionuclide bone scan of the pelvis in a 68-year-old man with hip pain. Bilateral central area of diminished uptake surrounded by a zone of increased uptake in the femoral head consistent with avascular necrosis.

Currently, MRI is the technique of choice for the diagnosis of avascular osteonecrosis in the early stages. This technique has been proven to be a highly accurate method both for early diagnosis (changes can be seen early in the course of disease when other studies are negative) and for staging of the disease (Malizos et al., 2007). MRI is far more sensitive than plain radiographs or bone scanning, with an overall reported sensitivity of 91% (Jones, 2011; as cited in Chang et al., 1993). Nevertheless, 99mTc bone scintigraphy also plays an important role in the early diagnosis of avascular necrosis and whole body bone scan is useful in patients with suspected polytopic osteonecrosis. The characteristic distribution of the radiopharmaceutical in the affected area (cold area surrounded by a hyperfixation rim) enables early diagnosis, before the appearance of anatomical changes, which only show up later with radiography (Jones, 2011; as cited in Feggi et al., 1987 and Maillefert et al., 1997). The presence of this tipical pattern may increase the diagnostic accuracy to distinguish between osteonecrosis and transient osteoporosis, which usually has a diffuse pattern of tracer uptake, with no cold area. The accuracy of scintigraphy can be improved by using SPECT in patients with suspected avascular necrosis of the femoral head but have concomitant changes that may show up as false positives, such as severe acetabular osteoarthritis (Jones, 2011; as cited in Collier et al., 1985). It also may help us to avoid overlooking a subchondral fracture.

6.1 Transient osteoporosis

Transient osteoporosis of the hip, also called transient marrow edema syndrome, is characterized by the presence of intense radionuclide uptake in the femoral head, which may extend to the femoral neck, to the intertrochanteric region, or to proximal femoral diaphyseal region. It is also typical to find hyperactivity at the images of flow phase and blood pool phase. Ischemia of the femoral head, that has not caused necrosis, has been suggested as a possible cause of this process. The reactive hyperemic response to this ischemic phenomenon, with a repair process, would explain scintigraphic changes. Insufficiency fractures in this location can provide similar scintigraphic imaging (Schneider, 2006).

7. Reflex sympathetic dystrophy

Reflex sympathetic dystrophy (RSD) is a complex physiologic response of the body to an external stimulus resulting in pain sympathetically mediated, usually nonanatomic pattern, which is out of proportion to the inciting event or expected healing response (Fournier & Holder 1998). It is a syndrome affecting an extremity after a minor trauma or surgery, but the particular mechanism remains uncertain. The diagnosis of RSD relies on clinical evaluation, scintigraphy or MR imaging, and routine radiographs. In the spontaneous course of this syndrome three phases can be distinguished: Stage I is the warm or hypertrophic phase, stage II is called the cold or atrophic phase and the third stage corresponds to stabilization or, in rare instances, to healing (Driessens et al., 1999; Ornetti & Maillefert, 2004).

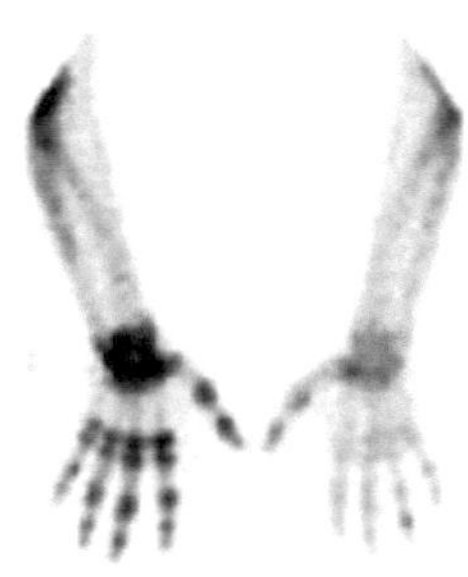

Fig. 4. Bone scanning: Diffusely increased uptake in the distal right upper extremity in reflex sympathetic dystrophy.

Three-phase scintigraphy has been widely utilized in both the diagnosis and monitoring of treatment (Murray, 1998). Scintigraphy imaging (**Fig. 4**) shows increased perfusion during the angiographic and vascular pool phases and widespread increases in radiophosphonate bone uptake in the late stage (Colamussi et al., 2004). The highest diagnostic accuracy is provided by the combination of three signs: Increase activity ratio in the blood pool phase performed at 5-15 min, diffuse uptake in the carpus o tarsus and periarticular uptake in all the small joints (Murray, 1998). Decreased radiotracer accumulation has also been described, especially in children and adolescents (Driessens et al., 1999; Love et al., 2003). Bone scintigraphy is of major importance for the diagnosis in order to clearly differentiate from other conditions which are incorrectly diagnosed and treated as RSD. If the bone scan is not suggestive of RSD, the clinical picture, radiological examination and vascular scan may lead to the correct diagnosis. This may be a pseudodystrophy, in which a hypovascularization is found right from the start, while in true RSD there is initially a hypervascularization. Other conditions which may be confused with RSD are causalgia, neurotic compulsive postures, hysterical conversion, malingering and even self-mutilation (Driessens et al., 1999). Bone scintigraphy has a high sensitivity in the initial stage of Sudeck's syndrome, but after 26 weeks, it loses accuracy (Benning & Steinert, 1988; Lee & Weeks, 1995).

8. Metabolic bone disorders

8.1 Osteoporosis

Osteoporosis is defined as a systemic skeletal disease characterized by low bone density and microarchitectural deterioration of bone tissue, with an increase in bone fragility and susceptibility to fractures. Despite an increase in bone turnover that is usually present in osteoporosis, the bone scan has no role in the diagnosis of uncomplicated osteoporosis, but the Tc-99m-MDP bone scan is most often used in established osteoporosis to diagnose fractures, particularly at sites that are difficult to image with plain film radiography (eg, sacrum, ribs), and may be particularly useful in the diagnosis and timing of vertebral fractures. It also has an important role in assessing suspected fractures where radiography is unhelpful, either because of poor sensitivity related to the anatomical site of the fracture (eg, sacrum **Fig. 5**) or because adequate views are not obtainable because of the patient's discomfort (Fogelman & Cook, 2003). The characteristic appearance of these fractures is discussed elsewhere in this chapter. If a patient complains of back pain with multiple previous vertebral fractures noted on

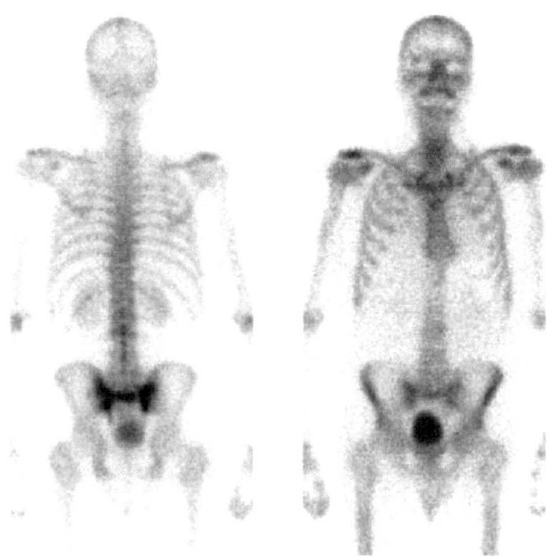

Fig. 5. Posterior and anterior Tc-99m-MDP bone scan showing a typical "H-shaped" pattern in the sacrum, indicating a sacral insufficiency fracture.

radiographs, and the bone scan is normal, then this essentially excludes recent fracture as the cause of symptoms and other causes of pain should then be considered.

8.2 Paget

Paget's disease is a localized disease of bone remodeling characterized by an increased bone resorption mediated by osteoclasts and a compensatory increase in bone formation. The result is a disorganized mosaic of woven and lamellar bone at affected skeletal sites. This structural change produces bone that is expanded in size, less compact, more vascular and more susceptible to deformity and fracture than in normal bone. It can affect any bone, but is more common in skull, hip, pelvis, legs and back. Paget's disease may be monostotic, but the majority of patients have a polyostotic disease (80-90%). Most patients are asymptomatic, but they can experience a variety of symptoms such as bone pain, bone deformity, secondary arthritic problems, excessive warmth over bone area and different neurological complications caused by compression of adjacent neural tissues.

Bone scintigraphy, combined with radiology, is the technique of choice for assessing the location and extent of the pagetic bone lesions. It allows of evaluating the entire skeleton and is more sensitive than radiography in identifying metabolically active lesions (Fogelman & Carr, 1980): there is no radiological correspondence over 10% of scintigraphic hot spots (Devogelaer & De Deuxchaisnes, 2003). Symptomatic lesions are usually characterized by an increased uptake. Characteristically, affected bones show a striking increase in metabolic activity that starts at one edge of the bone and extends distally or proximally, often showing a "V" or "flame - shaped" leading edge. Both osteolytic and osteoblastic lesions are associated with and increase in radiotracer uptake on bone scan (**Fig. 6**). Scintigraphic pagetic bone features are usually characteristic, presenting as "hot spots". Whole bone may be affected, especially at pelvis, scapula and vertebrae. Abnormal tracer accumulation throughout the vertebra, affecting the body and posterior elements, is the characteristic finding in this localization. The skull may show a different pattern with a ring of increased activity only in the margins of the lesion (Fogelman & Cook, 2003). The intensity of radiactive tracer uptake, usually Tc-99m-MDP, depends on the metabolic activity of Paget's disease. In later stages, the disease may go into a period of inactivity and bone scan shows little or no uptake. Therefore, bone scintigraphy is complementary to the use of biochemical markers (e.g. serum alkaline phosphatase, urine hydroxyproline) for the assessment of bone turnover and may be useful in assessing therapeutic efficacy, since a good correlation between bone scintigraphy uptake and clinical and biochemical markers has been found (Cook et al., 2010). Cases of scintigraphic evidence of pagetic activity in the setting of normal serum alkaline phosphatase have been reported. In these cases, bone scintigraphy is the main technique in the evaluation of the effectiveness of the treatment. Bone scan can be performed 3-6 months after treatment with bisphosphonates, although scintigraphic images may respond in a heterogeneous way (after intravenous bisphosphonate therapy, some bones may become normal, most bones show some improvement, and a small proportion remain unchanged), and even lead to infrequent images that sometimes mimic those of bone metastases. In these cases, knowing the medical history of the patient is essential (Fogelman & Cook, 2003). The superior quantitative accuracy of PET using 18F-fluoride ion has been described in the evaluation of pagetic bone (Cook et al., 2002), and this method has also been described to measure response to bisphosphonate treatment. An increase in 18F-FDG uptake has also been reported in pagetic bone (Cook et al., 2010; as cited in Cook et al., 1997), correlating also with disease activity. Bone scintigraphy can also identify complications (**Fig.

6) of Paget's disease like fractures (shown as a linear area of increased activity perpendicular to the cortex) or sarcomatous degeneration. The latter should be suspected in patients with persistent pain. The most common scintigraphic sign in the setting of sarcomatous degeneration is a cold area inside an area of increased uptake. The scan may also show heterogeneous and irregular uptake in the study area or adjacent soft-tissue uptake. The evaluation of the lesion should always be completed with x-ray and, even if doubts persist, with an MRI, which could allow a more precise diagnosis (Fransen et al., 1998).

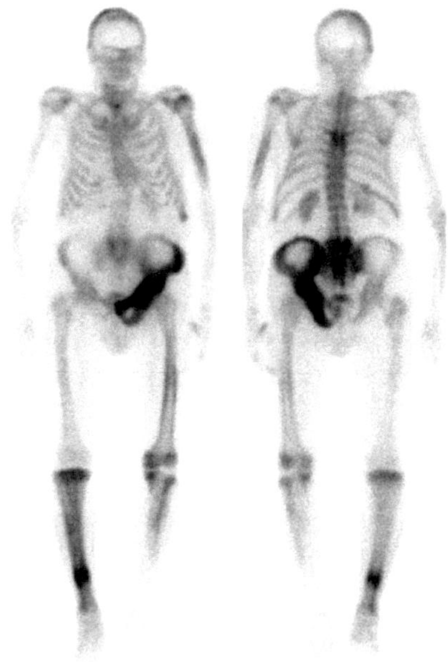

Fig. 6. A Tc-99m-MDP bone scan showing Paget's disease affecting the left humerus, mid-thoracic and lower lumbar spine, sacrum, right 11th rib, left pelvis, left femur and tibia, and the right tibia. Focal linear activity in the right tibia indicates an incremental fracture

8.3 Hyperparathyroidism

Most cases of primary hyperparathyroidism are asymptomatic and are unlikely to be associated with changes on bone scintigraphy. The diagnosis is made biochemically and the use of bone scintigraphy does not make sense with this goal. But bone scan may be useful to differentiate the causes of hypercalcemia, in particular, hyperparathyroidism vs malignancy, so that typical features of metabolic bone disorders may be recognized. There is increased skeletal turnover in hyperparathyroidism, commonly seen as part of renal osteodystrophy, and in the more severe cases, this will be evident scintigraphically. A bone scan may show several features in hyperparathyroidism, but the most important is the generalized increased uptake throughout the skeleton that may be identified because of increased contrast between bone and soft tissues. This is commonly termed the metabolic superscan to differentiate from superscans caused by widespread bone metastases. Other typical features that have been described in this context include a prominent calvarium and mandible, beading of the costochondral junctions, and a "tie" sternum (Fogelman & Carr, 1980). Severe forms of hyperparathyroidism may be associated with uptake of bone radiopharmaceuticals into soft tissue, related with ectopic calcification. Focal skeletal abnormalities may represent associated Brown tumors, although these are relatively uncommon.

8.4 Renal osteodystrophy

Renal osteodystrophy is secondary to a combination of bone disorders as a consequence of chronic renal dysfunction, and often shows the most severe cases of metabolic bone disease. It may include osteoporosis, osteomalacia, adynamic bone, and secondary hyperparathyroidism in varying degrees. The most frequent bone scan imagings are similar to a superscan from other metabolic bone disorders, and uptake of diphosphonate in areas of ectopic calcification also may be seen. A lack of bladder activity (secondary to the renal failure) may help in identification and differentiating this type of scintigraphic pattern from others. Aluminum toxicity from hemodialysis, rarely seen now, causes a poor quality bone scan with reduced skeletal uptake and increased soft-tissue activity, as aluminum blocks mineralization and hence the uptake of tracer, resulting in a pattern applicable to all forms of adynamic bone disease. Quantitative measurements of bone metabolism in renal osteodystrophy using 18F-fluoride have been compared with bone histomorphometry and have shown a close relationship between the net plasma clearance of 18F-fluoride to bone mineral and the histomorphometric indices of bone formation. The method was able to differentiate low turnover from high turnover states of renal osteodystrophy (Cook et al., 2010; as cited in Messa et al., 1993).

8.5 Osteomalacia

Patients with osteomalacia usually demonstrate similar features of a bone scan as described in hyperparathyroidism, although in the early stages of the disease it may appear normal (Cook et al., 2010). The reason that osteomalacia shows these features is not fully understood. Tracer avidity may reflect diffuse uptake in osteoid, although more likely, it is due to the degree of secondary hyperparathyroidism that is present. In addition, the presence of focal lesions may represent pseudofractures or true fractures. Pseudofractures are characteristically found in the ribs, the lateral border of the scapula, the pubic rami, and the medial femoral cortices. Although osteomalacia is usually a biochemical and/or histologic diagnosis, the typical bone scan features can be helpful in suggesting the diagnosis. The detection of pseudofracutures with this technique is more sensitive than that with radiography (Cook et al., 2010; as cited in Fogelman et al., 1977, 1978).

9. Bone tumors

For the diagnosis study of primary bone tumors prevails the importance of the morphological study to characterize the lesion and, in many cases, the initial plain films guides the diagnosis. In these cases, the usefulness of bone scintigraphy is lesser, but may be useful for detecting a lesion that is difficult to assess radiologically because of its location, and supporting the suspicion about the benignity or malignancy of the lesion. Characteristic patterns of uptake have been described in some primary bone tumors, but they are not reliable enough, given that there is an overlap in the scintigraphic characteristics of the benign and malignant bone lesions. The differential diagnosis of a solitary bone lesion usually depends more on morphologic imaging techniques, including radiographs, CT, and MRI, and on expert histologic analysis. In contrast, a larger role is developing for 18F-FDG-PET/CT for staging and response assessment of several bone tumors. Three-phase bone scintigraphy offers information about the vascularity of the bone lesion: Malignant tumors tend to be more vascularized and be uptake in all three phases of the scan, while benign bone tumors often do not show changes in the first two phases of the scintigraphy. Normal uptake, even in the third stage, is a sign for the mildness of the bone lesion. Osteoid osteoma is a benign bone tumor that constitutes an exception to this statement: It is highly vascular and provides uptake images in all three phases of the scan. In fact, a normal bone scan excludes its diagnosis. Aneurysmal bone cyst may show similar features. In patients with a benign tumor and a bone scan showing intense uptake, a fracture should be suspected.

9.1 Benign bone tumors and tumor- like disorders

In benign bone tumors, the uptake of radiopharmaceuticals (e.g. 99mTc) varies by type of tumor and may be normal, mild or severe. Bone scintigraphy is useful for the diagnosis of osteoid osteoma, especially when it is located at the spine, pelvis or hip, where radiological studies are usually not diagnosed. The typical scintigraphic finding is a round focal uptake lesion. CT is always necessary to confirm the diagnosis and surgical treatment. Most enchondromas appear like hot spots at bone scan study. This technique can locate these tumors in multiple enchondromatosis, but it can not differentiate between enchondroma and chondrosarcoma. The scintigraphic feature of the giant cell tumor is increased tracer uptake in all phases of this study, and the image of donut of the lesion, with a rim of uptake surrounding a central area of low uptake. Nevertheless, this image may also appear in other bone tumors. In fibrous displasia, characterized by replacement of normal bone tissue by abnormal fibro-osseous tissue with a high bone turnover, bone scan also display areas of increased uptake. In other bone lesions such as Langerhans cell histiocytosis, hemangiomas and aneurysmal bone cysts, the sensitivity of this technique is variable (Schneider, 2006).

9.2 Soft tissue tumors and primary malignant bone tumors

Musculoskeletal sarcomas represent a heterogeneous group of malignancies involving bone and soft tissue. Multiple myeloma is the most common primary malignancy of bone in adults, with an incidence of 3 per 100,000 in the USA. It may affect any bone with hematopoietic red marrow. Patients affected are usually over 50 years of age with the most common age group being between 60 and 65 years of age. Excluding myeloma and lymphoma, malignant primary bone tumors constitute only 0.2% of all malignancies in adults and approximately 5% of childhood malignancies, and, excluding mieloma in adults, the overwhelming majority of cases consist of osteosarcoma or Ewings' sarcoma (Green, 2009). Both are more common in the pediatric than the adult population. Osteosarcoma is the most frequent primary bone malignancy in children and second in adults following multiple myeloma. The Ewing's sarcoma family of tumors is the second most frequent primary bone malignancy in children and young adults and it is the most lethal bone tumor. The most common presenting symptom for primary bone tumors is a painful swelling arising in the bone. The presentation may be similar to acute or chronic osteomyelitis with systemic symptoms of fever, malaise, weight loss, and leukocytosis. Approximatly 15% of patients have clinically evident metastasic disease at diagnosis. Metastatic spread is mainly hematogenous, and the lungs are the most common site of metastases, followed by bone and bone marrow. Anatomic imaging techniques including radiography, US, CT and MRI, currently play a dominant role in the evaluation of suspected and known sarcomas of both soft tissue and bone. Nuclear medicine techniques such as scintigraphy, Thallium-201, and 67Ga imaging have all been used in the assessment of primary bone tumors. However, PET is becoming the most imporant modality for assessing biologic characteristics of the tumor, for primary staging, and for determining response to treatment. Although imaging studies may be highly suggestive of the diagnosis, they cannot reliably differentiate among the various types of malignant bone tumors, and even among malignant and benign conditions. Histopathologic confirmation, therefore, is required. The sites for biopsy are critical for accurate histological diagnosis and staging because biopsy of a small site may not represent the overall character of the tumor, missing high-grade areas, and non-diagnostic biopsies may also occur (Howman-Giles et al., 2006).

The diagnosis of indeterminate bone lesions is limited with 18F-FDG-PET, but in general the greater the level of uptake, the more likely a lesion is malignant in nature. However, it has been reported that some giant cell tumors and fibrous dysplasia may show uptake equivalent to osteosarcomas and that some other benign bone lesions may show high 18F-FDG accumulation (Aoki et al., 2001). Despite this, 18F-FDG-PET has a high specificity for excluding malignant bone tumors (Cook et al., 2010). Recently, dual time point imaging and calculation of a retention index for 18F-FDG have shown improved discrimination of benign and malignant bone lesions compared with static measures, but that some overlap was still present (Tian et al., 2009). Lodge et al observed difference in time-activity curves between benign and low-grade malignant tumors that show peak activity within the first 30 minutes post-injection and high-grade sarcomas, which reach peak activity 4 hours after injection. This quantitative approach cannot separate low-grade sarcomas from benign lesions. MRI is the modality of choice to define the extension of tumors to surrounding soft tissue as well as to estimate the local tumor infiltration into bone marrow. However, in the pediatric population, 18F-FDG-PET is valuable for detection of skip metastases in cases of equivocal MRI findings due to the physiological red blood marrow in long bones (Even-Sapir, 2007; as cited in Wuisman P, Enneking WF, 1990). With the new hybrid imaging, it is now possible to take advantage of the metabolic and morphologic information from 18F-FDG-PET/CT to enhance discrimination between benign and malignant bone lesions by dedicated interpretation of the CT characteristics (Strobel et al., 2008). 18F-FDG-PET data can also assist in optimizing the biopsy site of heterogeneous masses by guiding sampling to active tumor sites and avoiding errors due to biopsy of necrotic tumor areas (Even-Sapir, 2007; as cited in Pezeshk et al., 2006). In general, 18F-FDG-PET or PET/CT would appear to have a complementary role to conventional staging procedures (Cook et al., 2010; as cited in Kleis et al., 2009, Kneisl et al., 2006 and Völker et al., 2007). After a diagnosis of a malignant primary bone lesion is made, the use of bone scintigraphy to define the extent of tumor before surgical resection is controversial: good correlation between increased bone tracer uptake and true anatomical extent that has been reported (Cook et al., 2010; as cited in Goldmann et al., 1975, McKillop et al., 1981, and Papanicolou et al., 1982), has not been supported by other studies (Chew & Hudson, 1982). These discrepancies may be due to peritumoral reactive changes overestimating extent or underestimations due to inability to detect marrow and soft-tissue involvement. For these reasons, MRI is the most accurate noninvasive assessment of tumor extent. On the other hand, several studies have reported the ability of bone scintigraphy to predict histological response to preoperative chemotherapy in patients with primary malignant bone tumors. Ozcan et al have reported a study of 27 patients with osteosarcoma, Ewing's sarcoma, and malignant fibrous histiocytoma, which has displayed a reduction in hyperemia and extension as the most notable findings on three-phase bone scintigraphy. A reduction in tumor blood flow of 58.7% was found in 15 responding patients compared with 19.9% in the nonresponders. A higher accuracy in assessing response was possible using all the information from three-phase scintigraphy (88%), compared with static imaging alone (74%) where the blood flow and blood pool images showed a reduction in vascularity and extension. These are consisting features with the results published in previous studies (Cook et al., 2010; as cited in Knop et al., 1990, and Sommer et al., 1987). The sensitivity of 18F-FDG-PET in staging primary bone tumors appears to vary between different tumor types and location of metastases. Spiral CT is the modality of choice for detection of relatively small lung metastases. Franzius et al compared the detection lung metastases of sarcoma by CT and 18F-FDG-PET, showing a higher sensitivity for the former modality especially in lesions <9 mm. 18F-FDG-PET may, however, assist in differentiating nonspecific lung nodules from metastases detected by CT in case of larger lung lesions, within the size range of PET resolution. 18F-FDG-PET may also identify unexpected extra pulmonary metastases. Serial 18F-FDG-PET assessment of primary bone tumors (predominantly osteosarcomas, Ewing's sarcomas, or both) is a good non-invasive method to predict pathologic neoadjuvant chemotherapy response (Cook et al., 2010; Even-Sapir, 2007). Another earlier study also showed a correlation with pathologic response but described high 18F-FDG uptake in granulation and/or fibrotic tissue and in the fibrous pseudocapsule of treated tumors (Cook et al., 2010; as cited in Jones et al., 1996).

Multiple myeloma hardly triggers osteoblastic reaction and therefore scintigraphy is less sensitive than plain radiography and CT. FDG-PET indicates active myeloma and CT shows bone destruction. Therefore hybrid whole-body PET/CT is an excellent method to evaluate myeloma. Currently whole-body and spinal MRI and PET/CT are considered the imaging techniques of choice for initial evaluation and follow-up of these patients. Durie et al assessed the role of 18F-FDG-PET in 66 patients with multiple myeloma and monoclonal gammopathy of undetermined significance. Their results suggested that a positive 18F-FDG-PET reliably indicates the presence of active myeloma, whereas a negative study strongly supports the diagnosis of monoclonal gammopathy of undetermined significance. 18F-FDG-PET has also been reported to identify unexpected medullar and extramedullar sites of myelomatous disease not appreciated on X-ray, CT, or scintigraphy (Even-Sapir, 2007). In a recent report on 28 patients with multiple myeloma, 18F-FDG-PET/CT and MRI of the spine were shown to have complementary roles. Although the former modality detected more lesions, all of which were located outside the field of view of MRI, the latter modality was found superior for diagnosing an infiltrative pattern in the spine (Nanni et al., 2006). In another recent report, 18F-FDG-PET was found to be valuable in detecting infection in patients with multiple myeloma (Even-Sapir, 2007).

Osteosarcoma represents only 0.1% of all tumors, but it is the second most frequent malignant primary bone tumor after myeloma. The diagnosis of osteosarcoma is based on characteristic histologic features in combination with typical radiographic findings. MRI of the entire suspected bone is performed to define the degree of penetration of the tumor surrounding soft tissue as well as to estimate the local tumor infiltration into bone marrow. Furthermore, CT of the chest and conventional bone scan are necessary for early detection of metastases. MRI and scintigraphy are also used to distinguish postoperative changes from residual or recurrent tumor tissue after local surgical treatment. Because osteosarcoma metastases usually incorporate bisphosphonates, bone scanning can be used for follow-up examinations to detect both osseous and nonosseous metastases. High-resolution CT has been shown to be superior to 18F-FDG-PET for detecting lung metastases. Data on the benefit of 18F-FDG-PET for detecting skeletal metastases in osteosarcoma patients are still very sparse, but successful detection of all sites of bone involvement by 18F-FDG-PET has been reported recently (Even-Sapir, 2007; as cited in Franzius et al., 2002). Nevertheless, in children there may be an exception for primary staging, where there may be an indication for 18F-FDG-PET to detect intraosseous skip metastases in cases of unequivocal MRI findings, although no data are yet available to support this hypothesis. PET scans will not obviate the need for biopsy and tissue diagnosis in soft-tissue and bone masses, but it is remarkably helpful to guide biopsy. Non-PET–guided biopsy might miss the most biologically significant region, resulting in a false low pre-therapeutic tumor grading. 18F-FDG-PET imaging data has shown reliability for prediction of tumor response to preoperative, neoadjuvant chemotherapy. On the other hand, for differentiation between benign residual mass lesions caused by post-therapeutic tissue changes and residual tumor tissue or local relapse, 18F-FDG PET is considered to be highly sensitive and more accurate than CT or MRI (Brenner et al., 2003). A high baseline uptake of 18F-FDG in osteosarcoma has been reported as showing an inverse correlation with prognostic indicators and is associated with a poor outcome with similar results for patients with high post-treatment FDG activity (Cook et al., 2010; as cited in Costelloe et al., 2009; Franzius et al., 2002).

Ewing's sarcoma is a highly malignant primary bone tumor that is being derived from red bone marrow. It accounts for approximately 5% of biopsy-analyzed bone tumors and approximately 33% of primary bone tumors. No single morphologic or functional imaging method provides findings for a specific diagnosis of Ewing's sarcoma, but the results do contribute to tumor staging. Because the clinical symptoms of Ewing's sarcoma are nonspecific and because they frequently suggest osteomyelitis, an initial conventional radiographic and/or MRI examination is performed. With static bone scintigraphy, Ewing's sarcoma is usually depicted as a focal area of increased radionuclide activity. Whole-body bone scans can provide information about the primary lesion and depict skip lesions. Also, bone scintigraphy can be used to localize distant metastases during tumor staging. Three-phase dynamic bone scintigraphy can help in the assessment of treatment effects, with a reported accuracy of 88%. In cases that respond to treatment, a reduction of both flow and tracer uptake can be observed. 18F-FDG-PET may help to detect lesions that are not shown on conventional bone scans. It is the most sensitive modality for therapeutic follow-up, and this modality can reveal early changes in tumor metabolism, which is an indicator of the therapeutic effect.

Regarding the lymphomatous disease, primary skeletal involvement occurs in 3 to 5% of patients with non-Hodgkin's lymphoma, and secondary bone involvement occurs in up to 25% of patients. Moog et al have reported 18F-FDG-PET to be more sensitive and specific than Tc-99m-MDP bone scintigraphy for detection of osseous involvement by lymphoma. Early bone involvement may present as abnormal on 18F-FDG-PET with normal CT appearance, since detection of malignant bone involvement on CT depends on the presence of a considerable amount of bone destruction.

9.3 Metastases

Bone metastasis is the most common malignant bone tumor. It affects two thirds of cancer patients, and tumors that most often lead to metastases are breast, lung and prostate neoplasms. Bone involvement by cancer occurs most commonly by hematogenous spread, although tumor may occasionally extend directly from the soft tissue to the adjacent bone. The vast majority of bone metastases initiate as intramedullary lesions. The normal bone undergoes constant remodeling, maintaining a balance between osteoclastic (resorptive) and osteoblastic activity. As the metastatic lesion enlarges within the marrow, the surrounding bone undergoes osteoclastic and osteoblastic reactive changes. Based on the balance between the osteoclastic and osteoblastic processes, the radiographic appearance of a bone metastasis may be lytic, sclerotic (blastic), or mixed. The osteoblastic component of the metastasis represents reaction of normal bone to the metastatic process. The incidence of lytic, blastic, and mixed types of bone metastases is different in various tumor types. Lytic lesions may be seen in almost all tumor types. Bone metastases of bladder, kidney, and thyroid cancer and lesions of multiple myeloma are invariably lytic. Blastic lesions are frequently seen in prostate and breast cancer, occasionally in lung, stomach, pancreas, and cervix carcinomas, and infrequently in colorectal cancer (Beheshti et al., 2009; Even-Sapir, 2005). The most frequent distribution of metastasis in the human skeleton is usually 80% in the axial skeleton and ribs, 10% skull and 10% in long bones. Approximately 40% of patients with metastases have no pain at diagnosis (Diaz & De Haro, 2005). Symptoms occur mainly when the lesion increases in size, causing extensive bone destruction, which may lead to collapse or fracture, or in the presence of accompanying complications, such as spinal cord compression or nerve root invasion.

Bone scan is the primary tool for screening or monitoring bone metastases due to its high sensitivity, versus plain radiography (Brown, 1993), and plays an integral part in tumor staging and management, since early detection of skeletal metastases optimizes management (Even-Sapir, 2005). Scintigraphic image of metastases is one or more high uptake foci in 98% of the cases, and the usual pattern consists of increased radiotracer deposition in areas of osteoblastic reparative activity in response to tumor osteolysis. The presence of multiple, randomly, distributed areas of increased uptake of varying size, shape, and intensity is highly suggestive of bone metastases, specially at sternum, scapula and ribs. Although multiple foci of increased activity may be encountered in other pathologic conditions, it is often possible to distinguish metastatic disease from other entities by analyzing the pattern of distribution of the abnormalities. Traumatic injury, in contrast to metastatic disease, generally manifests as discrete focal abnormalities of similar intensity. Multifocal rib trauma has a characteristic linear distribution. In patients with osteoporosis, the presence of kyphosis and/or an H-shaped sacral fracture suggests the correct diagnosis. In older patients, osteoarthritis and degenerative changes may manifest as areas of intense activity on radionuclide bone images. These changes can be distinguished from metastatic disease by virtue of their characteristic location (eg, knees, hands, wrists). Involvement of both sides of the joint is common in arthritis but unusual in malignant conditions. The remaining 2% is mild uptake foci owing to preponderance of osteolytic activity. The possibility of an artifact should be ruled out in cases of well-defined cold spot. In cases of wide-spread metastases, the radiopharmaceutical can be almost completely captured and it may lead to a superscan image, where kidney or bladder silhouettes are not initially seen by the delay in urinary excretion of radiotracer. A superscan may also be associated with metabolic bone disease but, in this case, the uptake is more uniform in appearance and extends into the distal appendicular skeleton. Intense calvarial uptake that is disproportionate to that in the remainder of the skeleton is another feature of a metabolic superscan. SPECT is reported to detect 20 to 50% more lesions in the spine compared with planar scintigraphy, and it increases both the sensitivity and specificity. The new hybrid system, SPECT with multislice CT, improves diagnostic accuracy (Dasgeb et al., 2007). The most common radiotracer is Tc-99m-MDP but in patients with follicular thyroid carcinoma or in cases of neuroblastoma, iodine-131 (131I) and 123I-Metaiodobenzylguanidine (123I-MIBG) are more sensitive. Increased uptake of these radiotracers reflects the osteoblastic reaction of bone to the destruction of bone by the tumor cells, whereas increased 18F-FDG activity at the sites of bone lesions on PET study represents active tumor itself. Bone scintigraphy is more sensitive than FDG-PET for detection of blastic/sclerotic lesion, whereas FDG-PET is more sensitive for lytic lesions and bone marrow disease. The latter has the additional ability to assess extraskeletal metastatic disease. Hybrid PET/CT imaging improves the specificity of FDG-PET for skeletal metastases (Dasgeb et al., 2007; as cited in Even-Sapir, 2005). An additional finding from scanning the peripheries, particularly in patients with bronchogenic carcinoma, may be the observation of hypertrophic osteoarthropathy secondary to cortical periostitis, that typically appears as symmetrical, nonuniform, irregular cortical uptake involving the long bones, most often seen in the femora, tibiae and wrists, and giving rise to the "tramline sign" (Gnanasegaran et al., 2009; Love et al., 2003; as cited in Ernstoff & Meehan, 2000). In patients with bone metastases who have received chemotherapy, reparative osteoblastic reaction that occurs after this treatment may lead to the appearance of bone areas with intense uptake during the first 3 months (flare phenomenon). As healing progresses, uptake in the lesion disminishes and by 6 months it should generally be possible to differentiate response from progression (Love et al., 2003).

18F-FDG-PET has become a routine imaging modality for staging and monitoring the response to therapy in patients with lymphoma. There are accumulating data indicating that 18F-FDG-PET may detect early marrow infiltration and may add clinically relevant information when performed in patients with primary or secondary lymphomatous bone involvement. FDG-PET can detect early marrow infiltration and therefore is more sensitive than planar scintigraphy or CT for assessment of early skeletal involvement in lymphoma (Dasgeb et al., 2007). A pattern of heterogeneous patchy marrow activity should raise the suspicion of marrow involvement in an 18F-FDG-PET study prior to therapy, while a pattern of diffuse uptake, mainly in Hodgkin's Lynphoma, is more commonly associated with reactive hematopoietic changes or myeloid hyperplasia (Even-Sapir, 2007).

Metastatic disease occasionally manifests as a solitary abnormality, usually in the spine, although other causes such as fractures, avascular osteonecrosis, primary bone tumors and infections must be previously ruled out. The location and/or characteristics of the lesion may guide the diagnostic suspicion but, especially if it is a solitary lesion, it must be studied with other imaging techniques such as CT or/and MRI (Schneider, 2006). Approximately 50% of cases in which scintigraphy detect a solitary focal uptake in a patient with a history of cancer, it is a metastasis. In patients with breast cancer, the sternum is a relatively common site to be affected often as a solitary lesion and probably results from local spread from the involved internal mammary lymph nodes. If a sternal lesion is situated distant from the manubriosternal junction, is irregular, asymmetric, or eccentric, then malignant involvement should be suspected. In a retrospective study of patients with breast cancer, 3.1% presented with an isolated sternal lesion and 76% of these were found to represent metastatic disease (Gnanasegaran et al., 2009; as cited in Kwai et al., 1988). Vertebral body fractures have a characteristic appearance on bone scintigraphy, showing a horizontal linear pattern of increased tracer accumulation. However, it is usually not possible to differentiate fractures due to benign diseases, such as osteoporosis from malignant collapse. In such cases, further evaluation with MRI is often the most informative. However, multiple linear abnormalities of varying intensity favour a benign etiology with presumed osteoporotic fracture occurring at different time points. Also, a follow-up bone scan after a few months that shows reducing activity at a vertebral fracture site, suggests a benign cause and a healing fracture. SPECT technique improves the localization and characterization of the vertebral lesions, due to its ability to delineate the body, pedicles, and spinous process:

Lesions that extend from the vertebral body into the posterior vertebral elements or involve the pedicle are more likely to represent metastases than lesions confined to the facet joints, anterior vertebral body, or either side of a disc (Gnanasegaran et al., 2009).

10. Osteoarthritis

Osteoarthritis (OA) is the most prevalent chronic joint disease and it has the greatest health economic impact. Conventional radiography is still the first and most commonly used imaging technique for evaluation of a patient with a known or suspected diagnosis of OA (Guermazi, 2009). MRI is an appropriate tool for describing changes in cartilage volume and concomitant soft-tissue alterations. But for qualitative cartilage imaging, MRI has, to date, not been fully validated. Bone scan allows the differentiation of inflammatory from degenerative joint affections and may add information on the activity of the subchondral bone, which may develop to a prognostic marker of OA (Zacher et al., 2007). Another pronostic marker of slower progression that can help us deciding the most appropriate management is the imaging of the joints that show up as "cold" (Colamussi et al., 2004). Radionuclide joint imaging is more sensitive than clinical or radiographic techniques in detecting early joint involvement but usually it must be supplemented by other techniques to establish a specific diagnosis (Hoffer & Genant, 1976).

Usefulness of molecular imaging for early diagnosis of OA is still a challenge. Cartilage damage in OA is being recharacterized as having an earlier dynamic phase, where cartilage damage is potentially reversible, followed by an irreversible pathologic phase that ultimately leads to joint pain and immobility (Hu & Du, 2009). The point at which cartilage damage is deemed irreversible has not been defined but probably depends on the size of the lesion, age of the patient, underlying cause, comorbid factors, activity level, use of joint stabilizers, genetic predisposition, and other factors. To detect early cartilage damage, molecular imaging research has focused on the identification of better ways to either visualize extracellular matrix depletion or measure events that are associated with cartilage damage, such as chondrocyte death and the elaboration of matrix-degrading enzymes. In OA, there is general acceptance that abnormal chondrocyte apoptosis is a pivotal event in the eventual destruction of articular cartilage (Biswal et al., 2007). A method for the study of cell death in living subjets is based on an endogenous protein, annexin V, whose function is not clearly understood but which is thought to play a role in coagulation (Biswald et al., 2007; as cited in Reutelinsperger & Van Heerde, 1997). This protein has an extremely strong affinity for the cell membrane phospholipid phosphotidylserine, which is expressed to the outer surface of the cell membrane during the apoptotic cascade. The use of annexin V, labelled with either a radioisotope or a fluorescent marker, provides an excellent opportunity to image programmed cell death. To date, annexin V has been labelled with 99mTc, iodine (125I, 124I, 123I), 111In, 11C, gallium (Ga-67, Ga-68), and 18F, making it appropriate for either SPECT or PET imaging (Biswald et al., 2007; as cited in Blankenberg, 1998; Glaser, 2003; Lahorte, 2004; Russell, 2002; Zijlstra, 2003). However Annexin V imaging has yet to be applied to the assessment of human OA. Another event associated with cartilage damage is the elaboration of matrix-degrading enzymes. In OA damaged cartilage appears to activate hibernating proteases such as matrix metalloproteinases and cathepsins. Using a cathepsin B-sensitive near-infrared fluorescent probe, researchers have found significant amounts of signal arising from an arthritic knee compared with normal knees in an animal model of OA (Biswald et al., 2007; as cited in Lai, 2004).

11. Heterotopic ossification

Heterotopic ossification (HO) is defined by the presence of bone in soft tissue where bone tissue normally does not exist, and it usually takes place around large joints (Medina et al., 2008). Its etiology is unknown, but is frequently precipitated by trauma, spinal cord injury or central nervous system injury (Shebab et al., 2002). The incidence of HO varies widely between populations. The incidence after hip replacement ranges from 16% to 53%; among patients with spinal cord injury HO develops in 20-25% and in brain injury patients the incidence of HO ranges from 10 to 20% (Medina et al., 2008; as cited in Vanden & Vanderstraeten, 2005). Around 20% of the patients who have an HO will develop functional limitation and it will be severe in 8% to 10% (Medina et al., 2008; as cited in Buschbacher, 1992; Subbarao, 1999). HO may closely mimic the presentation of cellulitis, osteomyelitis, or thrombophlebitis. HO can even be confused with some bone tumors such as osteosarcoma or osteochondroma. To resolve such diagnostic uncertainty and to prevent functional limitations, clinicians often request bone scanning and other imaging studies for patients at risk (Shebab et al., 2002). Radiography, MRI and CT have low sensibility in early stages of HO and three-phase bone scintigraphy (**Fig. 7**) is the most sensitive imaging modality during this period. It is also useful for its monitoring (Vanden & Vanderstraeten, 2005).

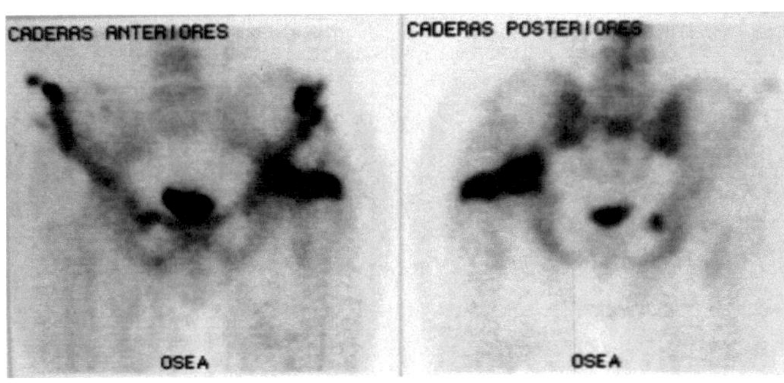

Fig. 7. Bone Scanning: increased uptake around the left hip consistent with Heterotopic Ossification.

First and second phases of three-phase bone scintigraphy are especially sensitive to detect incipient HO, which may be diagnosed 2.5 weeks after injury. Findings on the third phase may become positive approximately 1 week later. Radiographic studies do not show any change for at least 5- 8 weeks after initial injury (Shebab et al., 2002; as cited in Freed et al., 1982; Orzel & Rudd, 1985). Activity on the delayed bone scans usually peaks in a few months and after that the intensity of HO activity progressively lessens and thus the uptake of the radiotracer on the scans, which return toward normal within 12 months. However, in some cases activity remains slightly elevated even though the underlying HO has become mature (Shebab et al., 2002; as cited in Tibone et al., 1978). During the course of HO, bone scans made on follow-up may show radiotracer uptake on third phase even after flow and blood-pool images have returned to normal. Serial bone scans have been used successfully to monitor the metabolic activity of HO and determine the appropriate time for surgical resection, if needed, and to predict postoperative recurrence (Shebab et al., 2002; as cited in Freed et al., 1982; Muheim et al., 1973; Rossier et al., 1973; Tanaka et al., 1977). For the differential diagnosis of osteomyelitis complementary imaging with gallium-67 citrate (for spinal infection) or indium-111-labeled autologous leukocytes (for the appendicular

skeleton) may be necessary, as commented in that section. Gallium-67 citrate uptake in HO is proportional to the uptake of 99m Tc-diphosphonates, in contrast to the relatively greater gallium-67 citrate uptake characteristic of osteomyelitis (Shebab et al., 2002).
A diagnostic-treatment algorithm of heterotopic ossification has been proposed, and three-phase bone scintigraphy has been recommended, after clinical signs and laboratory test, for its diagnosis in patients without HO but with high risk factor. If clinical signs and symptoms are present but initial radiographic studies are normal, bone scan should be repeated after 4-6 weeks, and when scintigraphic studies have displayed the HO, it should be made every three months during the first year. Bone scan has also been proposed during the follow-up after HO removal to monitor possible recurrences (Medina et al., 2008).

12. Fractures

Following known injury, fractures are commonly demostrated by conventional radiography of most sites of trauma. In such circumstances bone scintigraphy has no major role, although unsuspected lesions may be identified. Acute fractures show increased perfusion on the radionuclide angiogram; intense, poorly marginated increased tracer accumulation representing relatively increased vascularity on the blood pool images; and intense poorly defined increased tracer accumulation on delayed images (Holder, 1993).

12.1 Occult fractures

Scintigraphy may be valuable in the diagnosis of occult fractures, which are true fractures not immediately obvious on clinical examination or plain radiography, and it is particularly useful to detect certain type of fractures that require urgent orthopedic treatment, such as femoral neck and intertrochanteric fractures, scaphoid fracture, and Lisfranc fracture. Occult femoral neck and intertrochanteric fractures are frequents in older females with continued hip pain following a fall. Shortly following the time of injury, there is an increase in perfusion to the fracture site which can be demonstrated during the rapid sequence flow study and blood pool phases of the so called three-phase bone scan. The time for first appearance of increased uptake on delayed 99mTc-diphosphonate images remains controversial, fluctuating between 24 hours and 2 weeks (Collier et al., 1993; as cited in Holder et al., 1990; Matin, 1979; Spitz, 1991). These problems are not encountered in the identification of scaphoid fracture which is readily visualized within 3 days of trauma. Bone scan demonstrates a focus of intense uptake usually centered in the scaphoid (Collier et al., 1993; as cited in Patel et al., 1992; Tiel-van-Buul et al., 1992). High-resolution bone scan images obtained with the wrist first in a neutral position and then in ulnar deviation are used to localize the scintigraphic abnormality to the scaphoid. With ulnar deviation there is movement and rotation of the scaphoid relative to adjacent bony landmarks such as the radial styloid (Collier et al., 1993). Premature imaging withing 48 hours must be avoided, particularly as the osseous scintigraphic changes may be obscured by the diffuse uptake resulting from superficial hyperemia or traumatic sinovitis. Prolonged delay of this study may also result in increased uptake associated with disuse and thus, masking the fracture (Murray, 1998). Scintigraphy is therefore of considerable value in identifying this lesion before X-ray change appears, especially as difficulty may be encountered in radiological diagnosis even after 2-3 weeks (Murray, 1998). Difficulties in identifying the exact anatomic localization of a focus of uptake can be overcome by the technique of a combined display of the scan and the X-ray (Murray, 1998; as cited in Hawkes, 1991). Other occult fracture that can require urgent treatment is Lisfranc fracture. This fracture presents a characteristic appearance on bone scan with a band of increased uptake extending across multiple tarsometatarsal joints, typically involving the first through fifth or the second through fifth tarsometatarsal joints (Collier et al., 1993; as cited in Fogelman & Collier, 1989).

12.2 Stress fractures

Stress fracture occurs when a bone breaks after being subjected to repeated tensile or compressive stresses, none of which would be large enough to cause individually the bone to fail, in a person who is not known to have an underlying disease that would be expected to cause abnormal bone fragility (De Weber, 2011). The incidence of stress fractures is less than 1 % in the general population. The reported incidence in athletic populations varies with the type of athlete. Among military recruits the incidence ranges from 1 to 31 %, among runners 13 to 52 %, and among participants in collegiate team sports 1 to 8 % (De Weber, 2011; as cited in Bennel, 1997). In most instances, the individuals who suffer stress fractures have been engaging in vigorous activity to which they have not yet become conditioned. The failure to recognize the characteristic clinical and imaging findings of a stress fracture and the continued excessive exercise by the athlete will occasionally lead to a complete fracture (Collier et al, 1993). Imaging is needed when high risk stress fractures are suspected or a definitive diagnosis is necessary. The sites at high risk complications are the pars interarticularis of the lumbar spine, femoral head, superior side of the femoral neck, patella, anterior cortex of the tibia, medial malleolus, talus, tarsal navicular, proximal fifth metatarsal, great toe sesamoids, and the base of the second metatarsal bone (De Weber, 2011).

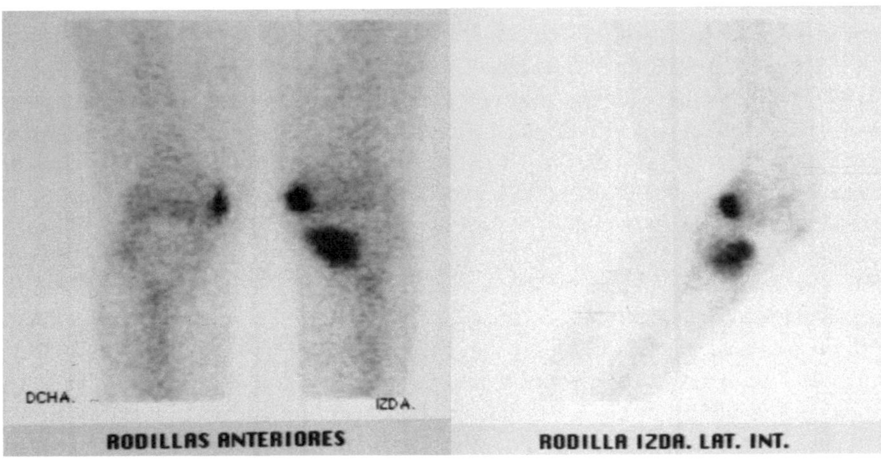

Fig. 8. Scintigraphy: localized uptake in tibial metaphysis and both internal femoral condyles.

Three-phase bone scan has traditionally been used for diagnosis of stress fractures because it can show evidence of stress fracture within 2 to 3 days of injury and has high sensitivity. Acute stress fractures appear as discrete, localized, sometimes linear areas of increased uptake on all three phases (angiographic, soft tissue, and delayed phases) of a Tc-99m-MDP bone scan (**Fig. 8**). However, the specificity of bone scan is low. Approximately 40 % of positive findings occur at asymptomatic sites (De Weber, 2011; as cited in Bennell et al., 1999). Bone scan can also be falsely positive with shin splints, despite shin splints are typically positive only during the delayed phase of the scan (De Weber, 2011; as cited in Deutsch, 1997). Areas of increased uptake may represent subclinical sites of bone remodeling or stress reactions. Increased uptake can also appear in the setting of bone tumors, osteomyelitis, or avascular necrosis. Although rare, there are reports of false-negative bone scans (De Weber, 2011; as cited in Gaeta et al., 2005; Spitz & Newberg, 2002). Because of these limitations, MRI is supplanting bone scan as the diagnostic tool of choice when plain radiographs are negative and confirmation of suspected stress fracture is needed.

12.3 Insufficiency fractures

Insufficiency fracture occurs when the mechanical strength of a bone is reduced to the point that a stress which would not fracture a healthy bone breaks the weak one (De Weber, 2011). Most commonly postmenopausal osteoporosis is the cause for insufficiency fractures. Additional conditions affecting bone turnover include osteomalacia, chronic renal failure, and high-dose corticosteroid therapy (Krestan et al., 2011). Insufficiency fractures occur most commonly in the pelvis, including the sacrum, followed by the proximal femur and the vertebral bodies, in particular in the lower thoracic and the lumbar spine. Other sites frequently affected by insufficiency fractures are the tibia, fibula, and calcaneus (Krestan & Hojreh, 2009; as cited in Soubrier, 2003). Radiographs are the basic modality used for screening of insufficiency fractures, but depending on the location of the fractures, sensitivity is limited. Thus, MRI and CT are both standard techniques when insufficiency fracture is suspected and initial radiological studies are negative. MRI is a very sensitive tool to visualize bone marrow abnormalities associated with insufficiency fractures and allows differentiation of benign versus malignant fractures. Multidetector CT depicts subtle fracture lines allowing direct visualization of cortical and trabecular bone (Krestan et al., 2011). Bone scintigraphy is also highly sensitive and specific when typical pattern of abnormality is present. One of those typical patterns of uptake is the classical H ('Honda' sign) or butterfly-shaped appearance in sacral insufficiency fracture in the elderly osteoporotic patient without definite trauma history. The vertical limbs of the H lie within the sacral ala, parallel to the sacroiliac joints, while the transverse limb of the H extends across the sacral body. Other sacral variant uptake patterns occur frequently and include the unilateral ala, incomplete H and horizontal linear dot patterns. Iliac fractures are seen as linear areas of increased radionuclide uptake. Pubic and supra-acetabular fractures produce areas of linear or focal uptake. Concomitant findings of two or more areas of increased uptake in the sacrum and at another pelvic site are considered diagnostic of insufficiency fractures of the pelvis. If a typical pattern of abnormality is not present, the radionuclide bone scan is much less specific. If abnormal or incomplete patterns of uptake are observed, findings may be mistaken for malignancy and other etiologies. PET–CT with hybrid-scanners has been the upcoming modality for the differentiation of benign from malignant fractures (Krestan et al., 2011).

12.4 Pathologic fractures

This type of fractures is due to a localized loss of strength secondary to an underlying disease process. Examples of pathologic fractures include those that occur at sites of bone tumors (primary or metastatic), bone cysts, and infections (De Weber, 2011). About 10% of patients with known bone metastases will sustain a fracture. Most patients with high-risk conditions for bone metastasis are followed serially with bone scan to detect occult metastasis. In general, lytic lesions are considered more prone to fracture than blastic ones. In the spine, CT or MRI are both indicated to quantify the extent of tumor infiltration, including any extension into the spinal cord and are useful in distinguishing osteoporotic vertebral collapse from pathologic fracture.

12.5 Non-union fractures

In the setting of impaired fracture healing we can distinguish three complications: the delayed union, non-union and pseudoartrhosis. Delayed union describes the situation where there are distinct clinical and radiological signs of prolonged fracture healing time (Panagiotis, 2005). Scintigrams demonstrate intense tracer concentration at the fracture site, as does a fracture undergoing normal or non-union. Therefore, differentiation of a normal or delayed union from nonunited fracture may not be possible by scintigram alone. Clinical findings along with roentgenograms are usually adequate to distinguish delayed healing from nonhealing (Desai et al., 1980). Non-union fracture is defined as the cessation of all reparative processes of healing without bone union 6 to 8 months following the fracture or by the absence of progressive repair that has not been observed radiographically between the third to sixth months following a fracture (Panagiotis, 2005). Two main types of non-union fractures are differentiated according to the viability of the ends of the fragments (Frölke& Patka, 2007; as cited in Weber & Cech, 1976): Avascular non-union and hypervascular non-union. In the first type the ends of the fragments are avascular or atrophic, inert and incapable of biologic reaction, and therefore bone scintigraphies indicate a poor blood supply at the edges of the fragments (Frölke& Patka, 2007). On delayed images atrophic non-union rim is seen as a photon deficient band between fracture ends (Holder, 1993). The main problem in this type is the poor quality of the bone ends and the significantly diminished potential for repair (Gelalis et al., 2011). In the second type the rims of the fragment are hypervascular or hypertrophic and are capable of biological reaction. Bone scintigraphy in the latter indicates a rich blood supply in the ends of the fragments (Frölke& Patka, 2007). The main problem in this type is inadequate fracture stability or reduction. The third complication, pseudoarthrosis, is a non-union fracture which may take years to develop and may occur without clinical symptoms. It is characterised by the formation of a false joint where a fibrocartilaginous cavity is lined with synovium producing synovial fluid (Panagiotis, 2005; as cited in McKee, 2000). Scans using Tc-99m-MDP show the presence of a synovial pseudoarthrosis (Csongradi & Maloney, 1989; as cited in Esterhai et al., 1984). Two types can be distinguished as in the non-union fractures: atrophic and hypertrophic pseudoarthrosis. The first one is characterized in the scintigraphy by the absence of peripheral accumulation in contrast with the intense uptake surrounding a hypertrophic pseudoarthrosis. Those finding in the bone scan are highly suspect for pseudoartrhosis after 12 months. The use of SPECT with bone scanning enhances the sensitivity and specificity, especially in the pseudoarthrosis of the spine after a lumbar spinal fusion (Collier et al., 1993; Lee & Worsley, 2006). SPECT identifies a more focal area of intense activity within the area of increased accumulation at the fusion site (Murray, 1998). Some authors have used radionuclide scans to determine whether the fracture has the biologic ability to respond to a specific therapy such as electrical stimulation. With mature nonunions, radionuclide scans can identify large hypovascular areas that have no potential for healing. In such cases, operative intervention is needed. In a case of nonunion, the possibility of infection must be considered. An increase in activity at the fracture site on the radionuclide scan is consistent with both bony healing and infection. Infection at the fracture site can also be a cause of persistent pain and contribute to the non-union (Csongradi & Maloney, 1989). Gallium scan is indicative of infection if 67Ga uptake exceeds 99mTc uptake on the bone scan. The most specific tracers for infection however are leukocytes labelled with indium-111 or 99mTc (Schelstraete et al., 1992).

13. Technical aspects and applications of bone scintigraphy in pediatric populations

13.1 Technical aspects of bone scintigraphy in pediatric populations

Technical considerations concerning care of the child, immobilization, dosing of radiopharmaceuticals, and instrumentation are of major importance in pediatric nuclear medicine. It is routine in many dedicated pediatric nuclear medicine departments to allow parents or siblings to remain in the imaging room to provide a sense of security and safety for the child. Similarly, the patient is allowed to hold a favorite toy or a prized possession and parents are instructed to bring such items with them for the test. Children are often most worried about the needle required for the injection. Many nuclear medicine departments now routinely use the application of topical anesthetic creams as part of the preparation for the examination (Nadel & Stilwell, 2001). Immobilization techniques to gain patient support in pediatric studies can vary from wrapping the patient to the use of sedation and general anesthesia. For neonates to age 2, it may suffice to hold the patient in place, deprive sleep, and feed the child while on the imaging table. Papoose techniques for bundling and entertainment including television, movies, music, or stories can be used to immobilize children older than 4 to 5 years of age. The cooperation of an older child can often be obtained if the procedure is carefully explained to them and their parents. Children between the ages of 2 and 5, or who are mentally retarded, or have severe attention deficit problems, are more likely to require sedation (Nadel & Stilwell, 2001). Guidelines from the American College of Radiology and the American Academy of Pediatrics can help in developing an appropriate institutional sedation protocol (Shammas, 2009; as cited in Gilday, 2003).

The correct dosing for administration of radiopharmaceuticals to children is available in standard pediatric nuclear medicine texts and can be based on either body surface area or the weight of the child relative to adult dosage (Nadel & Stilwell, 2001; as cited in Miller & Gelfand, 1994; Treves, 1995). 99mTc- MDP is the most commonly used radiopharmaceutical for bone scintigraphy. Scanning is usually performed as a three-phase bone scan with immediate blood flow and blood pool imaging of the site of symptoms obtained after injection, followed by delayed imaging 1.5 to 2 hours later. It is important that the children are well hydrated to have optimum visualization. Other radiopharmaceuticals are also useful in the evaluation of musculoskeletal disease, such as 67Ga citrate or labelled leukocytes using indium-111 or 99mTc for musculoskeletal infection or a bone marrow scan using a 99mTc-sulfur colloid for bone marrow infarction, particularly in sickle cell disease (Shammas, 2009; as cited in Connolly et al., 2007; Gilday, 2003; Nadel & Stilwell, 2001). 18F-FDG is the most common radiopharmaceutical used for PET or PET/CT. 18F-FDG accumulation occurs in inflammation and infection (Shammas, 2009; as cited in Love et al., 2005; Zhuang & Alavi, 2002). Imaging of inflammation with 18F-FDG PET relies on the fact that infiltrated granulocytes and tissue macrophages use glucose as an energy source. When they are activated in inflammation, metabolism and thus FDG uptake increases (Shammas, 2009; as cited in Kubota et al., 1992).

Proper positioning is important in pediatrics particularly in young infants, and although children are smaller, it does not imply that more of a child can be imaged on a single scintigraphic view. In fact, examinations take longer in children and infants because of the requirement of joint-to-joint images for detailed assessment. Although the new gamma camera systems often allow whole-body passes it is often necessary to supplement these images with magnified spot views or even pinhole imaging. Image magnification either with camera zoom, computer magnification, or collimation is essential when performing scintigraphic examinations in children. Magnification is either optical with collimation or electronic. Optical magnification uses either a pinhole or converging collimator, enlarges the image, and improves overall system resolution. Electronic magnification makes the image bigger without altering overall system resolution. The capability for SPECT imaging is essential in pediatric scintigraphy. SPECT allows for improved image contrast and hence improved diagnostic accuracy. It is helpful in localizing and further defining most musculoskeletal abnormalities to include the extremities and is essential when assessing a child with the clinical problem of back pain. Multiple head detector gamma camera systems are becoming more available in pediatric centers. The advantages of these systems include increased resolution and sensitivity and decreased time of examination in a child. Correlative imaging is essential to state of the art practice of pediatric nuclear medicine. Computer multimodality image fusion programs are becoming available and more sophisticated. They allow comparison of different isotope scintigraphic studies or serial studies in the same patient or comparison of scintigraphy with other imaging modalities, such as CT, MR imaging, and PET for better correlation of anatomy and function. New combined gamma camera and CT devices allowing direct anatomic and physiologic correlation are also being manufactured and will have further impact on the care of the pediatric patient.

The normal distribution in a pediatric bone scan may differ from adults (Shammas, 2009; as cited in Nadel, 2007). In children there is high physeal and apophyseal uptake due to their rich blood supply and active enchondral ossification. Absence of uptake in nonossified cartilaginous structures should not be mis- taken for avascular necrosis. Regions where this may be of concern in younger children include the femoral capital epiphysis, patella, and navicular bone. Before ossification, the ischiopubic synchondrosis appears as a discontinuity of the inferior pubic ramus. During ossification, increased uptake in ischiopubic synchondroses is a common normal variant and should not be misinterpreted as a pathological lesion (Shammas, 2009).

13.2 Applications of bone scintigraphy in pediatric populations

13.2.1 Infections

Acute osteomyelitis is a common pediatric disease that mostly affects children under 5 years old. It usually is the result of hematogenous spread of infection due to the rich vascular supply of the growing skeleton. Typically, bone scan become positive 24 to 72 hours after the onset of infection, while plain films do not manifest evidence of infection until 3 to 4 weeks after. Therefore, three-phase bone scintigraphy is the most sensitive imaging modality for early diagnosis. The sensitivity of a three-phase bone scan has been estimated as 94% with a specificity of 95% (Shammas, 2009; as cited in Schauwecker, 1992). Ideally, scintigraphic imaging should be obtained before joint aspiration, and a delayed whole-body scan on skeletal phase should be obtained because osteomyelitis in childhood can be multifocal or present with referred pain. In addition, malignant disease such as leukemia and sarcoma may mimic acute osteomyelitis (Shammas, 2009; as cited in Connolly et al., 2007; Ma et al., 2007). All three phases of the bone scan show focally high uptake in the affected bone. Occasionally, the affected bone in children shows low uptake or a photopenic defect (cold osteomyelitis) (Shammas, 2009; as cited in Pennington, 1999). This is most likely due to reduced tracer delivery by increased intraosseous pressure from inflammation, oedema, and joint effusion (Shammas, 2009). Cellulitis may be differentiated from osteomyelitis because the former typically demonstrates diffuse increased activity in the soft tissues on the first two phases, without focal osseous abnormality on the third phase (Shammas, 2009; as cited in Wegener & Alavi, 1991). Although chronic recurrent multifocal osteomyelitis (CRMO) and acute osteomyelitis share a common histopathologic feature, namely chronic inflammation, they are different in important ways (Nadel & Stilwell, 2001). CRMO occurs most frequently in the latter half of the first decade and the first half of the second decade of life, and it is more common in girls, differently from acute osteomyelitis that occurs in children under 5 years old (Shammas, 2009). A predisposing cause is not found for CRMO in contrast to conventional osteomyelitis (Nadel & Stilwell, 2001). Bone scintigraphy is helpful in identifying the multifocal bone lesions and characteristically displays high uptake in both symptomatic and asymptomatic lesions (Shammas, 2009, as cited in Connolly, 2007). Other infection typical of children under 3 years of age is septic arthritis. Monoarticular involvement is the most common pattern. The more affected joints are the knees and the hips. As in the osteomyelitis, there is an increased uptake on all three phases of three-phase bone scan, but in septic arthritis there is a symmetric uptake in both sides of the joint (Diaz& De Haro, 2005). Transient synovitis is the most common condition that mimics septic arthritis. In this case, three-phase bone scan may be normal or may show diffuse increased activity on the first two phases. Delayed images may displa periarticular increased activity in the affected joint (Shammas, 2009).

13.2.2 Legg-Calve Perthe disease

Legg-Calve Perthes disease is an idiopathic ischemic necrosis of the femoral head that occurs characteristically in children between 5 to 8 years. Bone scintigraphy is more sensitive than radiography for early diagnosis, and comparable to MRI (Shammas, 2009; as cited in Ma et al., 2007). Studies performed early after the onset of clinical symptoms show absence of activity in the capital femoral epiphysis and it may precede radiographic changes (Shammas, 2009; as cited Connolly & Treves, 1998). Later scans may demonstrate increased activity due to revascularization and remodeling. Bone scintigraphy has also a pronostic value and can be used in routine management to identify patients at high risk for a poor outcome (Shammas, 2009; as cited in Comte et al., 2003): Persistent absence of bone uptake in the proximal femoral epiphysis after 5 months or metaphyseal hyperactivity is highly correlated with more severe disease and a poorer prognosis. The early formation of a lateral column of tracer uptake in the capital femoral epiphysis, even before radiography, is associated with a good prognosis due to early revascularization (Shammas, 2009; as cited in Conway, 1993 and Tsao et al., 1997).

13.2.3 Slipped capital femoral epiphysis

Slipped capital femoral epiphysis is characterized by a displacement of the capital femoral epiphysis from the femoral neck through the physeal plate with medial and posterior rotation of the epiphysismost commonly in the adolescence. Bone scintigraphy is useful for assessing the vascularity of the femoral head. In the absence of avascular necrosis, the bone scan findings in slipped capital femoral epiphysis are nonspecific and consist of mildly increased activity with widening and blurring of the growth plate activity (Shammas, 2009; as cited in Connolly et al., 2006, 2007).

13.2.4 Sickle cell disease

Sickle cell disease is the most common hereditary blood disorders. It occurs almost exclusively among black americans and black africans, related with the presence of a mutated form of hemoglobin, hemoglobin S. Bone and joint problems are the most common manifestations. Distinguishing sickle cell crisis with possible bone marrow infartion from osteomyelitis is a challenge (Shammas, 2009; as cited in Connolly et al., 2007). Bone marrow scan with 99mTc-sulfur colloid plus conventional bone scan may be used in the evaluation of sickle cell disease, but it should be done within the first 7 days after the pain onset to be helpful in the differential diagnosis (Shammas, 2009). If the bone marrow scan is abnormal at the site of pain, followed by normal or decreased uptake on conventional bone scan, infarction is the likely diagnosis. Increased uptake in blood pool and delayed images on conventional bone scan is more suggestive of osteomyelitis (Shammas, 2009; as cited in Gilday, 2003).

13.2.5 Reflex sympathetic dystrophy

Reflex sympathetic dystrophy has also been described elsewhere in this chapter. The typical findings on three-phase bone scan are hyperemia on the first two phases with intense periarticular activity in the affected extremity. In children, a cold variant has been reported, which is characterized by decreased activity in the three phases of the scintigraphy in the affected limb, compared with the nonaffected limb (Shammas, 2009; as cited in Nadel, 2007).

13.2.6 Fractures

The occult fracture more common in children is the Toddler's fracture, which is a spiral or oblique fracture that can occur from pelvis to feet but mostly involves the tibia (Shammas, 2009). Radiographic findings are often subtle and fractures may not be apparent, for that reason bone scan is a valuable tool for detecting this injury. Scintigraphy shows diffuse increased uptake in the tibial diaphysis or the bone affected. A linear or spiral pattern of high uptake may be seen in some children (Shammas, 2009; as cited in Connolly et al., 2006; Gilday 2003).

Among stress fractures, spondylolysis is the more important in children with back pain, which represent a stress fracture of the pars interarticularis of the vertebra, commonly in the lower lumbar spine secondary to repetitive minor trauma such as hyperextension (Shammas, 2009). Clinical signs and symptons and radiographies are normally used for the diagnosis. A bone scan or a MRI may be necessary to determine if the spondylolysis is active or inactive. Bone scintigraphy shows little or no abnormality on blood pool images, but it typically demonstrates focally high uptake in the region of the pars interarticularis on delayed images. SPECT imaging is more sensitive than planar studies and detects abnormalities in about a third of individuals with normal planar examinations and so, it is recommended in the evaluation of low back pain in young athletes (Shammas, 2009; as cited in Sty, 1993).

Scintigraphy has also an important role to provide a quick assessment for defining and characterizing the extent and severity of trauma in the setting of child abuse, complementary to other radiologic investigations. Its major advantage is the increased sensitivity in detecting evidence of soft-tissue and bone trauma (25%to 50%), and in the documentation of specific and characteristic sites of abuse, such as in the ribs or the diaphyses of the extremities (Nadel & Stilwell, 2001; as cited in Conway et al., 1993, Sty & Wells, 1994).

13.2.7 Primary bone tumors in childhood

Benign bone tumors are by far the most common type of tumors that grow within the skeleton. Nonossifying fibromas, osteochondromas and simple bone cysts are the types most often found in children and teenagers. Children between the ages of 6 and 12 are the most likely to develop benign bone tumors, although the tumors sometimes show up in children as young as age 2. Exostosis tumors are slightly more common in boys than girls. Nonossifying fibroma usually is in the actively growing sections of long bones such as the thighbone (femur). Exostosis (osteochondroma) contains both bone and cartilage and usually grows in the thighbone, the shinbone (tibia) or the bone in the upper arm (humerus). Unicameral (simple) bone cysts are holes in the bone that fill with fluid and tissue. They usually occur in the bone in the upper arm or in the upper part of the thighbone. In some cases, a benign bone tumor can cause problems while it grows. It can weaken the child's bone and make it more likely that the bone will break. Tumors also can press on nerves and cause pain. In cases like these, surgery may be necessary. Malignant primary bone tumors make up 5% of childhood malignancies, and osteosarcoma is the most commonly isolated malignant bone tumor in children, followed by Ewing's sarcoma. These bone neoplasms usually begin during childhood and adolescence, when bones are growing quickly and they often are taking part in sports and other physical activities. Langerhans cell histiocytosis is also more common in the pediatric population. A smaller number of patients have other diagnosis such as malignant fibrous histiocytoma, angiosarcoma and chondrosarcoma, but these conditions are very rare in paediatric population. The use of nuclear medicine techniques in the diagnosis, staging and monitoring of the different bone tumors has been detailed in a previous section of this chapter. FDG-PET has become to be one of the best tools for the baseline evaluation and follow-up, although some benign bone lesions may show high 18F-FDG accumulation, equivalent to osteosarcomas. Despite this, 18F-FDG-PET has a high specificity for excluding malignant bone tumors (Cook et al., 2010). FDG- PET has been shown to help determine the presence and extent of sarcomas and even may allow the noninvasive estimation of the histologic grade of some tumors, although the biopsy remains necessary. This technique allows targeted biopsies, which can reduce the likelihood of underestimation of tumor grade and inadequate therapy. Furthermore, 18F-FDG-PET is useful in the pediatric population for detection of skip metastases in cases of equivocal MRI findings (Even-Sapir, 2007).

14. Therapeutic alternatives with radionuclides: Radiosynoviorthesis

In the treatment of inflammatory rheumatic diseases with chronic course, operative and respectively arthroscopic synovectomy on the one hand and synoviorthesis on the other hand come into question. Synoviorthesis by corticosteroids has a very large indication if the corresponding measures of precaution are heeded. Chemical synoviorthesis, mainly by osmium tetroxide, is applied above all in exudative inflammatory diseases, whereas radiosynoviorthesis with the nuclides used at present is mainly applied in proliferative diseases. The cytotoxic effects intrinsic to the beta radiation emission from some radionuclides have been exploited by nuclear medicine and, as well as treating several forms of neoplasia, this method can also be used to treat a number of benign articular pathologies in the field of rheumatology. Carry out a 'radiosynovectomy' procedure is possible after intra-articular administration of suitable radiopharmaceuticals. The direct irradiation of the synovial membrane can produce a therapeutic effect on persistent synovitis that is resistant to traditional drug treatment. The radiopharmaceuticals that have been used to date for radiosynovectomy are made up of small colloidal particles labelled to β-emitting isotopes (yttrium-90, rhenium-186, erbium-169, samarium-153). These compounds release their radiation energy within a radius of a few millimetres from the uptake sites. These substances are phagocytized by synoviocytes localised in relation to the synovia and it creates a radiation source that can act locally and reduce inflammatory and proliferative elements (Colamussi et al., 2004; as cited in Gumpel et al., 1975). The availability of new radiopharmaceuticals, created by replacing the colloid vector with hydroxyapatite crystals, has allowed the main undesired effect of these substances (radiation to other organs such as drainage lymph nodes, liver, spleen and bone marrow, due to the passage of the radio compound from the articular cavity to the lymphatic and then to the blood flow systems) to be avoided (Clunie et al., 1996). In the absence of side effect, this technique of low cost may be useful, not only in the treatment of advanced stage and drug-resistant arthropathies, but also to manage pain and improve articular function in the first stages of rheumatoid arthritis (Colamussi et al., 2004; as cited in Uyeo et al., 1978). A fundamental element to the success of radiosynovectomy therapy is that treatment is started early in the disease's history. This is because while radiation therapy can successfully control proliferation of the inflamed synovial membrane, it is not effective in joints that have suffered advanced osteo-cartilage damage and where the synovitic component is virtually non-existent (Franssen et al., 1989). Cases reported would further suggest its use in a wider spectrum of rheumatic disorders ranging from spondylitis to Paget's disease and from hæmophiliac synovitis to pigmented villonodular synovitis. Nevertheless, despite abundant anecdotal evidence of its efficacy, there is a paucity of controlled trials and those that have been done have produced conflicting results (Dos Santos et al., 2009, 2011) and/or have been of insufficient sample size. Two meta-analyses have been published. The first one (Jones, 1993) was made in order to assess the evidence on yttrium-90 therapy for chronic synovitis of the knee. It found out that Yttrium was superior to placebo (OR 2.42, 95% CI 1.02-5.73), although possible publication bias limited the interpretation of this result. Yttrium was not superior to triamcinolone (OR 1.89, 95% CI 0.81-10.55) or other active modalities (OR 1.04, 95% CI 0.72-1.52). The second one and most recent (Van der Zant et al., 2009) has been published with the objective to perform a systemic review and meta-analysis on the effectiveness of radiosynoviorthesis. It has shown high success rates of radiosynoviorthesis, but differences in effect with glucocorticoid injection are less evident, although there is marked heterogeneity in study design of a small number of comparative studies. Therefore the efficacy of radiosynovectomy alone or in combination with steroid therapy must be assessed by other sufficiently powered randomised controlled studies.

15. Conclusion

Nuclear medicine techniques supply physiological information that is complementary to that provided by radiological techniques and can play a fundamental role not only for the examination and treatment of articular disorders but also in overall patient evaluation.

Though scintigraphical examination is ideal in the early stages of diseases, it also plays a complementary role to radiographical investigations in more advanced disease stages. An assessment as complete as possible which includes different complementary studies must be performed to achieve the best diagnostic and prognostic accuracy. In this context, conventional scintigraphy is still a major test in a limited number of rheumatological diseases such as Paget, reflex sympathetic dystrophy and osteonecrosis, and can be a useful complementary study in other diseases. New molecular imaging tools for the evaluation of musculoskeletal diseases are now available and these particular tools will advance the understanding and management of several chronic musculoskeletal diseases. In the next decade, PET/CT and SPECT/CT will be the major workhorses for molecular imaging, with the advantage that PET-based technologies have high sensitivity and the ability to use biologic molecules that can be radiolabelled.

Despite the important role of the anatomic imaging techniques in the evaluation of primary bone tumors and metastases, radionuclide imaging techniques have all been used in the assessment of these disorders. PET and hybrid PET/CT imaging are becoming the most important modalities in this field.

B-radiation emission from some radionuclides has been exploited by nuclear medicine and has been used to treat benign joint pathologies, as well as treating several forms of neoplasia. It is of interest in the field of rheumatology, since it is as a safe procedure and, after intra-articular administration of suitable radiopharmaceuticals, is able to control proliferation of the inflamed synovial membrane in the treatment of chronic arthropathies, particularly in the initial stages of the disease.

16. References

Aoki J, Watanabe H, Shinozaki T, Takagishi K, Ishijima H, Oya N, Sato N, Inoue T & Endo K. (2001). FDG PET of primary benign and malignant bone tumors: Standardized uptake value in 52 lesions. *Radiology;* 219: 774-777.

Bálint G & Szebenyi B. (1996). Diagnosis of osteoarthritis. Guidelines and current pitfalls. *Drugs;* 96; 52 Suppl 3:1-13.

Beheshti M, Langsteger W & Fogelman I. (2009). Prostate cancer: Role of SPECT and PET in imaging bone metastasis. *Semin Nucl Med;* 39 (6): 396-407.

Benning R & Steinert H. (1988). Diagnostic criteria of Sudeck's syndrome. *Rontgenblatter;* 41 (6): 239-45.

Biswal S, Resnick DL, Hoffman JM & Gambhir SS. (2007). Molecular imaging: integration of molecular imaging into the musculoskeletal imaging practice. *Radiology;* 244 (3): 651-71.

Blockmans D, de Ceuninck L, Vanderschueren S, Knockaert D, Mortelmans L & Bobbaers H. (2006). Repetitive 18F-fluorodeoxyglucose positron emission tomography in giant cell arteritis: a prospective study of 35 patients. *Arthritis Rheum;* 55: 131–137.

Brenner W, Bohuslavizki KH & Eary JF. (2003). PET Imaging of Osteosarcoma. *J Nucl Med;* 44: 930–942.

Brown ML, Collier BD, Fogelman Jr & Fogelman I. (1993). Bone Scintigraphy: Part 1. Oncology and Infection. *J Nuci Med;* 34: 2236-2240.

Buckland-Wright C. (1997). Current status of imaging procedures in the diagnosis, prognosis and monitoring of osteoarthritis. *Baillieres Clin Rheumatol;* 11 (4): 727-48.

Chew FS & Hudson TM. (1982). Radionuclide bone scanning of osteosarcoma: Falsely extended uptake patterns. *AJR Am J Roentgenol*; 139: 49-54.

Clunie G, Lui D, Cullum I, Ell PJ & Edwards JC. (1996). Clinical outcome after one year following samarium-153 particulate hydroxyapatite radiation synovectomy. *Scand J Rheumatol*; 25: 360–366.

Colamussi P, Prandini N, Cittanti C, Feggi L & Giganti M. (2004). Scintigraphy in rheumatic diseases. *Best Pract Res Clin Rheumatol*; 18 (6): 909–926.

Collier D, Fogelman I & Brown ML. (1993). Bone Scintigraphy: Part 2. Orthopedic Bone Scanning. *J Nuci Med*; 34: 2241-2246.

Cook GJ, Blake GM, Marsden PK, Cronin B & Fogelman I. (2002). Quantification of skeletal kinetic indices in Paget's disease using Dynamic 18F-fluoride positron emission tomography. *J Bone Miner Res*; 17: 854-859.

Cook GJR, Gnanasegaran G & Chua S. (2010). Miscellaneous Indications in Bone Scintigraphy: Metabolic Bone Diseases and Malignant Bone Tumors. *Semin Nucl Med*; 40: 52-61.

Csongradi JJ & Maloney WJ. (1989). Ununited lower limb fractures. *West*; 150 (6): 675-80.

Dasgeb B, Mulligan MH, Kim CK. (2007). The current status of bone scintigraphy in malignant diseases. *Semin Musculoskelet Radiol*; 11 (4): 301-11.

De Gersem R & Jamar F. (2010). Nonspecific human immunoglobulin G for imaging infection and inflammation: what did we learn? *Q J Nucl Med Mol Imaging*; 54 (6): 617-28.

De Leonardis F, Orzincolo C, Prandini N & Trotta F. (2008). The role of conventional radiography and scintigraphy in the third millennium. *Best Pract Res Clin Rheumatol*; 22: 961- 979.

De Weber K. (2011). Overview of stress fractures, In: *Uptodate*. Eiff P & Grayzel J.

Desai A, Alavi A, Dalinka M, Brighton C & Esterhai J. (1980). Role of bone scintigraphy in the evaluation and treatment of nonunited fractures: Concise communication. *J NuclMed*; 21: 931-934.

Devogelaer JP & de Deuxchaisnes CN. (2003). Paget´s disease of bone. In: *Rheumatology* Hochberg MC, Silman AJ, Smolen JS, Weinblatt ME & Weishman MH (ed SV Mosby). 3rd edn. pp. 2139-2147. Toronto.

Diaz C & De Haro FJ. (2005). Estudios isotópicos del sistema musculoesquelético y densitometría ósea, In: *Técnicas de exploración en Medicina Nuclear*. (Ed) Masson, pp 131 - 148. ISBN 84-458-1420-6, Barcelona, Spain.

Dos Santos MF, Furtado RN, Konai MS, Castiglioni ML, Marchetti RR, Silva CP & Natour J. (2011). Effectiveness of radiation synovectomy with Yttrium-90 and Samarium-153 particulate hydroxyapatite in rheumatoid arthritis patients with knee synovitis: a controlled, randomized, double-blinded trial. *Clin Rheumatol*; 30 (1): 77-85.

Dos Santos MF, Furtado RN, Konai MS, Castiglioni ML, Marchetti RR & Natour J. (2009). Effectiveness of radiation synovectomy with samarium-153 particulate hydroxyapatite in rheumatoid arthritis patients with knee synovitis: a controlled randomized double-blind trial. *Clinics (Sao Paulo)*; 64 (12): 1187-93.

Driessens M, Dijs H, Verheyen G & Blockx P. (1999). What is reflex sympathetic dystrophy? *Acta Orthop Belg*; 65 (2): 202-17.

Durie BG, Waxman AD, D'Agnolo A & Williams CM. (2002). Whole-body 18F-FDG PET identifies high-risk myeloma. *J Nucl Med*; 43: 1457-1463.

El-Maghraby TA, Moustafa HM & Pauwels EK. (2006). Nuclear medicine methods for evaluation of skeletal infection among other diagnostic modalities. *Q J Nucl Med*; 50 (3): 167-92.

Elzinga EH, van der Laken CJ, Comans EF, Boellaard R, Hoekstra OS, Dijkmans BA, Lammertsma AA & Voskuyl AE. (2011). 18F-FDG PET as a tool to predict the clinical outcome of infliximab treatment of rheumatoid arthritis: an explorative study. *J Nucl Med*; 52 (1):77-80.

Even-Sapir E. (2005). Imaging of Malignant Bone Involvement by Morphologic, Scintigraphic, and Hybrid Modalities. *J Nucl Med*; 46:1356-1367.

Even-Sapir E. (2007). PET/CT in Malignant Bone Disease. *Semin Musculoskelet Radiol*; 11 (4): 312 - 321.

Fogelman I & Carr D. (1980). A comparison of bone scanning and radiology in the assessment of patients with symptomatic Paget's disease. *Eur J Nucl Med*; 5: 417-421.

Fogelman I & Cook GJR. (2003). Scintigraphy in Metabolic Bone disease. In: *Primer on the Metabolic Bone Diseases and Disorders of Mineral Metabolism.* Murray J. Favus (5th ed.) pp. 189 - 195. ISBN 0-9744782-0-2.

Frölke JP & Peter P. (2007). Definition and classification of fracture non-unions. *Injury*; 38 (2): 19-22.

Fournier RS & Holder LE. (1998). Reflex sympathetic dystrophy: diagnostic controversies. *Semin Nucl Med*; 28 (1): 116-23.

Fransen P, Mestdagh C & Dardenne G. (1998). Pagetic sarcoma of the calvarium: report of two cases. *Acta Neurol Belg*; 98: 352–355.

Franzius C, Daldrup-Link HE, Sciuk J, Rummeny EJ, Bielack S, Jürgens H & Schober O. (2001). FDG-PET for detection of pulmonary metastases from malignant primary bone tumors: comparison with spiral CT. *Ann Oncol*; 12: 479–486.

Franssen MJ, Boerbooms AM, Karthaus RP, Buijs WC & van de Putte LB. (1989). Boerbooms AM, Karthaus RP et al. Treatment of pigmented villonodular synovitis of the knee with yttrium-90 silicate: prospective evaluations by arthroscopy, histology, and 99mTc pertechnetate uptake measurements. *Ann Rheum Dis*; 48: 1007–1013.

Gelalis ID, Politis AN, Arnaoutoglou CM, Korompilias AV, Pakos EE, Vekris MD, Karageorgos A & Xenakis TA. (2011). Diagnostic and treatment modalities in nonunions of the femoral shaft. *Injury*, doi: 10.1016/j.injury.2011.06.030.

Gemmel F, Dumarey N & Palestro CJ. (2006). Radionuclide imaging of spinal infections. *Eur J Nucl Med Mol Imaging*; 33 (10): 1226-37.

Glaudemans AW, Dierckx RA, Kallenberg CG & Fuentes KL. (2010). The role of radiolabelled anti-TNFα monoclonal antibodies for diagnostic purposes and therapy evaluation. *Q J Nucl Med Mol Imaging*; 54(6): 639-53.

Gnanasegaran G, Cook G, Adamson K & Fogelman I. (2009). Patterns, Variants, Artifacts, and Pitfalls in Conventional Radionuclide Bone Imaging and SPECT/CT. *Semin Nucl Med*; 39: 380-395.

Gotthardt M, Bleeker-Rovers CP, Boerman OC & Oyen WJG. (2010). Imaging of Inflammation by PET, Conventional Scintigraphy, and Other Imaging Techniques. *J Nucl Med*; 51: 1937–1949.

Green RAR. Nuclear Medicine. (2009). In: *Imaging of Bone Tumors and tumor-like lesions: Techniques and Applications*. Davies AM, Sundaram M & James SLJ (Ed) pp. 53- 93. ISBN 978-3-540-77982-7, Berlin, Germany.

Guermazi A, Burstein D, Conaghan P, Eckstein F, Hellio Le Graverand-Gastineau MP, Keen H & Roemer FW. (2008). Imaging in osteoarthritis. *Rheum Dis Clin North Am*; 34 (3): 645-87.

Guermazi A, Eckstein F. Hellio Le Graverand-Gastineau MP, Conaghan PG, Burstein D, Keen H, Roemer FW. (2009). Osteoarthritis: current role of imaging. *Med Clin North Am*; 93 (1): 101-26, xi.

Hang LW, Hsu WH, Tsai JJ, Jim YF, Lin CC & Kao A. (2004). A pilot trial of quantitative Tc-99m HMPAO and Ga-67 citrate lung scans to detect pulmonary vascular endothelial damage and lung inflammation in patients of collagen vascular diseases with active diffuse infiltrative lung disease. *Rheumatol Int*; 24 (3): 153-6.

Haugeberg G. (2008). Imaging of metabolic bone diseases. *Best Pract Res Clin Rheumatol*; 22 (6): 1127–1139.

Hautzel H, Sander O, Heinzel A, Schneider M & Müller HW. (2008). Assessment of large-vessel involvement in giant cell arteritis with 18F-FDG PET: introducing an ROC-analysis-based cutoff ratio. *J Nucl Med*; 49: 1107–1113.

Herranz R, Pons F & Del Río L. (1990). Exploraciones isotópicas del sistema musculoesquelético, In: Imágenes en medicina nuclear. Diagnóstico morfológico y funcional, Idepsa, pp.126-153, ISBN: 8485600754, Madrid, Spain.

Hoffer PB & Genant HK. (1976). Radionuclide joint imaging. *Semin Nucl Med*; 6 (1): 121-37.

Holder LE. (1993). Bone scintigraphy in skeletal trauma. *Radiol Clin North Am*; 31(4):739-81.

Horwich P. (2011). Approach to imaging modalities in the setting of suspected osteomyelitis, In: *UpToDate*, Sexton DJ, Hochman M &Baron EL.

Howman-Giles R, Hicks RJ, McCowage G & Chung DK. (2006). Primary bone tumors. In: *Practical Pediatric PET imaging*. Martin Charron (Ed), pp: 267 - 301. ISBN-10: 0-387-28836-8. Toronto, Japan.

Hu J & Du N. (2009). Early evaluation of osteoarthritis using objective diagnostic methods. *Zhongguo Gu Shang*; 22 (5): 402-4.

Jones G. (1993). Yttrium synovectomy: a meta-analysis of the literature. *Aust N Z J Med*; 23 (3): 272-5.

Jones LC. (2011). Osteonecrosis. In: *UpToDate*, Goldenberg DL.

Kim EE, Haynie TP, Podoloff DA, Lowry PA & Harle TS. (1989). Radionuclide imaging in the evaluation of osteomyelitis and septic arthritis.*Crit Rev Diagn Imaging*, 29(3):257-305.

Krestan CR, Nemec U & Nemec S. (2011). Imaging of insufficiency fractures. *Semin Musculoskelet Radiol*; 15 (3): 98-207.

Krestan C & Hojreh A. (2009). Imaging of insufficiency fracture. *Eur J Radiol*; 71 (3): 398-405.

Lalani T. (2011). Overview of osteomyelitis in adults. In: *UpToDate*, Sexton, DJ & Baron EL.

Lee E & Worsley DF. (2006). Role of radionuclide imaging in the orthopedic patient. *Orthop Clin North Am*; 37 (3): 485-501.

Lee GW & Weeks PM. (1995). The role of bone scintigraphy in diagnosing reflex sympathetic dystrophy. *J Hand Surg Am*; 20 (3): 458-63.

Lodge MA, Lucas JD, Marsden PK, Cronin BF, O'Doherty MJ, Smith MA. (1999). A PET study of 18FDG uptake in soft tissue masses. *Eur J Nucl Med*; 26: 22-30.

Love C, Din AS, Tomas MB, Kalapparambath TP & Palestro CJ. (2003). Radionuclide bone imaging: an illustrative review. *Radiographics*; 23 (2): 341-58.

Love C, Marwin SE & Palestro CJ. (2009). Nuclear medicine and the infected joint replacement. *Semin Nucl Med*; 39 (1): 66-78.

Love C, Tomas MB, Marwin SE, Pugliese PV & Palestro CJ. (2001). Role of nuclear medicine in diagnosis of the infected joint replacement.*Radiographics*; 21 (5): 1229-38.

Malizos KN, Karantanas AH, Varitimidis SE, Dailiana ZH, Bargiotas K & Maris T. (2007). Osteonecrosis of the femoral head: etiology, imaging and treatment. *Eur J Radiol*; 63 (1): 16-28.

Malviya G, Conti F, Chianelli M, Scopinaro F, Dierckx RA & Signore A. (2010). Molecular imaging of rheumatoid arthritis by radiolabelled monoclonal antibodies: new imaging strategies to guide molecular therapies. *Eur J Nucl Med Mol Imaging*; 37: 386–398.

McQueen FM & Ostergaard M (2007). Established rheumatoid arthritis: new imaging modalities. *Best Pract Res Clin Rheumatol*; 21: 841–856.

Meller J, Sahlmann CO, Gürocak O, Liersch T & Meller B. (2009). FDG-PET in patients with fever of unknown origin: the importance of diagnosing large vessel vasculitis. *Q J Nucl Med Mol Imaging*; 53: 51–63.

Moog F, Kotzerke J, Reske SN. (1999). FDG PET can replace bone scintigraphy in primary staging of malignant lymphoma. J Nucl Med; 40: 1407–1413.

Murray IPC (1998). Bone scintigraphy: the procedure and interpretation. In: Nuclear Medicine in clinical diagnosis and treatment, Livingstone, pp 1125 - 1152, ISBN 044305861X, Edinburgh, Scotland.

Murray IPC. (1998). Bone scintigraphy in trauma, In: Nuclear Medicine in clinical diagnosis and treatment, Livingstone C; 1241-1267, 044305861X, Edinburgh.

Murray IPC. (1998). Vascular manifestations, In: Nuclear Medicine in clinical diagnosis and treatment, Livingstone C; 1223-1239, 044305861X, Edinburgh.

Naddaf SY, Collier BD, Elgazzar AH & Khalil MM. *(2004)*. Technical Errors in Planar Bone Scanning. *J Nucl Med Technol*; 32: 148-153.

Nadel HR & Stilwell ME. (2001). Nuclear medicine topics in pediatric musculoskeletal disease: techniques and applications. *Radiol Clin North Am*; 39 (4): 619-51.

Nanni C, Zamagni E, Farsad M, Castellucci P, Tosi P, Cangini D, Salizzoni E, Canini R, Cavo M & Fanti S. (2006). Role of 18F-FDG PET/CT in the assessment of bone involvement in newly diagnosed multiple myeloma: preliminary results. *Eur J Nucl Med Mol Imaging*; 33: 525–531

Ornetti P & Maillefert JF. (2004). Reflex sympathetic dystrophy: still a poorly defined entity. *Rev Prat*; 31; 54 (2): 123-30.

Ostendorf B, Mattes-György K, Reichelt DC, Blondin D, Wirrwar A, Lanzman R, Müller HW, Schneider M, Mödder U & Scherer A. (2010). Early detection of bony alterations in rheumatoid and erosive arthritis of finger joints with high-resolution single photon emission computed tomography, and differentiation between them. *Skeletal Radiol*; 39:55–61.

Ozcan Z, Burak Z, Kumanlioglu K, Sabah D, Başdemir G, Bilkay B, Cetingül N & Ozkiliç H. (1999). Assessment of chemotherapy induced changes in bone sarcomas: Clinical experience with 99mTc-MDP three-phase dynamic bone scintigraphy. *Nucl Med Commun*; 20: 41-48.

Palestro CJ. (1998). Radionuclide diagnosis of the painful joint replacement, In: Nuclear Medicine in clinical diagnosis and treatment, Livingstone C; 1209-1221, 044305861X, Edinburgh.

Palestro CJ & Torres MA. (1997). Radionuclide imaging in orthopedic infections. *Semin Nucl Med*; 27 (4): 334-45.

Palestro, CJ & Torres, MA. (1997). Radionuclide imaging in orthopedic infections. Semin Nucl Med; 27 (4): 334-45.

Panagiotis M. (2005). Classification of non-union.Injury, 36 (4): 30-7.

Pape D, Seil R, Kohn D & Schneider G. (2004). Imaging of early stages of osteonecrosis of the knee. *Orthop Clin North Am*; 35 (3): 293-303.

Reinartz P. (2009). FDG-PET in patients with painful hip and knee arthroplasty: technical breakthrough or just more of the same. *Q J Nucl Med Mol Imaging*; 53 (1): 41-50.

Schelstraete K, Daneels F& Obrie E. (1992). Technetium-99m-diphosphonate, gallium-67 and labeled leukocyte scanning techniques in tibial nonunion. *Acta Orthop Belg*; 58 (1): 168-72.

Schneider R. (2006). Radionuclide techniques. In: *Bone and joint imaging*. Resnick & Kransdorf, pp 88 – 119. ISBN 84-8174-883-8. Spain.

Shammas A. (2009). Nuclear medicine imaging of the pediatric musculoskeletal system. *Semin Musculoskelet Radiol*; 13(3): 159-80.

Song IH, Carrasco-Fernández J, Rudwaleit M & Sieper J. (2008). The diagnostic value of scintigraphy in assessing sacroiliitis in ankylosing spondylitis: a systematic literature research. *Ann Rheum Dis*; 67 (11): 1535-40.

Strobel K, Exner UE, Stumpe KD, Hany TF, Bode B, Mende K, Veit-Haibach P, von Schulthess GK & Hodler J. (2008). The additional value of CT images interpretation in the differential diagnosis of benign vs. Malignant primary bone lesions with 18F-FDG-PET/CT. *Eur J Nucl Med Mol Imaging*; 35: 2000-2008.

Strobel K & Stumpe KD. (2007). PET/CT in musculoskeletal infection. Semin Musculoskelet Radiol; 11 (4): 353-64.

Termaat MF, Raijmakers PG, Scholten HJ, Bakker FC, Patka P & Haarman HJ. (2005). The accuracy of diagnostic imaging for the assessment of chronic osteomyelitis: a systematic review and meta-analysis. *J Bone Joint Surg Am*; 87 (11): 2464-71.

Tian R, Su M, Tian Y, Li F, Li L, Kuang A & Zeng J. (2009). Dual-time point PET/CT with F-18FDG for the differentiation of malignant and benign bone lesions. *Skeletal Radiol*; 38: 451-458.

Van der Laan L & Goris RJ. (1997). Reflex sympathetic dystrophy.An exaggerated regional inflammatory response? *Hand Clin*; 13 (3): 373-85.

Van der Zant FM, Boer RO, Moolenburgh JD, Jahangier ZN, Bijlsma JW & Jacobs JW. (2009). Radiation synovectomy with (90)Yttrium, (186)Rhenium and (169)Erbium: a systematic literature review with meta-analyses. *Clin Exp Rheumatol*; 27(1): 130-9.

Zacher J, Carl HD, Swoboda B & Backhaus M. (2007). Imaging of osteoarthritis of the peripheral joints. *Z Rheumatol*; 66 (3): 257-8, 260-4, 266.

6

Role of the Radionuclide Metrology in Nuclear Medicine

Sahagia Maria
Horia Hulubei National Institute for R&D in Physics and Nuclear Engineering, IFIN-HH, Romania

1. Introduction

Nuclear medicine practices rely on the use of radiopharmaceuticals, for diagnosis and therapy purposes. Their use is based on the incorporation in the human body through a medical procedure: intravenous injection, ingestion, or inhalation. The quality of the administration procedure is tightly influenced by the following determining factors: the administration of the right activity to the patient, such as prescribed by the medical doctor, and the quality of the radiopharmaceutical product. The full control of these parameters is obtained by using high quality measurement equipment and following well established procedures for the measurement and application of the radiopharmaceutical.

The radiopharmacy units, the measurement equipment providers and the nuclear medicine units can fulfill these requirements only by using calibrated instrumentation and following validated measurement methods. The technical support is offered by the Radionuclide Metrology Laboratories (RML) which can assure the continuity of the metrological traceability chain of measurement up to the highest, primary radioactivity standards. The metrological traceability and its chain are defined by the document: *"BIPM, JCGM 200:2008 – International vocabulary of metrology – Basic and general concepts and associated terms (VIM)"*, as:

- *"Metrological traceability – property of a measurement result whereby the result can be related to a reference through a documented unbroken chain of calibrations, each contributing to the measurement uncertainty"*
- *"Metrological traceability chain – sequence of measurement standards and calibrations that is used to relate a measurement result to a reference"*

From these definitions one can deduce the role of the RMLs: to develop activity standards, to validate them in relation with the International System of Units (SI) and to disseminate them as radioactive standard sources and solutions, or calibration services to the implied entities.

This chapter of the book presents the following aspects:

- Measurement requirements in radiopharmacy, in measurement instrument calibration process, and in nuclear medicine units;
- Role of the Radionuclide Metrology Laboratory in the practical accomplishment of these requirements

2. Radiopharmaceutical products and their characterization by measurements

2.1 Types of radiopharmaceutical products

A radipharmaceutical (RPM) product contains a radionuclide in an adequate chemical form, the transporter, which conducts it towards the organ or tissue of interest, when it is administrated to the patient "in vivo" by ingestion, inhalation or intravenous injection. In the case of diagnosis the radionuclide is used as a "tracer", while in therapy it is employed due to the cytotoxic effect of the emitted ionizing radiations. The radiopharmaceuticals are presented as ingerable gelatin capsules (or solutions), injectable solutions and inhalation gases.

2.1.1 Transporters

Various types of transporters are used, formulated such as to assure a maximum localization of the radiopharmaceutical in the zone of interest while exposing the neibouring area to minimum detriment (Kornyei.2008, Mikolajczak. 2008). The types of transporters are generally similar for both of nuclear medicine procedures, diagnosis and therapy; some formulations are presented as follows:

- Simple inorganic compounds such as salts, containing the radionuclide in an ionic form: $Na^{99m}TcO_4$, ^{131}INa, $^{89}SrCl_2$, $Na^{186,188}ReO_4$
- Simple gas molecules: $^{11}CO_2$, $^{15}O_2$, ^{81m}Kr
- Labeled organic molecules: ^{18}F-DG; ^{67}Ga-cytrate
- Metal-ligand complexes: ^{99m}Tc-MDP, DTPA; ^{188}Re-HEDP; ^{177}Lu-EDTMP
- Colloids, labeled micro and nano spheres: ^{99m}Tc-fytate
- Labeled biomolecules:
  i. Monoclonal antibodies (mAb): ^{90}Y-anti-CD20; ^{188}Re-anti-VEGF
  ii. Meta Iodo Benzil Guanidine (MIBG)-^{131}I
  iii. Peptide Receptor Radionuclide, somatostatin analogous: Pentetroid-DTPA-^{111}In, TOC-HYNIC-^{99m}Tc. ^{188}Re-DOTA-Lan and ^{188}Re-Lan.

The detailed description of these compounds is outside the scope of the chapter.

2.1.2 Radionuclides

In contrast with the transport molecules, the choice of the radionuclides differs for the two types of nuclear medicine procedures: diagnosis and therapy.

Radionuclide diagnosis principle: The incorporated radiopharmaceutical product, localized at the interest zone emits gamma-rays, which cross the body and are detected by the gamma cameras, containing a detection system, based on the use of scintillation detectors and a network of photomultipliers. A bi-dimensional image, called scintigram, is obtained; if the computer tomography principle is applied, a 3D image appears. In principle it is necessary to use as much as possible of the emitted radiation for detection and to avoid the unnecessary irradiation of the body; the irradiation detriment is expressed in terms of committed effective dose per activity unit, *E/A*. For this reason, the choice of radionuclides is focussed on the use of radionuclides with short half life and emitting low energy and intensity electrons and abundant gamma-rays, not much absorbed inside the body, and situated in the optimal energy detection interval, 100 - 600 keV. Two types of diagnosis procedures are in use:

- Single Photon Emission Tomography (SPET) is based on the use of a single detector and of radionuclides decaying by isomeric transition, such as ^{99m}Tc, and by electron capture, ^{123}I. As an exception, ^{131}I emitting beta-gamma radiations, is still used in some special procedures, like the iodine uptake in thyroidal investigations.

- Positron Emission Tomography (PET), sometimes associated with x-ray tomography, PET/CT. In this case, radionuclides decaying by positron emission are used. The stopped, or in flight, positron annihilates with a neighbouring electron, and two 511 keV annihilation quanta at an angle of 180^0 are emitted. These quanta can be detected in coincidence, using two detectors situated at 180^0. The procedure allows a much better resolution and consequently a more precise diagnosis, due to the measurement of coincident radiations. The positron emitters used for PET systems have short half life and for this reason the *E/A* value is low, although they emit positive electrons, absorbed inside the body. The most used radionuclide is ^{18}F.

Table 1 presents a list of radionuclides used for the production of radiopharmaceuticals, in terms of production mode, nuclear decay data and *E/A*. Referring the *E/A* value, it is strongly dependent on the type of radiopharmaceutical, diagnostic procedure and the age of the patient; only for a rough information, the comparative dose values due to the ingestion of radionuclides by the adult public (ICRP 1996c) are given, in order to emphasize the strong dependence of the dose on the characteristics of the nuclear decay scheme.

The values of *E/A* from Table 1 are based on the Medical Internal Radiation Dose (MIRD) model, while at present time the calculation models use the "voxel phantom", defined in international documents as *"a computational anthropomorphic phantom based on medical tomographic images where the anatomy is described by small three dimensional volume elements (voxels) specifying the density and the atomic composition of the various organs and tissues of the human body"*. A special attention is paid to the radionuclide ^{99m}Tc, used nowadays in about 80% of the world diagnosis procedures. Its widespread use is due to several properties:

i. Its committed effective dose of activity unit is *E/A* =0.022mSv/MBq and the corresponding doses in the diagnostic procedures are generally within the limits (1 -2) mSv, due to the short half-life and to the small content of low energy electrons.
ii. The 140.5 keV quanta are emitted with a high intensity, being situated near the maximum detection efficiency of the usual scintillators.
iii. It can be extracted from a ^{99}Mo generator (2.75 d,) a reasonable life time for transport and use for a period of two weeks, or can be prepared in a pharmaceutical unit and delivered to the neighboring hospitals in the same day.
iv. It is carrier free and due to its position in the Mendeleev Table, the VII-b group, with 7 valence electrons, it can be used for binding in various chemical compounds, with various valence states.

Radionuclide (targeted) therapy principle. The incorporated radiopharmaceutical is localized in the biological formation to be destroyed by irradiation. In this case, the entire energy of particles must be transferred to the matter. Consequently, low range radiations, such as: alpha particles and electrons - beta radiation, Auger and conversion electrons, are useful. This is the reason for which alpha, strong beta with high energy, electron capture and conversion decaying radionuclides are used. Lately a special attention is given to the beta-gamma triangular decay scheme radionuclides, with strong beta and weak gamma - ray energies and intensities, due to the ability to be monitored by a gamma camera during the treatment procedure. The half life can be from hours up to tens of days, in order to assure the prescribed dose to the biological formation to be destroyed. The choice of the radionuclides takes into account their chemical properties, as well as their radiations range in the tissue, which must be comparable with the dimensions of the biological formation to be destroyed. Table 2 presents a list of therapeutical radionuclides, with their modes of production, nuclear decay parameters and the tissue range.

Type of Diagnostic	Radio nuclide	Obtaining	Half life	Emitted radiations			*E/A, mSv/MBq* adults, ingestion
				Type	Energy, keV	Intensity %	
SPET	^{131}I	NR*: ^{130}Te (n,γ)^{131}Te, β decay, ^{131}I, or ^{235}U fission	8.02 d	β^- γ	248-606 max 364.5	100 81.6	22
	^{123}I	Cyclotrone: ^{123}Te(p,n)^{123}I	13.2 h	e X γ	127-158 27-32 159	3.36 85.6 83.3	0.22
	^{67}Ga	Cyclotrone: ^{67}Zn(p,n)^{67}Ga	3.26 d	e γ	84-93 91 -393	35 87	0.19
	^{201}Tl	Cyclotrone: ^{203}Ta(d,4n)^{201}Pb. E.C.^{201}Tl	3.04 d	e X Y	16-153 12-82 167.5	51.8 140 10	0.095
	^{99m}Tc	NR: ^{99}Mo generator (2.75 d) ^{98}Mo(n, γ)^{99}Mo or ^{235}U fission	6.007 h	e X γ	120-138 18.3-20.7 140.5	11 7.6 89	0.022 / diagnostic 0.005-0.029 (Toohey & Stabin. 1996)
	^{111}In	Cyclotrone: ^{111}Cd(p,n)^{111}In	2.80 d	e X γ	145-219 23-27 171.3 245.4	13.6 3.2 90.6 94	0.29
	^{81m}Kr	Cyclotrone: ^{81}Rb generator (4.25 h) ^{79}Br(α,2n)^{81}Rb	12.8 s	e X γ	176 -188 12.6-14.1 190.3	32.1 16.8 67.1	0.00004 inhallation
PET	^{18}F	Cyclotrone: ^{18}O(p,n)^{18}F; ^{16}O(α,pn)^{18}F; ^{20}Ne(d,α)^{18}F	110 min	β^+ $\gamma^\pm$	634 max, tissue range 2mm 511	96.9 194	0.049
	^{11}C	Cyclotrone: ^{14}N(p, α)^{11}C	20.4 min	β^+ $\gamma^\pm$	960 max 511	100 200	0.024
	^{68}Ga	^{68}Ge generator (270.83 d) Cyclotrone: ^{66}Zn(α,2n)^{68}Ge	67.7 min	β^+ $\gamma^\pm$	1899 max 511	88 178	0.10
	^{64}Cu	NR:^{63}Cu(n,γ)^{64}Cu Cyclotrone: ^{64}Zn(d,2p)^{64}Cu	12.70 h	$\beta^\pm$ $\gamma^\pm$	653 max 511	56.9 35.7	0.12

NR* = Nuclear Reactor. In the future, most of NR produced radionuclides is expected to be obtained from high neutron flux sources, based on the use of a proton accelerator and the emission of neutrons by the accelerated protons reaction with a mercury target. ^{99}Mo can be produced also at a linear accelerator: $^{100}Mo(\gamma,n)^{99}Mo$

Table 1. The most used radionuclides for diagnosis. Monographie BIPM-5 (Bé et al. 2004), ICRP1996c (1996).

Type	Radio nuclide	Obtaining	Half life	Type of radiations	Energy, keV; Intensity	Tissue range Max./Mean
Alpha emitters	^{211}At	Cyclotrone ^{209}Bi (α,2n)^{211}At	7.21 h	α	5868-7448; 100%	80 μm
	^{213}Bi ^{225}Ac (10 d) generator	^{225}Ac is in ^{237}Np decay chain or cyclotrone: ^{226}Ra(p,2n)^{225}Ac	45.6 min	α β	5869; 2% 987-1426; 97%	70 μm 2.5 mm
	^{212}Bi ^{212}Pb (10.64h) generator	^{212}Pb is in natural ^{232}Th chain, or Cyclotrone: ^{210}Po (t, p)^{212}Bi	Bi-212 60.54 min	α β	6050-6090 ; 35.8% 1527-2250 ; 64.2%	80 μm 4.0 mm
Electron capture (EC) radio nuclides	^{125}I	NR: ^{124}Xe (n, γ) ^{125}Xe, EC, ^{125}I	59.90 d	Auger L Auger K	3.7; 79.3% 22.7 - 34.5; 33.9%	Tens of nm about 47μm
	^{117m}Sn	NR: ^{116}Sn(n, γ)^{117m}Sn	13.6d	Internal conversion electrons	127 keV 152 keV	210 μm 290 μm
Pure beta emitters	^{32}P	NR: ^{32}S(n,p)^{32}P	14.28 d	β	Max 1710, mean 695.5; 100%	9.8 mm/ 2.8 mm
	^{90}Y	NR: ^{89}Y(n,γ)^{90}Y; or ^{235}U fission: Generator: ^{90}Sr (28.15 y):	2.67 d	β	Max 2284, mean 939; 100%	12 mm/ 4.0 mm
	^{89}Sr	NR: ^{88}Sr (n,γ)^{89}Sr or ^{235}U fission	50.65 d	β	Max 1492, mean 584; 100%	8 mm/ 2.5 mm
Beta - gamma emitters	^{131}I	NR: ^{130}Te(n, γ)^{131}Te, β decay, ^{131}I or ^{235}U fission	8.023 d	β	Max 338-605, mean 97-192 ; 100%	4mm/ 0.8 mm
	^{153}Sm	NR: ^{152}Sm(n, γ) ^{153}Sm	1.956 d	β	Max 634-807 , mean 200-263 ;100%	5 mm/ 1.2 mm
	^{177}Lu	NR: ^{176}Lu (n, γ)^{177}Lu or: ^{176}Yb(n, γ)^{177}Yb, β decay, ^{177}Lu	6.734 d	β	Max 175.8-497.1, mean 47-149 ;100%	1.6 mm/ 0.7 mm
	^{186}Re**	NR: ^{185}Re(n, γ)^{186}Re	3.775 d	β	Max 939.4-1077, mean 309-362; 93.1%	5.0mm/ 1.7 mm

Type	Radio nuclide	Obtaining	Half life	Type of radiations	Energy, keV; Intensity	Tissue range Max./Mean
	^{188}Re**	NR: $^{187}Re(n, \gamma)^{188}Re$ or $^{186}W(n, \gamma)^{187}W$ $(n, \gamma)^{188}W$ (69.4 d) Generator	16.98 h	β	Max 1962-2118. mean 706-784;100%	11 mm/ 3.5 mm

**) When a natural Rhenium target is irradiated, a mixture ^{186}Re+^{188}Re is obtained. It can be used in this composition, for the short time irradiation of the external part of large dimension tumors by ^{188}Re and for the long time irradiation of their cores by ^{186}Re. Otherwise, after a week period ^{188}Re decays and almost pure ^{186}Re is obtained. ^{186}Re and ^{188}Re are very important for the obtaining of therapy pharmaceuticals, due to their similar chemical behavior (VII b group) with ^{99m}Tc, very extensively studied.

Table 2. Radionuclides used for therapy radiopharmaceuticals.

2.2 Technical parameters of radiopharmaceuticals and control methods

One radiopharmaceutical product is characterized by several types of parameters, whose determination requires a very good knowledge of the physico-nuclear parameters of the radionuclide and the use of adequate methods and equipment for measurements. Their accepted limit values and methods of determination are described in international and national technical regulatory documents, such as the European Pharmacopoeia (2002). It is considered that the radiopharmaceuticals are products with a high pharmaceutical risk. The parameters are determined first of all in the radiopharmacy, which must dispose of control laboratories in full compliance with the requirements for Good Laboratory Practice (GLP) and accredited according to the international standard *"General Requirements for the Competence of Testing and Calibration Laboratories"*, ISO/IEC 17025:2005. Their determined values are confirmed by the national control laboratories, or are internationally recognized by conventions. Some parameters are controlled only in radiopharmacy, while others are compulsory for the nuclear medicine units, mainly when supplementary operations are carried. A detailed description of the requirements and of their accomplishment mode, regarding quality assurance in radiopharmaceutical measurement is presented in the document *Technical Report Series 454 (TRS 454)*, elaborated by the International Atomic Energy Agency (IAEA) (2006).

Three types of radiopharmaceuticals' parameters are generally defined and controlled: radiometrologic, physico-chemical and biological-microbiological parameters.

2.2.1 Radiometrologic parameters and their determination

(i) Activity, Bq, and derived quantity Radioactive Concentration (Massic Activity), expressed in Bq g^{-1} of solution, or Bq mL^{-1}. These are basic parameters of a radiopharmaceutical product, as the precise determination of the activity administrated to the patient, in full compliance with the prescriptions of the medical doctor, determines his/her committed effective dose, mSv, in radionuclide diagnosis and absorbed dose in the organ/tissue, mGy, in radionuclide therapy, and assures the safety and effectiveness of the medical procedure. Due to this reason, the special requirements regarding the reporting of total activity of a radiopharmaceutical product, on a reference time, are specified by the *Basic Safety Standards*

(1996), para.II.19, such as follows: *"the calibration of sources used for medical exposure shall be traceable to a Standard dosimetry laboratory"* and *"unsealed sources for nuclear medicine procedures shall be calibrated in terms of activity of the radiopharmaceutical to be administrated, the activity being determined and recorded at the time of administration"*. The conclusion of these assertions is that the activity must be precisely measured and the metrological traceability up to the primary level must be assured.

In radiopharmacy and nuclear medicine units, the activity is usually determined using Radionuclide Activity Calibrators, or Dose Calibrators. They contain a reentrant (well type) ionization chamber under pressure, connected to an electrometric system. The manufacturers perform the calibration of the equipment in terms of calibration factors, introduced in dial settings, established for a list of the most used medical radionuclides. The calibrations are performed using sets of standard solutions, provided by the radionuclide metrology laboratories or by commercial producers, having metrological traceability to a primary activity standard declared. Usually, these factors are determined for various types of recipients used in hospitals, such as: P6 or Schott 10-R vials, syringes, gelatin iodide capsules, etc.

The pharmacopoeias impose the uncertainty limits in the measurement of activity, as: <5% for therapy and <10% for dignosis. The activity is measured in radiopharmacy, but it must be measured also in the hospital, as several operations, such as portioning, administration with a syringe, are carried by the involved staff. Due to the crucial importance of these measuremens, the radionuclide calibrator precision in the calibration and maintenance of its corresponding technical condition, together with the correct method of activity measurement in the nuclear medicine units are matters of concern at international level. The IAEA initiated a program aimed to improve and harmonize the quality of activity measurements. In November 2002 a group of consultants had a meeting in the IAEA Vienna headquarters, giving advice on the Methodology of Radioactivity Standardization. The Coordinated Research Project (CRP) codified as: E2.10.05, entitled: *"Harmonization of quality practices for nuclear medicine radioactivity measurements"* was started in 2004. Following the recommendations of the first meeting, a second consultants meeting was held and recommended to develop a set of procedures in the form of a draft Code of Practice in radioactivity measurement. Among other results of the CRP deployment, the elaboration of the above named document TRS454: *Quality Assurance for Radioactivity Measurement in Nuclear Medicine* was very important. The document presents in detail (Table 4, page 69) the types of tests and acceptance criteria for radionuclide activity calibrators to be performed upon the initial acceptance in the unit or after repair, daily checks in the hospital, monthly and annually. As for accuracy of measurement, an upper limit of 5% is imposed. In this respect, a radionuclide metrology laboratory is the entity providing assurance of metrological traceability chain directly, by providing standards, by performing calibrations and by organizing proficiency tests among the personnel doing measurements in radiopharmacy, in the control authorities, at the calibrators' producers and the nuclear medicine staff.The requirement of accuracy in the metrology laboratory is 2%. It can be primary activity standard, or a secondary one, metrologically traceable to a primary activity standard, disposing of a calibrated reentrant ionisation chamber, such as described by (Schrader, 1997).

(ii) Specific activity, expressed in units, Bq g^{-1} of solid mass. It defines the activity of the mass unit of the chemical element or solid compound and determines the capacity of labeling, mainly for biomolecules, and also the radiopharmaceutical's toxicity for human body. Two situations must be taken into consideration:

- Obtaining of the radionuclide. If the radionuclide is obtained in the nuclear reactor by neutron activation, generally it contains a mass of inactive carrier, which is determined by spectrophotometry, or by calculation from irradiation data. The accuracy of these calculations rely on the precision of irradiation data: neutron flux Φ, activation section σ, irradiation time t, but also on the target data such as mass M, isotopic composition η, radionuclide half life, $T_{1/2}$. In the case of radionuclides obtained by irradiation at cyclotrone, or separated from a radionuclide generator, or when the radionuclide of interrest is different from the irradiated target, as for example ^{131}I obtained by irradiation of ^{130}Te, the obtained radionuclide is carrier free.
- Obtaining of the radiopharmaceutical product. In this case, the specific activity depends on the labeling yield, such as the labeling of various kits with ^{99m}Tc in the hospital, under the use of stanous chloride as catalist.

2.2.2 Physico-chemical parameters

(i) Radionuclidic purity, expressed as the ratio between the activity of the base radionuclide and total activity. This parameter is important from two points of view:

i. influence of impurities on accuracy of activity measurements and
ii. their contribution in the committed effective dose of the patient, mainly when the impurities have values of the E/A higher than the main radionuclide. One relevant example is the (^{99}Mo- ^{99m}Tc) generator, where $(E/A)_{Mo\text{-}99}$ =1.2 *mSv/MBq*, 55 times higher than for ^{99m}Tc; a 2% ^{99}Mo impurity will duplicate the committed effective dose. For this reason the ^{99}Mo impurity in ^{99m}Tc elute, known as "molybdenum breakthrough", is restricted at 0.1%. The precise determination of impurity level depends on the knowledge of the decay parameters, such as presented in the Monographie BIPM-5 (2004): half life, type and intensity of emitted radiations for all impurities and also on the precision of the method used in determination. In the simple case, when the involved radionuclides are gamma-ray emitters, the well-known gamma-ray spectrometry method, based on spectrometers provided with high resolution HPGe or Ge(Li) detectors, multichannel analyzers (MCA) and sets of software for processing of data, is used (Debertin & Helmer.1988). The energetic resolution is expressed in terms of full width at half maximum (FWHM) and reflects the ability of the system to distinguish two close energy full absorption peaks. Their calibration contains two components:

- The energy calibration is expressed in terms of number of energy units per MCA channel (generally keV/channel) allowing the identification of all radionuclides contained in a sample;
- The full absorption peak efficiency calibration consists in the determination of a calibration curve, generally expressed in terms of efficiency versus the logarithm of energy, used for the measurement of individual activities; it is established for a determined measurement geometry (distance detector - source) and for each type of measured recipient. The calibrations are performed by using sets of monoenergetic standard sources, covering the whole 50 keV - 3000 keV energy interval. The sets of standard sources are provided by a RML and are certified with uncertainties of (1- 5) %. The spectrometry systems are also provided with dedicated software sets,

allowing the determination of full absorption peak areas and for performing corrections for: geometry, matrix and sample volume, coincidence summation for multigamma emitting radionuclides. The determination of purity consists from the following steps: identification of the main radionuclide and of the impurities in the sample, according to the energy calibration; measurement of the areas of all full absorption peaks; calculation of individual activities, using the efficiency calibration curve and the gamma-ray emission intensity from the radionuclide decay scheme; calculation of the ratios between the activity of the main radionuclide and the sum (main radionuclide plus radio impurities). Generally, the impurity level is controlled only in the radiopharmacy, but in the case of molybdenum breakthrough, it must be controlled also in the hospital, due to the possible deterioration of molybdenum retention in the alumina column along its use. On this purpose, the radionuclide calibrators are usually provided with a lead shield, which absorbs the ^{99m} Tc, 140.5 keV gamma-rays. The detection of sole ^{99}Mo gamma-rays and use of ^{99}Mo calibration factor, corrected for the absorption of its gamma-radiations in the shield, allows the determination of the impurity level, expressed as the ratio between ^{99}Mo and ^{99m}Tc activities. The problem is more complex when pure beta or alpha-ray emitters are used. Some relevant examples:

a. Determination of ^{90}Sr content in ^{90}Y when a ^{90}(Sr+Y) generator is used. In this case, only liquid scintillation spectrometry (Grau Malonda et al. 1994) or counting is used (Wyngaardt. 2006).
b. Determination of alpha and beta impurities in ^{99m}Tc, due to fission ^{99}Mo used for generator production. In this case, the restrictive limits for alpha impurities are of the order of 10^{-9} and for beta emitters of the order of 10^{-6}. This level of impurities is possible to be measured only after the complete decay of the ^{99m} Tc elute by using the liquid scintillation counting, alpha/beta discrimination (Terlikowska et al. 2000).

(ii) Radiochemical purity or ratio between the activity of the main compound and sum of all chemical compounds. The determination is compulsory in the radiopharmacy, but it is advisable also in the hospital, when operations like the preparation of labeled kits is performed. For example, the determination of radiochemical purity of Labeled ^{99m}TcMDP, expressed as the ratio: ^{99m}TcMDP/(^{99m}TcMDP+Na^{99m}TO_4). This purity determination is important, as the tropism of the compound to the target organ/tissue is affected, resulting in the dangerous irradiation of other organs. The imposed limits are generally of 97-98%. The radiochemical purity is determined by using the radiochromatographic methods: either thin layer chromatography (TLC) or more sophisticated - high purity liquid chromatography (high pressure liquid chromatography)-HPLC. The determination consists of the measuring the activities of the two fractions and calculating the ratio between the activity of the main fraction and the sum of main and impurity fractions. The precision of measurement depends mainly on the linearity of the measurement instrument, which must be verified by using two standard sources with activity ratio of about 100, similar with the ratio of measured activities. The counting rates ratio must be equal with the ratio of sources activities, which must be certified with uncertainties <5%.

(iii) Chemical purity, defined by the existence of some nonradioactive elements. The chemical impurities can be: alumina, cooper, ions types $(NH_4)^+$ or $(NO_3)^-$ in ^{99m}Tc elutes from a generator. Their presence can produce the toxicity of the radiopharmaceutical, or can deteriorate the labeling yield of the kits. They are usually determined in the radiopharmacy, but in some cases, the medicine units can dispose of the necessary equipment for control. The methods are specific to the analytical non radiation chemistry, such as spectrophotometry or colorimetry.

2.2.3 Biological and microbiological parameters

These parameters are of maximum importance mainly when the radiopharmaceutical is administrated as an injection, but they are beyond the scope of this chapter and will not be further presented.

3. Primary standard radionuclide metrology laboratory

From the content of section 2, one can conclude that the nuclear medicine applications of radionuclides raise many challenges to the nuclear physicists, from several points of view:

- A very long list of radionuclides is used for the production of radiopharmaceuticals. Other new radionuclides, presenting convenient physico-nuclear and chemical properties, are discovered and introduced in the radiopharmaceutical use.
- The quality requirements can only be accomplished by the very precise determination of the activity of radiopharmaceuticals and by a very deep knowledge of their physico-nuclear characteristics, generally defined as the decay scheme parameters. These two aspects are interconnected, each one depending strongly on the other.

The adequate solutions of these tasks are offered by the Radionuclide Metrology Laboratories, generally responsible national entities, which assure the continuity of the metrological traceability chain from the international level up to the nuclear medicine units.

General Metrology uses the basic terms which are defined according to the *International vocabulary of metrology – Basic and general concepts and associated terms (VIM), JCGM 200: 2008*:

Primary reference measurement procedure, Primary reference procedure = *Reference measurement procedure used to obtain a measurement result without relation to a measurement standard for a quantity of the same kind.*

Calibration = *Operation that, under specified conditions, in a first step, establishes a relation between the quantity values with measurement uncertainties provided by measurement standards and corresponding indications with associated measurement uncertainties and, in a second step, uses this information to establish a relation for obtaining a measurement result from an indication.*

Measurement uncertainty = *Non-negative parameter characterizing the dispersion of the quantity values being attributed to a measurand, based on the information used.*

Metrological traceability = *Property of a measurement result whereby the result can be related to a reference through a documented unbroken chain of calibrations, each contributing to the measurement uncertainty.*

3.1 Activity measurement

The national metrology laboratories dispose of two modalities to assure traceability in activity measurement. In many cases, they are Secondary Standard Laboratories (SSL), transferring the activity unit, Becquerel, from the well know and internationally recognized primary standard laboratories, like NIST (USA), LNHB (France), NPL (UK), PTB (Germany), etc. Alternatively, a national primary standard laboratory, recognized at the international

level, by demonstrating the equivalence of its standards to the International System (SI), can solve entirely this task.
Figure 1 presents the equivalence and traceability chain to be established in activity measurement, from the International System (SI), assured by the International Bureau of Weights and Measures (Bureau International des Poids et Mesures-BIPM) through primary standard laboratories which disseminate the standards to the SSLs and end users, in our case the nuclear medicine units. In order to accomplish its duties, one primary laboratory has to solve the following tasks: it must set up the installations for absolute standardization of radionuclides, demonstrate its international equivalence and assure traceability to the lower levels.

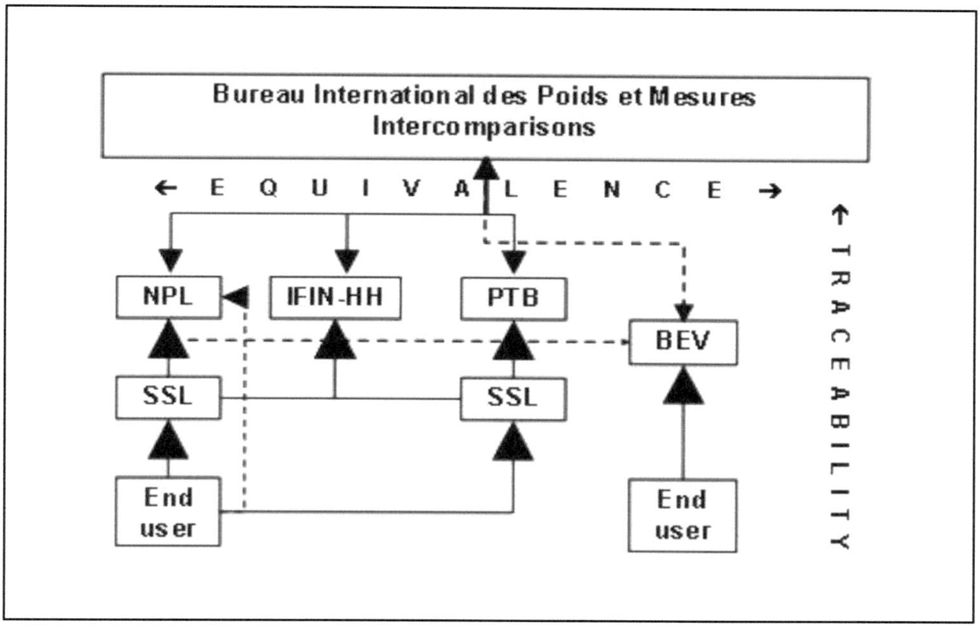

Fig. 1. Dissemination pathways for SI values of activity (From Woods & Sahagia. 2008).

3.1.1 Methods and installations for primary (absolute) standardization

The distinction between the radionuclide metrology and other metrology branches consists of the necessity to elaborate specific standardization methods almost for each radionuclide, due to the variability of decay schemes, and in the impossibility to construct an immuable standard, due to the radioactive dizintegration.
In radionuclide metrology, an absolute standardization is done by the following procedure: one detects the radiations emitted by a radioactive source and the method for establishing an adequate relation between the counting rate and the activity of the source is elaborated. A general relation is expressed as:

$$N_{rad} = \varepsilon\, s A = \varepsilon s N_0 \quad (1)$$

N_{rad} is the counting rate, s^{-1} (impulses per second) for the detected radiation; ε is the detection efficiency of the system; s, denoted also as (I, p) is the intensity of detected

radiations and A, or (N_0) is the activity of the source, Becquerel (Bq). Every standardization operation aims to determine as precisely as possible the quantity ε, or to find a method to eliminate it from relation (1)
Two basic methods are used, NCRP58 (1978). Methods based on the detection in a well-defined geometry (defined solid angle), the most used being the 4πsr geometry, applicable for radionuclides emitting a single type of radiations, and coincidence methods used for those emitting coincident radiations.

3.1.1.1 Methods based on determined geometry

Solid angle method is based on the precise calculation of the solid angle, of the absorption in air and in detector window, and of the radiations scattering correction. The method is used for the standarization of the alpha sources, in vacuum chambers, provided with Si barrier surface detectors; in other cases, for example beta radiations, it is not satisfactory precise.
Methods based on 4πsr geometry use a detection system assuring the quasi total detection of the radiations emitted by the source, which are used for measurement, what means that the following condition is fulfilled:

$$\varepsilon \approx 1 \quad (2)$$

The method of the 4π proportional counter, known as the method $4\pi PC$, is the most known. It is applicable to solid sources, or to radioactive solutions gravimetrically dropped on very thin solid supports, from pure beta emitters with high maximum energy, generally > 150 keV. The remaining corrections to be applied are due to: beta rays absorption in source mass (selfabsorption) and in its support. The method is frequently used for the standardization of the radioactive gases and is known as „gas fillig counter" (Stanga et al.2002). The corrections are due to the wall nondetection, mainly the extremity of counters. Another applied method is the sum peak counting, based on the use of a large NaI(Tl) well type crystal, with a thin window (Nedjadi et al.2007). It is used for radionuclides emitting gamma radiations with high energies and intensities, as for example: ^{124}Sb, ^{222}Rn decay chain, etc. The corrections are done by using Monte Carlo programs.
Liquid scintillator methods. The method is applicable to the radioactive solutions or gases, which are dissolved in a liquid scintillator. The detection geometry is 4πsr. The self-absorption and source support absorption are eliminated but other processes occur: the quenching and non-detection of low energy radiations. It is applicable to pure alpha emitters, for which $\varepsilon = 1$, and high energy pure beta emitters.

3.1.1.2 Coincidence methods

The methods are generally applicable for the radionuclides decaying with the emission of mixed radiations, such as: $a - \gamma$; $\beta - \gamma$; x, $e_A - \gamma$. It is extended to the pure beta or electron capture radionuclides.
Coincidence method and installation $4\pi PC\text{-}\gamma$. A classical coincidence installation contains: a proportional counter (PC), one or two NaI(Tl) detectors and electronic modules, allowing the individual recording of the impulses provided by the two detection channels, and the coincidences recorded by a coincidence selector. The principle of the method is the following: the relations between the counting rates on the three channels: proportional counter - N_{PC}, gamma ray counting - N_γ, coincidence - N_c , the activity N_0 and the corresponding detection efficiencies ε_{PC} and ε_γ , are:

$$N_{PC} = \varepsilon_{PC} N_0; \quad N_\gamma = \varepsilon_\gamma N_0; \quad N_c = \varepsilon_{PC} \varepsilon_\gamma N_0 \tag{3}$$

Relations (3) are equivalent with:

$$N_{PC} N_\gamma / N_c = N_0 \tag{4}$$

Relation (4) shows that the efficiencies of the two detectors are eliminated and consequently the activity can be determined directly from the three counting rates. Relations (3) and (4) were written in very simplifying assumptions, which in reality can not be reached: the radiouclides have a simple decay scheme - an alpha or beta decay, followed by a gamma transition to the daughter ground level; the detectors are fully specialized; no perturbations due to the installation, such as background counting rate, dead times, resolution time of the coincidence circuit modifies the counting rates. The coincidence relations are more complex, and were written by (Gandy.1961) and (Baerg.1973). For decay scheme corrections the coincidence method is applied associated with an efficiency extrapolation variant, and for the instrumental corrections various formulae were deduced by (Grigorescu.1973) and (Smith.1978). Many specific methods were elaborated in the primary activity standard laboratories, among them being the Radionuclide Metrology Laboratory from the Horia Hulubei National Institute for Research & Development in Physics and Nuclear Engineering (IFIN-HH, RML) Bucharest, the Romanian owner of the primary activity standard. A coincidence installation was set up in the sixties and was continuously updated in this laboratory. The variant of the efficiency extrapolation, allowing to accomplish the decay scheme corrections, was developed and applied for many types of radionuclides. The classical extrapolation coincidence method was applied for the beta-gamma medical radionuclide ^{131}I, for which the whole traceability chain was established (Sahagia et al.2008a). The therapy radionuclides ^{153}Sm, ^{177}Lu and ^{186,188}Re, strong beta - weak gamma-ray emitters, have a "triangular" decay scheme and were standardized by a special extrapolation procedure (Sahagia et al.2005a,2005b,2002). For the radionuclide ^{99m}Tc, decaying by isomer transition in competition with internal conversion, a new type of coincidence scheme was applied, based on the coincidence between 119.5-138 keV conversion electrons and Tc x-rays (Sahagia.2006). Radionuclide ^{125}I is an electron capture gamma emitter; it was standardized by the x - x, γ coincidence method (Sahagia et al.2008b). The positron emitters, used for PET, PET/CT systems, like ^{68}(Ge + Ga) generator, or other radionuclides decaying by electron capture in competition with positron emission, were standardized by the positron-annihilation-ray coincidence, or combinations of radiations (Grigorescu et al.2004; Grigorescu et al.1996). In the present time, in many laboratories, the classical, analog, coincidence set up is replaced by the Digital Coincidence Counting (DCC) (Buckman et al.1998). At the same time, instead of the PC, a liquid scintillation counter (LSC), associated with a NaI(Tl) detector is used for coincidence measurement (Chylinski & Radoszewski.1996)

Efficiency tracer method is an extension of the coincidence method applied for the standardization of pure beta decaying radionuclides. The solution to be standardized is mixed with a standard solution from a beta-gamma emitting radionuclide, preferable with a simple decay scheme, with a beta spectrum close to that of the radionuclide to standardize and chemically compatible with it. For the two radionuclide's mixture, relation (3) becomes:

$$N_{PC} = \varepsilon_{PC1} N_{01} + \varepsilon_{PC2} N_{02}; \quad N_\gamma = \varepsilon_\gamma N_{01}; \quad N_c = \varepsilon_{PC} \varepsilon_\gamma N_{01} \tag{5}$$

Index *1* refers to the tracer and *2* to the pure beta emitter. By an extrapolation procedure, a relation is established between the two ε_{PC1} and ε_{PC2} efficiencies, allowind the calculation of activity N_{02} of the pure beta radionuclide.The method is applied for therapeutic pure beta radionuclides, like ^{89}Sr, or other important radionuclides as ^{137}Cs (Razdolescu et al.2002a, Sahagia.1981) ^{32}P, ^{90}Y.

3.1.1.3 Advanced methods based on the liquid scintillation counting

The method consists of mixing the radioactive solution with a liquid scintillator (LS). The energy of the radiations is transferred to the LS; it emits light photons, which produce photoelectrons, multiplied in a photomultiplier (PMT). Electron impulses are collected at the PMT anode. The detection efficiency is superior to that of proportional counters, but it depends strongly on the radiations energy. A calculation model, known as the „Free parameter principle" was developed, leaving from the idea that the sum of fenomena: luminous photons emission in LS, their arrival at PMT photocathode and emission of a photoelectron as result of interaction, is described by a Poisson distribution law. Another influence of LS is the quenching; it can be due to its chemistry, but the most important is the ionization quenching, $Q(E)$, which is described by an empirical relation, written by (Birks.1964). Taking into account all these fenomena, a relation connecting the detection efficiency, ε, equal to the probability of producing a photoelectron, $P(\lambda,E)$, with the counter parameters and ionizing radiation energy, E was deduced. (Broda et al.2007; Pochwalski&Radoszewski.1979):

$$\varepsilon = P(\lambda,E) = 1 - e^{-\frac{EQ(E)}{\lambda R}} \qquad (6)$$

λ is called the free parameter and R is the number of photomultipliers in the system. In relation (6) it is important to adjust the free parameter such as to reflect the measurement conditions. On this purpose, two main models were developed.

CIEMAT/NIST method consists of the use of a LS counter provided with two PMTs in coincidence, in order to diminish the influence of background; commercial counters can be used. The adjustment of the free parameter is achieved by using an efficiency tracer, consisting of a tritium standard solution. The model contains several steps: a relation is established between the tritium detection efficiency and a quantity equivalent of the free parameter, known as quenching indicator parameter (QIP) (Grau Malonda.1999), measured by using the Compon radiation of an external source; a theoretical relation is calculated between the efficiency of tritium and that of the nuclide to standardize, for different QIP values, based on the beta spectra characteristics. Using a determined QIP value, one calculates the nuclide efficiency from the theoretical efficiency relation, corresponding to that QIP.

Triple to double coincidence ratio (TDCR) method makes use of a special counter, provided with three PMTs, connected in double and triple coincidences. Leaving from the general equation (6), the efficiencies, equal to the probabilities of registration for the logical sum of double, ε_d , and respectively triple, ε_t , coincidences were written by (Broda et al.2007; Pochwalski&Radoszewski.1979):

$$\begin{aligned} \varepsilon_d = d(E) &= 3\left(1 - e^{-\frac{EQ(E)}{3\lambda}}\right)^2 - 2\left(1 - e^{-\frac{EQ(E)}{3\lambda}}\right)^3 \\ \varepsilon_t = t(E) &= \left(1 - e^{-\frac{EQ(E)}{3\lambda}}\right)^3 \end{aligned} \qquad (7)$$

These relations are calculated theoretically, from the radionuclide spectrum, by itteration for a big number of values of the free parameter λ, by using computer programs, like SPEBETA; TDRCB-1, 2, 7; DETECSZ, etc., elaborated at LNHB-France and RC Poland. On the other hand, an experimental ratio between the counting rates of the two types of coincidences, equal to the efficiencies' ratio, is determined. They depend on the activity N_0 and efficiencies, as:

$$R_D = N_0 \varepsilon_d \,;\; R_T = N_0 \varepsilon_t \tag{8}$$

The theoretical ratio of efficiencies, corresponding to the adjusted free parameter is the optimum, when:

$$\frac{\varepsilon_d}{\varepsilon_t} = \frac{R_D}{R_T} \tag{9}$$

In this manner, the efficiencies are determined, and the activity N_0 is calculated from relations (8)
A TDCR system was set up in IFIN-HH,RML, with the assistance of Dr. Philippe Cassette from LNHB. It was used for the standardization of radionuclides as ^{3}H, ^{89}Sr, ^{63}Ni and was validated by international comparisons (Razdolescu et al.2004; 2006). Recently, a new counter was set up in RML, replacing the three PMTs with 6 channel photomultipliers (CPM) and designing a new optical chamber (Ivan et al.2010). It has the advantage of being compact and portable.

3.2 Validation of the primary installations and methods; international equivalence

3.2.1 The International System

The International Committee for Weights and Measures (CIPM) coordinates the metrology branches through the Consultative Committees, as the Comité Consultatif des Rayonnements Ionisants - CCRI. CCRI is divided in three sections. The Section II, CCRI(II) - Measurement of Radionuclides, coordinates the Radionuclide Metrology. The Bureau International des Poids et Mesures-BIPM, Sèvres, http://www.bipm.org France, has the custody of the international standards. The equivalence of the primary standards is assured at this level by absolute methods of standardization. At the regional level, the Regional Metrology Organizations (MRO) are operational. In Europe there exist: EURAMET - European Association of National Metrology Institutes and COOMET - Euro-Asian Cooperation of National Metrology Institutes. The connection between BIPM and MROs is assured by the Joint Committee of the Regional Metrology Organizations and the BIPM - JCRB. At this level one assures the traceability also by using secondary (relative) standardization methods. The CIPM-MRA, Mutual Recognition Arrangement (1999), defines the recognition of the calibration and measurement certificates issued by the National Metrology Institutes. For example, Romania is part of CIPM-MRA. The document contains four annexes: Annex A - List of signatories; the Romanian signatory is the Romanian Bureau of Legal Metrology - National Institute of Metrology (BRML-INM); Annex B - Key Comparison Data Base (KCDB) per Institute; Annex C- Calibration and Measurement Capabilities (CMC); Annex D - Key Comparison Data Base. The condition for the applicability of CIPM-MRA by the signatory countries is the demonstration of the equivalence of the primary standards, or of the traceability for the others, such as presented in figure 1. The equivalence is demonstrated only by the participation at international comparisons. IFIN-HH, RML, has participated at international comparisons since 1962. *The Key Comparison Data Base (KCDB) Annex B of the CIPM – MRA,* can be found at the address: http://kcdb.bipm.org/AppendixB/KCDB_ApB_search.asp. The participants in CIPM-MRA are the National Institutes of Metrology (NMIs), but for specialized metrology branches as the ionizing radiations, the participants can be the Designated Institutes. In Romania, according to the protocol concluded between BRML-INM and IFIN-HH it is established that IFIN-HH is designed as the owner of the primary activity (Becquerel) and derived quantities standard, with national and international responsibilities in the field:

- Designed Institute as responsible for participation in the CIPM-MRA, included in *Annex A of the CIPM-MRA, List of signatories.*
- Associated Institute to EURAMET, responsible for the Technical Committee of Ionizing Radiations, TC-IR

Due to its scientific authority, IFIN-HH became also: Member of the International Committee for Radionuclide Metrology (ICRM) in 1980 and Member of the Consultative Committee Section II, CCRI(II), in 2004

3.2.2 Validation of methods and establishment of equivalence by key comparisons

Definition of the Key Comparisons, according to VIM: *Selected comparisons taken formally into account for the establishment of equivalence.* CCRI(II) may approve also supplementary comparisons, initiated by other organizations, to be used for establishment of equivalence: EURAMET, COOMET, IAEA, JRC-IRMM, etc. Relative methods may be used at this level, in order to extend the applicability of the CIPM-MRA, Annex C.

The Comparisons are of the categories:

- *Comparisons type « CCRI(II)-K2. Radionuclide (Ex. Am-241)".* They are organized at worldwide scale. A single batch of radioactive solution is used for the preparation of all the samples which are sent to the participants, who measure and send to the BIPM the filled-in Reporting Form, containing the results. The reports are evaluated at BIPM and the Draft reports are drawn up. The Draft B is submitted to the approval of the CCRI(II) and published. For example, IFIN-HH, RML is registered with such comparisons in the KCDB with the radionuclides: ^{241}Am, ^{109}Cd, ^{139}Ce, ^{134}Cs, ^{137}Cs, ^{152}Eu, ^{55}Fe, ^{3}H, ^{125}I (2), ^{192}Ir, ^{177}Lu, ^{54}Mn, ^{32}P, ^{75}Se, ^{89}Sr, ^{204}Tl, ^{65}Zn.
- *Comparisons: "BIPM.RI (II)-K1.Radionuclide".* BIPM disposes of two reentrant (well type) ionization chambers, CENTRONIC IG11/20A, as the basis for creation of the International Reference System - SIR, for gamma-ray emitters (Ratel. 2007). The key comparison is carried out by the individual preparation and certification of an ampoule with standard solution by the participant laboratory, which is then sent to the BIPM with the Comparison filled-in Form. It is re measured at BIPM and the two results are compared. IFIN-HH, RML is registered with the radionuclides: ^{110m}Ag; ^{133}Ba; ^{60}Co (1983 and 2007); ^{134}Cs; ^{131}I; ^{57}Co; ^{137}Cs
- Supplementary Comparisons

Type: "EURAMET.RI(II)-S5.Radionuclide". These comparisons are deployed as Decay Data Evaluation Projects-DDEP. The first step of comparisons is similar to the CCRI(II)-K2. The second step consists of the measurement of the emission intensities for *x* and gamma-rays. IFIN-HH, RML is registered with: ^{169}Yb; ^{65}Zn; ^{124}Sb.

"IAEA-CCRI(II). Matrix content. Radionuclides". These comparisons are organized within the frame of the International Atomic Energy Agency (IAEA) - Coordinated Research Projects

(CRPs) and are approved by the CCRI(II); they refer to special types of samples and relative methods are accepted. IFIN-HH, RML is registered as *"CCRI(II)-S6.Radionuclide"*, for the radionuclides ^{57}Co and ^{131}I, of interest in nuclear medicine.

Establishment of the SI Activity Unit (Becquerel) by key comparisons.

The Activity Unit is established individually for each radionuclide, after the evaluation of the key comparison result, which is expressed as the Key Comparison Reference Value – KCRV.
Four methods are used to calculate the KCRV (Ratel.2007): arithmetic and weighted mean, median and weighted median. The most adequate variant is selected; in most cases, the arithmetic mean is preferred. The outliers are established after applying the exclusion criteria. The KCRV and its uncertainty are approved by the CCRI(II) and may be modified in time, after accumulating new results for the respective radionuclide. The "outliers" are not eliminated from KCDB, but their difference from KCRV must be taken into account when reporting the calibration uncertainties.
When both the *SIR-BIPM.RI(II)-K1.Radionuclide* and the *CCRI(II)-K2. Radionuclide* comparison results are registered for the gamma-ray emitters, a link is established between the two types of comparisons, through the measurement in the BIPM ionization chamber of the ampoules sent for the *K2* comparison.
Equivalence. An equivalence matrix is calculated. Two main quantities are reported and compared: Difference between the individual result and KCRV, (D_i) and its uncertainty (U_i), for a coverage interval k =2. The ratio of these quantities is the measure of degree of equivalence. The CCRI(II) approved "Draft B" is published in the KCDB and in *Metrologia, Technical Supplement issues.* IFIN-HH, RML, is registered in KCDB with 28 radionuclides.
Equivalence validity. A validity interval was adopted by consensus. Consequently, in order to maintain the equivalence for some radionuclides, IFIN-HH repeated the comparison. It participated in 1983 and in 2007 at the *SIR-BIPM.RI(II)-K1*.Co-60 comparisons. As for ^{134}Cs, the participations were: *CCRI(II)-K2* in 1978 and *SIR-BIPM.RI(II)-K1* in 2006 and for ^{137}Cs, the participations were: *CCRI(II)-K2* in 1982 and *SIR-BIPM.RI(II)-K1* in 2009.
Example: *Analysis of the IFIN-HH, RML result at the medical ^{131}I key comparison SIR-BIPM.RI(II)-K.1.I-131, 2007* (Ratel et al.2008). *KCRV* = (40400 ±40) *MBq; IFIN-HH* value = (40371 ± 139) *MBq*; *D*i =0.07%; *U*i=0.65% . Consequently, the IFIN-HH, RML's result was taken into account in the calculation of the *KCRV.*

SI Activity Unit (Becquerel) for other radionuclides.

A matrix of radionuclides, codified by colors, according to the standardization difficulty by method, was established by the CIPM-CCRI(II) Key Comparison Working Group (KCWG), within the document Grouping Criteria Radionuclides for Supporting CMCs (Karam.2007). It can be used as follows. A red coded radionuclide measured by LSC, such as ^{3}H, supports ^{89}Sr, ^{90}Y, LSC measured, and green color coded.

3.3 Implementation and recognition of the Quality Management System – Approval of CMC files

An international agreement for the practical use of the results obtained by the National Metrology Institutes (NMI) in assurance of the traceability chain and recognition of the measurements and certificates was concluded through the document: *"Joint statement by the CIPM and ILAC on the roles and responsibilities of national metrology institutes and national recognized accreditation bodies"*. At the level of EURAMET, the implementation of the Quality

Management System (QMS) is monitored by the EURAMET, Technical Committee – Quality, TC-Q.
At the level of CIPM - MRA, the statement is practically applied by the use of the Annex C of the CIPM-MRA, Calibration and Measurement Capability files – CMCs. The approval and publication of CMCs for a NMI is the result of two types of evaluation components for the international recognition: (i) Approval of the international equivalence for primary and of the traceability for secondary standards; (ii) Implementation of the QMS and recognition by the MRO's, TC-Q.

i. *Approval of equivalence and traceability.* The NMI, member of one MRO, draws up the primary or secondary CMC files. The statement is compared with the KCDB for primary, or in our case EURAMET for secondary standards. After the inter MROs' peer review process, they are submitted for the approval of the JCRB.
ii. *Implementation and approval of the QMS.* The EN/ISO/IEC 17025:2005, referential *"General requirements for the competence of testing and calibration laboratories"* is applied. A complete documentation and its implementation are presented at the annual meetings of the EURAMET, TC-Q. The technical experts monitor the documents and after the first approval, the QMS is annually reconfirmed. This is a prerequisite condition to maintain the CMCs in the published in Annex C of MRA. *Example, IFIN-HH, RML situation.* 34 CMC files, Radioactivity standards, passed the peer review process; the QMS was approved in 2007 and annually reviewed. All CMCs were approved by the JCRB in April 2008 and published in CIPM-MRA, Annex C. http://kcdb.bipm.org/AppendixC/default.asp

4. Setting up of the activity secondary standard systems

Realisation of the activity secondary standards.

Such as presented in figure 1 and as pointed in the references TRS 454 (2006) and (Zimmerman & Judge. 2007), the practical realization of the metrological traceability chain is possible by using the activity secondary standards. They are transfer instruments of the activity unit from the primary to the lower order, working standards, for the end users, through standard (reference) products or calibration services. They consist of installations for the secondary (relative) standardization; their calibration is done with sources and solutions absolutely standardized with the primary standards. In the case of the primary laboratories they use their own primary standards. In the case of the secondary standard laboratories (SSL), the standards leave from another primary laboratory, the traceability route being declared. The practical work at IFIN-HH, RML was described in (Sahagia & Woods.2008).

4.1 Secondary standards for high activity radiopharmaceutical solutions

The secondary standard for high activity solutions is a reentrant (well type) ionization chamber, filled with an inert gas as nitrogen or argon, at high pressure, of a special construction, largely described by H. Schrader in Monographie BIPM-4 (1997), or a commercial radionuclide calibrator. It is calibrated with standard solutions absolutely standardized, from the radionuclides of interest. The ionization current, registered by the associated electrometric circuit, is due to the radiations entering in the sensitive volume of the chamber and ionizing the filling gas. This chamber is mainly used for the measurement of activity for gamma-ray, but also for strong beta-ray emitters, when the ionization current is produced by the bremsstrahlung radiations. Usually, the calibration factor is expressed in terms of absolute or relative efficiency, or in ionization current per activity unit, $pA\ MBq^{-1}$. The calibration must be performed for several geometries of the recipients containing radioactive solution, or gelatin capsules in the case of iodine radioisotopes, as the calibration factor depends on the geometrical dimensions. For example, the IFIN-HH, RML well type ionization chamber is of the type CENTRONIC IG12/20A, filled with argon at a pressure of 2MPa (20Atm); its construction was first described in (Grigorescu et al. 2003). Recently, the old electrometric system was replaced with an electrometer Keithley E6517A. The validation of the calibration factors was done by several comparisons: (i) with the measurements performed at PTB-Braunschweig-Germany with PTB standard solutions; (ii) with the IFIN-HH, RML results obtained in international comparisons; (iii) respectively with the value of the KCRV (Sahagia et al. 2010). The calibration factors are determined for the radionuclides: ^{241}Am, ^{57}Co, ^{99m}Tc, ^{186}Re, ^{188}Re, ^{153}Sm, ^{177}Lu, ^{75}Se, ^{169}Yb, ^{131}I, ^{133}Ba, ^{51}Cr, ^{192}Ir, ^{134}Cs, ^{137}Cs, ^{54}Mn, ^{65}Zn, ^{60}Co, ^{152}Eu and for three geometries: (i) Solid sources; (ii) ^{131}I gelatin capsules; (iii) Solutions of volumes: 2 mL (PTB), 3.6 mL (SIR-BIPM), 5 mL (P6 used for radiopharmaceuticals). From the above list one may notice that the calibration is assured for the majority of medical radionuclides. The determined calibration factors allow the measurement and certification of the radiopharmaceutical solutions or capsules to be used for: (a) the calibration of the radionuclide calibrators, including those belonging to the radiopharmaceutical unit from IFIN-HH, (b) to be distributed to the interested laboratories, or (c) to be used for organization of national comparisons. The chamber operation is in compliance with the QMS rules, established in agreement with the requirements of the EN ISO/IEC 17025:2005 and TRS 454 document. The calibration uncertainty is in all cased less than 2.0%.

4.2 High resolution spectrometric system

In the field of nuclear medicine, spectrometric systems are used for the measurement of the radionuclide impurity level in radiopharmaceuticals (RPMs); in order to perform an adequate check of the requirements imposed to the RPMs, the system must have a high resolution, to allow the identification of the main radionuclide and impurities, and to be sensitive enough (to have a low background) in order to detect impurities content of the order of <0.1%, such as it is required for ^{99}Mo content in ^{99m}Tc.

IFIN-HH, RML disposes of a system containing a high resolution HPGe detector: relative efficiency 29%; energy interval 35 *keV* - 3 *MeV*; resolution: 0.85 *keV* (122 *keV*) and 1.74 *keV* (1.332 *MeV*) and a computer driven, software GAMMA VISION, V 6.01 spectrometric analyser. The specialized program GESPECOR (Sima & Arnold. 2002), for geometry, matrix and coincidence summation corrections is implemented. An efficient shield, consisting from: 10 cm old lead; 1 *mm* tin; 2 *mm* electrolytic cooper, assures a maximum integral background rate on the whole energy interval of 1.4 s^{-1}. The system is calibrated in terms of energy and efficiency with standard sources, in various geometries from point sources up to volume recipients, prepared from standard solution absolutely standardized, by the coincidence method. Various distances, from zero, up to 44.3 *cm* from the detector surface are used in measurements, depending on the activity interval. The calibration of the system was also validated by the participation at international NPL-UK or IAEA exercises for the measurement of various volume samples, containing mixtures of radionuclides (Luca et al. 2010). The system is taken as reference for the dedicated HPGe spectrometer used in the radiopharmacy unit.

Another use of the IFIN-HH, RML's spectrometric system is the precise determination of the emission intensity of gamma-rays for radionuclides of medical use. These parameters are of maximum importance for activity standardization by primary methods, as in most of measurements they are basic parameters in activity calculation. On the other hand, the efficiency and safety of the medical procedure depends directly on their precise knowledge. The precise value of half life is directly used in nuclear medicine units for the calculation of activity at the moment of administration. The calculation of patients' doses is based on the values of: activity, half life, radiations - types, energies and emission intensities. On the international scale, projects of the type: *"EURAMET.RI(II)-S5.Radionuclide"* are organized, for the experimental determination of emission intensities and evaluation projects coordinated by the Decay Data Evaluation Program (DDEP) are deployed. IFIN-HH, RML participates in both types of programs. For example, recently the laboratory participated at the exercise, organized for the new PET radionuclide ^{64}Cu, EURAMET project 1085 (Bé et al. 2011). RML standardized absolutely solutions from ^{64}Cu and ^{68}Ga by the coincidence method (Sahagia et al. 2011). Point solid sources from standard solution were prepared gravimetrically, and were used for the determination of their decay parameters: gamma-rays emission intensities with the calibrated HPGe spectrometric system and half life by the use of the CENTRONIC IG12/20A ionization chamber (Luca et al.2011).

5. The Radionuclide Metrology Laboratory support to the nuclear medicine

A primary/secondary standard laboratory is the entity which can assure the continuity of the metrological traceability in the measurement and characterization of radiopharmaceuticals in radiopharmacy units, national control authorities and hospitals from the top level, SI, up to the end user, the patient, by the following standards delivery and calibration operations (Zimmerman et al. 2007):

- Radioactive standards to be used in the interested entities;
- Calibration or Metrological Check of the Radionuclide Calibrators;
- Organization of national comparisons and proficiency tests.

These activities need to be accomplished under the regime of national accreditation, as a Calibration and Testing Laboratory, according to the provisions of the standard EN ISO/IEC 17025:2005 *"General requirements for the competence of testing and calibration laboratories"*. For example IFIN-HH, RML obtained the accreditation for both types of activities, from the Romanian accreditation body, RENAR, member of the European Accreditation (EA), for the products and services for clients, after implementing a Quality Management System (QMS). The QMS consists of the documentation and practical realization of the documents' provisions. The main documents, covering the Chapters 4 and 5 of the EN ISO/IEC 17025:2005 standard, are: RML Manual-containing the basic statement of the QMS, an Organizational procedure and two sets of procedures: System (Management) procedures (MP) and Work procedures (WP) and instructions (WI). The accreditation was obtained in 2009, for a 4-year period; annual survey audits of RENAR representatives are done. In contrast with other calibration or testing laboratories, where the accreditation refers to some well-defined activities, in our quality of primary standard laboratory, we have first of all the responsibility for the quality of primary, absolute standardizations, on the top of traceability chain, not in direct connection with customers' requirements. The first consequences are: (i) The traceability chain must be well defined and demonstrated in the laboratory. (ii) An internationally recognized expert must conduct the technical evaluation of the laboratory. On the other hand, as a national provider of radioactive standards, the RML must meet quality requirements in their production.

(i) *Definition of Activities and Establishment of Traceability Chain.* Clear distinction of the two types of activities in relation with the RENAR accreditation was defined: Calibration activities and Testing activities. (a) The calibration branch required a sharp definition of the traceability chain and activities deployed in regime of quality management. The declared activities under accreditation are: (I) Attestation of the installations for the absolute (direct) standardization, mainly used for international comparisons, in order to prove the international equivalence of the Romanian standards, and for the preparation of standard sources and solutions used for the calibration of the secondary equipment. (II) Calibration and metrological check of the secondary installations for the relative (indirect) standardization. (III) Standardization of the radioactive standard sources and solutions. (IV) Preparation and relative or absolute standardization of radioactive sources and solutions, under the quality management system. The traceability chain continues outside the laboratory, in connection with the users, and implies: (V) The delivery of radioactive sources, with Calibration Certificates, under the quality management system. (VI) The calibration and metrological check of activity measurement installations. (VII) The organization of inter laboratory comparisons (ILCs) and proficiency tests (PTs) for the testing and calibration laboratories. (b) The testing branch of accredited activities refers at the Analysis of very low activity samples by the gamma-ray spectrometry. Another special aspect in the application of the requirements of the 17025:2005 Standard in our case is the responsibility of the National Nuclear Authority (CNCAN) regarding the radioprotection of the workers, public and patients. In this respect IFIN-HH, RML was CNCAN designed also as a notified calibration and testing laboratory for the nuclear field.

5.1 Radioactive standards for nuclear medicine

The calibration and metrological check of the equipment for measurement of the radioactivity imposed the development of technics for the preparation of a large variety of standard sources and solutions, to be used in-house, or delivered to the external customers which are performing radioactivity measurement. A general WP, coded AC-PL-LMR-10, describes the common operations and detailed WIs present the specific operations.

Radioactive Solutions. A large variety of radioactive solutions, physico-chemically stable, adequate as radioactivity standards, are prepared (Grigorescu et al.1975). Some of them, even for external users' delivery, are standardized absolutely, or alternatively, by the use of the calibrated ionization chamber. They are certified in terms of radioactive concentration, $Bq\ g^{-1}$, and in total activity, *Bq*, per recipient, flame or mechanically sealed in glass ampoules or P6 vials.

Point and Large Area Alpha and Beta Sources. These sources are of immediate interest, both for calibration of contamination monitors (contaminometers), as well as for the effective measurement of the so called "Gross Alpha" and "Gross Beta" radioactive content of environmental, industrial and food chain samples. Their preparation and measurement of the particle emission rate in a 2πsr geometry are described in (Sahagia et al. 1996a).

5.2 Calibration and metrological check of measurement equipment

The main requirements regarding the characteristics of the equipment for the measurement of activity and of the physico-chemical parameters were described in section 2. In order to satisfy them, a radionuclide metrology laboratory is asked to perform calibrations or other metrology checks over it. The radionuclide calibrators are the most used devices for the measurement of activity in radiopharmacy, control units and hospitals (Razdolescu et al.2002b). In some cases the National Metrology legislation imposes their metrological control, according to legal metrology norms, and in others it is required their calibration at defined time intervals, by a metrology laboratory, accredited for calibration. In our case, the legal metrological control was mandatory until 2009. Starting with 2010, the calibration-recalibration was preferred. In this respect, IFIN-HH, RML obtained the RENAR accreditation for these operations within its QMS. The WP codified as AC-PL-LMR-11 is applied. As a general remark from our calibration experience is that the Romanian hospitals staff increased in time its awareness regarding the quality of activity measurement and more and more nuclear medicine units benefit from our laboratory's services of calibration, at present time regarding the radionuclides: ^{99m}Tc and ^{131}I. The deviations of the calibration factors from the reference values are generally within ±5%. The IFIN-HH radiopharmacy is under the permanent metrological survey of the RML. As this unit has under study new radiopharmaceuticals, the laboratory was asked to assess calibration factors to the radionuclide calibrators for the new radiouclides: ^{186}Re, ^{188}Re, ^{153}Sm, ^{177}Lu.

The second important action is the calibration of the HPGe spectrometric system used in the radiopharmacy for the control of radionuclidic impurities. It is calibrated and regularly recalibrated in energy and efficiency by the representatives of RML, using standard solutions prepared in RML, under accreditation regime, and the calibration procedure WP code AC-PL-LMR-0100 is applied.

Other equipment, belonging the radiopharmacy unit, are the radiochromatographs used in the control of the radiochemical purity; for their calibration and linearity check, a set of solid point standard gamma-ray emitting sources are used; for the case of ^{131}I control, two ^{133}Ba standard sources are measured. The action is also under accreditation regime and the WP code AC-PL-LMR-12 is applied.

Each nuclear medicine unit, operating with open radioactive sources, is provided with contaminometers for the control of radioactive contamination of surfaces, devices, clothes, operator hands, etc., which can occur during the medical procedures. This equipment can be under the legal metrological control of the state as it is in Romania, or only is recalibrated at defined intervals. The Romanian secondary standard laboratories performing these checks use large area standard sources emitting beta radiations, in most cases ^{90}(Sr+Y) sources. IFIN-HH, RML is the provider of these standard sources and also performs their calibration (Sahagia et al. 1996b).

5.3 Organization of national comparisons and proficiency tests

The most significant test, recognized as relevant in the evaluation of the capability of a laboratory performing measurements, is the participation in proficiency tests. For example, even when the calibration factors of the radionuclide calibrators are correct, the measurement in a hospital implies also the skill of the operating staff. Non experienced people are possible to choose wrong calibration factors' values, to do wrong readings and activity calculation on the administration time. From our practical experience, one may conclude that the proportion of laboratories with unsatisfactory results in proficiency tests is higher than that of wrong calibrated equipment. This is the reason for which in some countries the participation in proficiency tests is mandatory, but in others like Romania, it is only voluntary. IFIN-HH, RML organized in the past several national comparisons mainly for a scientific output, in order to understand which explanations for noncorresponding results are. The comparisons regarded the measurement of ^{131}I (Sahagia et al.1996b) and the set ^{99m}Tc and ^{57}Co, (Sahagia & Woods. 2008c). Within the frame of the above cited *IAEA, CRP E2.10.05*, a series of international actions were deployed, in order to harmonize the measurements in the participant countries, all over the world. The actions were organized in two steps. The first step was the participation of the national reference laboratories (primary or secondary) in two comparisons organized by the IAEA, recognized also as supplementary CCRI(II) -S6 comparisons, on ^{131}I and ^{57}Co (used a as mock solution for ^{99m}Tc), intended to verify their calibration capability. The results were presented by the comparisons organizers in the papers (Zimmerman et al. 2008; Zimmerman & Palm. 2010). After the evaluation of the results, each national laboratory organized then two national comparisons, for the radionuclides ^{131}I and ^{99m}Tc. IFIN-HH, RML organized the comparisons according to the prescriptions of the WP code AC-PL-LMR-07, written in accordance with the international documents: ISO Guide 43 *„Proficiency testing by interlaboratory comparisons"* Part 1: *„Development and operation of proficiency testing schemes"* and Part 2: *„Selection and use of proficiency testing schemes by laboratory accreditation bodies"* and following also the recommendations from the *Protocols on the organization of national comparisons of radiopharmaceuticals*, established within the frame of the *IAEA CRP. E2.10.05*.The analysis of the results was reported in the papers (Sahagia et al. 2009; Sahagia et al. 2010b). As conclusions from these tests are the proportions of hospitals measuring satisfactory the activities of the two radionuclides. In the case of ^{131}I, from a total number of 15 reported values, a number of 11 results are within the difference limit from reference value <5%, and 12 results within the limit <10%, a proportion of 80% from participating units, being in compliance with the Pharmacopoeia; for ^{99m}Tc, from 7 reported values, a number of 5 results are within < 5 % difference from the reference value, and 7 results within the limit < 10 %, a proportion of 100% from participating units. Regarding ^{131}I comparisons, after finalizing the *IAEA CRP. E2.10.05*, an interesting paper, summarizing all 8 national laboratories comparisons' organization and results was published recently (Olsovcova et al. 2010); a similar paper is in preparation, for presentation of the ^{99m}Tc national comparisons.

6. Conclusions

- Nuclear medicine benefits from a very wide range of radionuclides, to be used as radiopharmaceuticals for diagnosis and therapy procedures.
- The radiopharmaceuticals are classified as high pharmaceutical risk products, and therefore they must be very carefully characterized in terms of the main parameters: metrological, physico-chemical, biological.
- The precise measurement of activity is of crucial interest, as it determines directly the committed effective dose of the patient in diagnostic and organ/tissue absorbed dose in therapy.
- Precise measurements of activity are also implied indirectly in the full characterization of the radiopharmaceuticals' parameters.
- The Radionuclide Metrology Laboratory can assure the metrological traceability chain for activity starting from the primary level, by demonstrating its international equivalence, or starting from the secondary one, the traceability route being necessary to be declared.

- The Radionuclide Metrology Laboratory can offer the necessary support to the nuclear medicine for the safe and efficient use of radiopharmaceuticals, by assuring the standards and the metrology services to the implied entities: radiopharmacy, control laboratories, equipment producers, nuclear medicine units.

7. Acknowledgements

Thanks are due to my granddaughter Laura Calinoiu for the revision of the text and to my colleagues from IFIN-HH, Radionuclide Metrology Laboratory: Dr. E.L. Grigorescu, Mrs. A.C. Wätjen, Dr. A. Luca, Dr. C. Ivan, Mr. A. Antohe for our common work.

8. References

Baerg, A.P. (1973) The efficiency extrapolation method in coincidence counting. *Nuclear Instruments and Methods*. Vol 112, pp 143-150, ISSN 0168-9002

Bé, M.-M., Chisté, V., Dulieu, C., Mougeot, X., Browne, E., Chechev, V., Kuzmenko, N., Kondev, F., Luca, A., Galán, M., Arinc, A., Huang, X. (2004-2010) *Table of Radionuclides (vols. 1- 5). Monographie BIPM-5.* Ed. Bureau International des Poids et Mesures, Pavillon de Breteuil, F-92310 Sèvres, France, ISBN-13 978-92-822-2234-8.

Bé, M-M. Kossert, K., Dryak, P., Johansson, L., Sahagia, M., Luca, A., Antohe, A., Ratel, G. (2011) Standardization, decay data measurements and evaluation of ^{64}Cu. *18-th International Conference on Radionuclide Metrology and its Applications, ICRM2011*, Tsukuba, Japan, 18-23 September 2011

Birks, B. (1964) TheTheory and Practice of Scintillation Counting. Pergamon Press, Oxford

Broda, R., Cassette, P., Kossert, K. (2007). Radionuclide metrology using liquid scintillation counting. *Metrologia* Vol 44 pp. S36-S52, ISSN 0028-1394 (Print); 1681-7575 (Online)

Buckman, S.M., Keightley, J.D., Smith, D., Woods, M.J. (1998) The validation of a digital coincidence counting system. *Applied Radiations and Isotopes*, Vol 49, pp 1135-1140, ISBN 0969-8043

Chylinski, A., Radoszewski, T., (1996) Generalized tracer method 4π(LS)-γ for standardization of pure beta emitters . *Nuclear Instruments and Methods A*, Vol 369, pp 336-339, ISSN 0168-9002

Debertin, K., Helmer, R. G. (1998) *Gamma- and X-ray Spectrometry with Semiconductor Detectors*. Elsevier, North Holland, Amsterdam

EUROEAN DIRECTORATE FOR THE QUALITY OF MEDICINES. (2002) *European Pharmacopoeia*, 4th edition, Council of Europe, Strassbourg, France

F.A.O., I.A.E.A., I.L.O., O.E.C.D. Nuclear Energy Agency, PAN. AM. H.O., W.H.O. (1996) *International Basic Safety Standards for Protection against Ionizing Radiation and for the Safety of Radiation Sources*, Safety Series No.115, IAEA, Vienna, Austria

Gandy, A. (1961) *Mesues absolues de l'activité des radionucleides par la methode des coïncidences bêta-gamma àl'aide des detecteurs de grande efficacité.* Monographie BIPM, France

Grau Malonda, A., Rodriguez Barquero, L., Grau Carles, A. (1994) Radioactivity determination of ^{90}Y, ^{90}Sr and ^{89}Sr mixtures by spectral deconvolution. *Nuclear Instruments and Methods A*, Vol 339, pp 31-37, ISSN 0168-9002

Grau Malonda, A. (1999) *Free parameter models in liquid scintillation counting.* Coleccion Documentos CIEMAT, ISBN 84-7834-350-4.

Grigorescu, E. L.(1973) Accuracy of coincidence measurements. *Nuclear Instruments and Methods,* Vol 112, pp 151-154, ISSN 0168-9002

Grigorescu, E.L., Sahagia, M., Lates, G., Topa, A. (1975) Prepararea si etalonarea solutiilor radioactive de ^{198}Au, ^{51}Cr, ^{24}Na, ^{95}Nb, ^{65}Zn. *Studii si Cercetari de Fizica.* Vol 27, pp 945-954, ISSN 1221-1451 43 822

Grigorescu, E.L., Sahagia, M., Razdolescu, A.C., Ivan, C. (1996) Standardization of some electron capture radionuclides. *Nuclear Instruments and Methods in Physics Research A,* Vol 369, pp 414-420, ISSN 0168-9002

Grigorescu, E.L., Luca, A., Sahagia, M., Razdolescu, A.C., Ivan ,C. (2003) 4π Gamma ionization chamber method for secondary standardization of radioactive solutions. *Romanian Journal of Physics,* Vol 48, pp 91-95, ISSN 1221-146

Grigorescu, E. L., Negut, C.D., Luca, A., Razdolescu, A.C., Tanase, M. (2004) Standardization of ^{68}(Ge+Ga). *Applied Radiations and Isotopes,* Vol 60, pp 429-431, ISBN 0969-8043

ICRP, 1996c Age - dependent doses to members of the public from intake of radionuclides: Part 5. Compilation of ingestion and inhalation dose coefficients. *International Commission on Radiation Protection Publication 72.* Ann. ICRP 26(1)

Ivan, C., Wätjen, A. C. Cassette, P., Sahagia, M., Antohe, A., Grigorescu, E. L. (2008) Participation in the CCRI(II)-K2.H-3 comparison and study of the new TDCR-LS counter with 6 CPMs. *Applied Radiations and Isotopes,* Vol 68, pp 1543-1545, ISBN 0969-8043

Karam, L.R. (2007) Application of the CIPM-MRA to radionuclide metrology. *Metrologia,* Vol 44, pp S1-S6, ISSN 0028-1394

Kornyei, J. (2008) Radiolabeled Biomolecules and their Competitors for Nuclear Medicine.*Radioisotopes and Biomolecules. A Partnership for the Early Diagnosis and Targeted Therapy of Radiotherapy of cancer* Workshop, 26-28 November 2008, Bucharest, Romania

Luca,A., Wätjen, A.C., Grigorescu, E.L., Sahagia, M., Ivan, C. (2010) Conclusions from the Participation at Proficiency Tests for Gamma-Ray Spectrometry Measurements. *Romanian Journal of Physics.* Vol 55, pp 724-732, ISSN 1221-146

Luca, A., Sahagia, M., Antohe, A. (2011) Measurement of ^{64}Cu and ^{68}Ga half life and gamma-rays emission intensities. *18-th International Conference on Radionuclide Metrology and its Applications,* ICRM2011, Tsukuba, Japan, 18-23 September 2011

Mikolajczak, R. (2008) Therapeutic potential of radionuclides ^{90}Y, ^{177}Lu, ^{188}Re. Production possibilities and applications in nuclear medicine. *Radioisotopes and Biomolecules. A Partnership for the Early Diagnosis and Targeted Therapy of Radiotherapy of Cancer,* 26-28 November 2008, Bucharest, Romania

Mutual recognition of national measurement standards and of measurement certificates issued by national metrology institutes. (1999, revised 2003) Bureau Intrenational des Poids et Mesures (BIPM), Sèvres, France,

Nuclear Commission for Radiation Protection (NCRP), USA, Report No.58. (1978) A handbook of radioactivity measurements procedures. ISBN 0-913392-41-3

Nedjadi, Y., Spring, P., Bailat, C., Decombaz, M., Triscone, G., Gostely, J.J., Laedermann, J.P., Bochud, F. (2007) Primary activity measurements with 4πγ NaI(Tl) counting and Monte Carlo calculated efficiencies. *Applied Radiations and Isotopes,* Vol 65, pp 534-538, ISBN 0969-8043

Olsovcova, V., Iwahara, A., Oropesa, P., Joseph, L., Ravindra, A., Ghafoori, M., Hye-Kyung Son, Sahagia, M., Tastan,S., Zimmerman, B. (2010) National comparisons of I-131 measurement among nuclear medicine clinics of eight countries. *Applied Radiations and Isotopes,* Vol 68, pp, 1371 - 1377, ISBN 0969-8043

Pochwalski, K., Radoszewski, T. (1979) *Disintegration rate determination by liquid scintillation counting using the triple to double coincidence ratio (TDCR) method.* Institute of Nuclear Research, Warsaw, Poland INR 1848/OPIDI/ E/A.

Ratel, G. (2005) Evaluation of the uncertainty of the degree of equivalence. *Metrologia,* Vol 42, pp S140-S144, ISSN 0028-1394 (Print); 1681-7575 (Online)

Ratel, G. (2007) Systeme International de Reference and its applications in key comparisons. *Metrologia,* Vol 44, pp S7-S16, ISSN 0028-1394 (Print); 1681-7575 (Online)

Ratel, G., Michotte, C., Sahagia, M., Park, T.S., Dryak, P., Sochorova, J., Maringer, F., Kreuziger, M.(2008) Results of the IFIN-HH (Romania), KRISS (Republic of Korea), CMI (Czech Republic) and BEV (Austria) in the BIPM comparison BIPM.RI(II)-K1.I-131 of activity measurements of the radionuclide I-131. *Metrologia Technical Supplement,* Vol 45 no. 06007

Razdolescu, A.C., Sahagia, M., Cassette, P., Grigorescu, E.L., Luca, A., Ivan, C. (2002a) Standardization of ^{89}Sr. *Applied Radiations and Isotopes,* Vol 56, pp, 435-439, ISBN 0969-8043

Razdolescu, A.C., Sahagia, M., Luca, A., Bercea, S., Dumitrescu, C., Schrader, H. (2002) Results obtained in the metrological certification of a commercially available radionuclide calibrator. *Applied Radiations and Isotopes,* Vol 56, pp, 957-958, ISBN 0969-8043

Razdolescu, A.C., Cassette, P. (2004) Standardization of tritiated water and ^{204}Tl by TDCR liquid scintillation counting. *Applied Radiations and Isotopes,* Vol 60, pp, 493-497, ISBN 0969-8043

Razdolescu, A.C., Broda, R., Cassette, P., Simpson, B. (2006) The IFIN-HH triple coincidence liquid scintillation counter. *Applied Radiations and Isotopes,* Vol 64, pp, 1510-1514, ISBN 0969-8043

Sahagia, M. (1981) Some practical applications of tracing and extrapolation methods in absolute standardization of radioactive sources and solutions. *Isotopenpraxis* (At present time: *Isotopes in Environmental and Health Studies)* 17, H5, pp 211-213

Sahagia, M., Razdolescu, A.C., Ivan, C. (1996a) Equipment and Standards for surface contamination measurements. *International Radiation Protection Association, IRPA9 Congress,* Vol 3, pp 34-36, ISBN 3-9500255-4-5, Vienna, Austria, April 1996

Sahagia, M., Razdolescu, A.C., Grigorescu, E.L., Ivan, C., Luca, A. (1996b) National comparison of I-131 solution measurements in Romanian Nuclear Units. *International Radiation Protection Association, IRPA 9 Congress,* Proceedings Vol 3, pp 497- 499.ISBN 3-9500255-4-5, Vienna, Austria, April 1996.

Sahagia, M., Razdolescu, A.C., Grigorescu, E.L., Luca, A., Ivan, C. (2002) Precise measurement of the activity of ^{186}Re, ^{188}Re pharmaceuticals. *Applied Radiations and Isotopes,* Vol 56, pp, 349-356, ISBN 0969-8043

Sahagia,M., Razdolescu, A.C., Campeanu, C., Grigorescu, E.L., Luca. A., Ivan, C. (2005a). Preparation and standardization of a $^{153}SmCl_3$ radiopharmaceutical solution. *International Conference "High Precision Atomic & Nuclear Methods", HIPAN02,* Proceedings, Ed. Romanian Academy, pp 101-107, ISBN 973-27-1181-7

Sahagia, M., Razdolescu, A.C., Grigorescu, E.L., Luca, A., Ivan, C., Lungu, V.(2005b) The standardization of ^{177}Lu solution and its use in nuclear medicine. *EUR Report EN22136*, Luxembourg, EC (2005b) 181-184

Sahagia, M. (2006) Standardization of ^{99m}Tc. *Applied Radiations and Isotopes,* Vol 64, pp 1234-1237, ISBN 0969-8043

Sahagia, M., Razdolescu, A. C., Ivan, C., Luca, A. (2008a) Assurance of the traceability chain for ^{131}I measurement. *Applied Radiations and Isotopes,* Vol. 66, pp 539-544, ISBN 0969-8043

Sahagia, M., Ivan, C., Grigorescu, E.L., Razdolescu, A. C. (2008b) Standardization of ^{125}I by the coincidence method and practical applications. *Applied Radiations and Isotopes,* Vol. 66, pp 895-899, ISBN 0969-8043

Sahagia, M., Woods, M. J. (2008c) The national dissemination of international measurements. *American Institute of Physics,* AIP Conf. Proc.1036, pp.12-25, ISBN 978-0-7354-0560-8

Sahagia, M., Wätjen, A.C., Ivan, C. (2009) Progress in organizing national and international comparisons for nuclear medicine measurements. *Romanian Journal of Physics,* Vol 54, pp 619-627, ISSN 1221-146

Sahagia, M., Wätjen, A.C., Luca, A., Ivan, C. (2010a) IFIN-HH ionization chamber calibration and its validation; electrometric system improvement. *Applied Radiations and Isotopes,* Vol 68, pp 1266 – 1269, ISBN 0969-8043

Sahagia, M., Wätjen, A. C., Luca, A., Ivan, C., Antohe, A. (2010b) National and international comparisons on radiopharmaceuticals' activity measurement. *Romanian Journal of Physics.* Vol 55, pp 733-740, ISSN 1221-146

Sahagia, M., Luca, A., Antohe, A., Ivan, C. (2011) Standardization of ^{64}Cu and ^{68}Ga by the 4πPC-γ coincidence method and calibration of the ionization chamber. *18-th International Conference on Radionuclide Metrology and its Applications, ICRM2011,* Tsukuba, Japan, 18-23 September 2011

Schrader, H. (1997) *Activity Measurements with Ionization Chambers,* Monographie BIPM-4, Bureau International des Poids et Mesurements, Sèvres, France

Sima, O., Arnold, D. (2002) Transfer of the efficiency calibration Gamma-ray detectors using the GESPECOR software. *Applied Radiations and Isotopes,* Vol 56, pp 71-75, ISBN 0969-8043

Smith, D. (1978) Improved correction formulae for coincidence counting. *Nuclear Instruments and Methods,* Vol 152, pp 505-519, ISSN 0168-9002

Stanga, D., Picolo, J.L., Coursol, N., Mitev, K., Moreau, L. (2002) Analytical calculations of counting losses in internal gas proportional counting. *Applied Radiations and Isotopes,* Vol 56, pp 231-236, ISBN 0969-8043

Technical Reports Series 454 (TRS 454) (2006) *Quality Assurance for Radioactivity Measurement in Nuclear Medicine.* pp.1-96. Contributors to drafting and review: Dondi, M., Herbst, C.P., Iwahara, A., Morengo, M., Mather, S., Norenberg, J.P., Olsovcova,V., Oropesa Verdicia, P., Otiz-Lopez, P., Joseph, L., Ghafoori,M., Onto, J.A., Ramamoorthy, N., Sahagia, M., Shortt, K.R., Tastan, S., Woods, M.J. , Zimmerman, B.E. ISSN 0074-1914 no.454 STI/DOC/010/454, ISBN 92-0-105306-1, IAEAL-06-00465

Terlikowska, T., Hainos, D., Cassette, P., Radoszewski, T. (2000) Application of α/β discrimination in liquid scintillation counting for the purity control of ^{99m}Tc medical solutions. *Applied Radiations and Isotopes,* Vol 52, pp 627-632, ISBN 0969-8043

Toohey, R.E., Stabin, M.G.(1996) Effective dose and effective dose equivalent in nuclear medicine. *Proceedings of International Radiation Protection Association, IRPA9 Congress,* Vienna, Austria. Vol 3, pp 475-477, ISBN 3-9500255-4-5, Vienna, Austria, April 1996.

Woods, M.J., Sahagia, M. (2008) The international framework for maintaining equivalence and traceability in radionuclide metrology. *American Institute of Physics,* AIP Conf. Proc 1036, pp.5-11, ISBN 978-0-7354-0560-8

Wyngaardt, W.M., Simpson, B.R.S. (2006) A simple counting technique for measuring mixtures of two pure beta-emitting radionuclides. *Nuclear Instruments and Methods A,* Vol 564, pp 339 -346, ISSN 0168-9002

Zimmerman, B. E., Judge, S. (2007) Traceability in nuclear medicine. *Metrologia,* Vol 44, pp S127 – S132, ISSN 0028-1394

Zimmerman, B. E., Megzifene, A., Shortt, K.R. (2008) Establishing measurement traceability for national laboratories: results of an IAEA comparison of ^{131}I. *Applied Radiations and Isotopes,* Vol 66, pp 954-959, ISBN 0969-8043

Zimmerman, B.E., Palm, S. (2010) Results of an international comparison of ^{57}Co. *Applied Radiations and Isotopes,* Vol 68, pp 1217-1220, ISBN 0969-8043

7

Breast Cancer: Radioimmunoscintigraphy and Radioimmunotherapy

Mojtaba Salouti and Zahra Heidari
Department of Biology, Faculty of Sciences, Zanjan Branch, Islamic Azad University, Zanjan, Iran

1. Introduction

Breast cancer is one of the most common diseases and a major public health problem in the world today. It is responsible for 32% of all cancers and 15% of cancer deaths in women (Dirisamer et al., 2010). Advances in diagnosis and treatment of breast cancer have led to decline in mortality. However, just about 60% of patients can now be cured by initial treatments, but the rest, in spite of receiving palliation with currently available therapy methods die. Therefore, tremendous amounts of time and efforts are dedicated to search toward earlier detection and more efficient treatment of this disease. Advances in molecular cancer biology achieved an increased understanding of the biologic factors that contribute to breast cancer pathogenesis and progression. This understanding has already led to both early diagnosis and more effective treatment. Among different imaging and therapy contribution modalities, nuclear medicine provides an important role to the clinical management of breast cancer. In this chapter, we highlight the uses, advantages, limitations and possible improvements of radioimmunoscintigraphy and radioimmunotherapy techniques as targeted molecular imaging and therapy methods, respectively.

2. Diagnosis of breast cancer

Breast cancer is currently the most common cancer in females and the second highest cause of cancer death in female population of the world. The majority of breast cancer deaths are due to metastasis (Costelloe et al., 2009). If breast cancer is detected prior to metastatic spread, it has considerably better prognosis than the cancer that has already spread. Therefore, the detection of cancer in an early stage is a major factor in the reduction of patient mortality and leading to less cancer costs and more successful treatments. The management of patients with a suspicious lesion includes confirming the diagnosis, identifying the stage of disease and choosing an appropriate treatment for each individual patient. Identifying the stage of a disease in any patient is a crucial step, because it determines the type of treatment that is appropriate for that particular person. Also, it is necessary to follow patients that need therapeutic procedures to assess their response to the treatment. There are a number of methods available for the detection of breast cancer. This section briefly points out some difficulties that encounter with these conventional imaging modalities and describes application of nuclear medicine techniques and targeted molecular imaging in the investigation of patients with breast cancer.

2.1 Mammography

Mammography is a gold standard imaging method for breast cancer screening, detection and diagnosis in women under forty with a relatively high sensitivity in the range of 85-90% (Berg et al., 2004). This method is a national screening program in the United Kingdom (Glasspool & Evans., 2000). Although mammography is an effective imaging tool, it is not without limitations like many other diagnostic modalities. First, the sensitivity of mammography decreases dramatically in young patients due to their dense breast tissues. On the other hand, its ability to detect malignant lesions in young female patients decreases to 68% (Nystrom et al., 2002, Kopans, 1992). As a result, some patients with breast cancer are missed and some others without a malignant tumor undergo unnecessary biopsies due to incorrect mammography findings. Secondly, mammography in patients evaluated following breast surgery or radiotherapy, is unreliable with a false negative rate of 25-45%, because it cannot always differentiate benign from malignant diseases (Fass, 2008). Many efforts have ever been taken to establish new tests to enable us to collect more complete information by non-invasive methods. These efforts minimize the use of breast biopsy in women who do not have breast cancer. Therefore, many other imaging modalities such as ultrasonography (US), magnetic resonance imaging (MRI), diffuse optical tomography (DOT), computed tomography (CT) and measurement of tumor markers in blood serum have been initiated to increase the diagnostic accuracy of mammography.

2.2 Ultrasonography

Ultrasonography is an important adjunct to mammography for both diagnosis and characterization of breast cancer and is routinely used in this role (Fass, 2009). It is non-invasive, easily available, relatively cheap and also recommended for pregnant or lactating women when ionizing radiation may not be recommended (Schueller et al., 2008). It has been found that ultrasonography, when combined with mammography, can prevent up to 22% of unnecessary biopsies (Zonderland, 2000). Although ultrasonography can reliably differentiate a cystic lesion from a solid lesion, it does not provide a high specificity to distinguish benign from malignant lesions (Balleyguier et al., 2008; Sauer et al., 2005). Another disadvantage of this method as a screening tool, when applied to general population, is low sensitivity and specificity and furthermore it is operator-dependent (Liberman, 2000).

2.3 Magnetic Resonance Imaging (MRI)

Breast cancer was one of the first that was examined using MRI (Ross et al., 1982). This method is very useful for further evaluation when mammography and ultrasonography are indeterminate to study the presence or location of a suspect abnormality (Glasspool et al., 2000). However, due to cost reasons, low access and high false positives, MRI is not yet considered as a screening exam for breast cancer except for special cases. MRI of breast cancer is recommended in the repeated screening of patients who have the increased risk of radiation induced DNA mutations (Fass, 2008). MRI is used to screen women with a family history of breast cancer, women with very dense breast tissues or women with silicone implants that can obscure pathology in mammography (Fass, 2008).

2.4 Diffuse Optical Tomography (DOT)

While breast cancer is still increasing in frequency, new diagnostic procedures must be available to challenge existing procedures to make diagnosis of breast cancer more accurate and reliable. DOT is one of the most important non-invasive and non-ionizing imaging modalities that are available for breast cancer diagnosis. DOT can be used to locate lesions within breast (Frangioni, 2008; Kepshire et al., 2007; Hawrysz et al, 2000). Despite promising results, there are several factors that limit the wide application of DOT for the imaging of breast tissue in clinic. First, the maximum depth of imaging in breast tissue is less than 15 mm. Secondly, the spatial resolution of DOT is less than one centimeter, that is not as good as mammography, ultrasonography or MRI. Because of these limitations, DOT is not a widely-accepted imaging modality for breast cancer (Kepshire et al., 2007; Hawrysz et al., 2000).

2.5 Computed Tomography (CT)

X-ray computed tomography (introduced into clinical practice in 1972) was the first of modern slice-imaging modalities. CT scan has several advantages including (1) unlimited depth penetration; (2) high spatial resolution; (3) short acquisition time (minutes); (4) moderately cheap and (5) ability of performing anatomical imaging. CT has some limitations including (1) sensitivity of CT scan decreases in early stage of breast cancer, (2) CT scan is associated with radiation exposure and should never be done in pregnant females because of radiation risk to the fetus, (3) CT is not very good at identifying pathology of soft tissues, (4) the dye used in CT is iodine based and is often a cause of allergy and (5) CT probably can not be used for molecular imaging and currently is just used for anatomical and functional imaging (Pysz et al., 2010).

2.6 Measurement of tumor markers in blood

Several biochemical compounds in the serum/plasma may act as the indicators of the presence, risk or prognosis of cancer. In patients with history of breast cancer, elevated tumor marker levels may represent cases of tumor relapse. It has been shown that increasing levels of tumor markers is associated with disease recurrence and may indicate the need for further investigations. Examples of tumor markers in blood including CA 15.3, CA 27.29, CA125, CEA and circulating tumor cells. While breast cancer blood marker tests are promising, they are not absolutely conclusive. When a breast cancer blood marker test comes back negative, it doesn't necessarily mean that the patient is free and clear of breast cancer and a positive result does not always mean that the cancer is growing (Merkle et al., 2009).

2.7 Nuclear medicine

As cited, each imaging method has strengths and weaknesses in terms of sensitivity, specificity, spatial and temporal resolution, contrast and cost. Therefore, the fundamental efforts for introduction and development of new methods for breast cancer diagnosis are requested. Nuclear medicine is defined as a branch of medicine that employs open radioactive sources, commonly referred to radionuclides, in diagnosis and treatment of diseases (Glasspool & Evans, 2000). The application of nuclear medicine techniques to study patients with breast cancer has recently raised its profile particularly in the investigation of indeterminate mammographic lesions and for overcoming limitations of MRI, US, CT and

DOT techniques (Berghammer et al., 2001). The differences in tumor biology such as blood flow, metabolism, concentration of specific receptors or differences in antigen expression are exploited in order to target radionuclides to the tumor tissue (Glasspool & Evans, 2000). The major advantage of nuclear medicine is that just picomolar concentrations of radiotracers are required to provide a measurable signal (Cook et al., 2003).

2.7.1 Scintimammography

Future developments in nuclear medicine are in the area of development of specialized imaging systems. One example of specialized gamma camera is scintimammography in imaging of breast and axillary nodes. Scintimammography term is given to radionuclide imaging of breast cancer (Schillaci et al., 2007). Scintimammography is performed after injection of the radiopharmaceutical into an arm vein contralateral to the suspected tumor or into a pedal vein and the subsequent imaging with right and left lateral, prone and supine views, covering both breasts and both axillae and later computer acquisition of data (Nguyen et al., 2009; Brem et al., 2005). Most studies evaluating the role of scintimammography, have compared it with mammography, ultrasound and MRI. Its sensitivity has ranged from 62% to 93% with specificity from 79% to 94% (Schillaci & Buscombe, 2004). Its sensitivity is greater for palpable lesions. Current recommendations for the use of scintimammography are (Fass, 2008):

1. As a general adjunct to mammography to differentiate between benign and malignant breast lesions in patients with palpable masses or suspicious mammograms.
2. In patients referred for biopsy when lesions are considered to have a low probability of malignancy.
3. In patients with probably benign findings on mammography, but are recommended for close follow-up (e.g. repeated mammography in 3–6 months).
4. In patients who have dense breast tissues and are considered difficult to evaluate on mammography.
5. For detection of axillary lymph node metastases in patients with confirmed breast cancer.

The main limitations of scintimamography are low sensitivity and high dose of radionuclide that is used for imaging. Currently, for overcoming the cited limitations, the researchers are studying on targeted molecular imaging methods.

3. Treatment of breast cancer

To understand the diagnostic needs for breast cancer, it is important to understand the range of approaches for breast cancer treatment. With the exception of early and late stage disease, almost all breast cancer therapy methods, involve a combination of locoregional and systemic treatments. Locoregional therapy includes surgery and radiotherapy and systemic therapy includes chemotherapy, hormone therapy and targeted therapy. Because the breast cancer, that is metastatic beyond the regional node, is rarely cured, systemic therapy is the primary treatment for metastatic disease with locoregional treatment reserved for symptom control and is used possibly in some patients with limited metastatic disease who may achieve prolonged remissions.

3.1 Surgery

Surgery is the oldest and still the most widely used treatment modality that is available for breast cancer patients and can be accomplished by mastectomy, removal of the entire breast or by breast-conserving surgery often termed lumpectomy of cancer. If the tumor is detected at early stage before spreading, surgery alone might be sufficient to reach complete remission. When the tumor is detected after spreading with distant metastases, surgery is frequently used in combination with radiotherapy or chemotherapy (Keshtgar et al, 2010).

3.2 Radiotherapy

In radiotherapy, also known as radiation therapy, high-energy ionizing radiation such as x or γ-rays is irradiated to the tumor tissues for killing the cancer cells. Radiation can be delivered via external radiation from a source outside the body directing to the tumor or by an internal radiation source (brachytherapy) which is positioned inside the body adjacent to or inside the tumor. Radiation must affect only cancer cells in the treated area and not normal cells. To treat secondary tumors and stopping growth of any remaining tumor cells, radiation therapy is often used in conjunction with other treatment modalities like chemotherapy and surgery (Luini et al., 2007).

3.3 Chemotherapy

The use of cytotoxic chemotherapy, in both advanced and early stage of breast cancer, has made significant progress in the last decade (Hassan et al., 2010). Chemotherapy is a systemic breast cancer therapy and compared to surgery and radiation therapy, it has one advantage. It is able to eliminate cancer cells throughout the entire body. Chemotherapeutic agents currently approved for treatment of breast cancer are: anthracycline, alkaloids, topoisomerase inhibitors, alkylating agents, and antimetabolites. The important disadvantage of chemotherapy is side effects of drugs such as nausea, vomiting, fatigue, sore mouth, diarrhea, constipation and decreased blood cells count. These side effects can impact patient ability to tolerate treatment, maintain a healthy diet, stay active and enjoy a good quality of life (Hassan et al., 2010).

3.4 Hormone therapy

Hormone therapy, also called "endocrine-based therapy", is a systemic treatment and plays an important role in breast cancer therapy. It is the first type of systemic treatment directed at a specific target, the hormone-dependent cancer cell, and may be referred to "targeted therapy" (Hind et al., 2007). The purpose of hormone therapy is to add, block or remove hormones. There are certain hormones that can attach to breast cancer cells and affect their ability to multiply such as tamoxifen, fareston, arimidex and so on (Jones& Buzdar, 2004). Hormone therapy may be used alone or in combination with radiation therapy. It is rarely used simultaneously, but is often used following chemotherapy. The benefits and side effects of the drugs relate only to the natural effects of the hormone itself and the hormone-cancer cell interaction. For that reason, the typical side effects seen with chemotherapy are not present with hormone or endocrine-based therapies (Hind et al., 2007).

3.5 Immunotherapy

Immunotherapy (also called biological therapy, biotherapy or biological response modifier therapy) of breast cancer uses patient body's natural ability (immune system) to fight the disease and/or to lesson treatment-related side effects (Diss et al., 1997b). The immunotherapy drugs are bound to specific proteins on breast cancer cells to slow or stop their growth. Currently, there are at least three FDA-approved antibodies for targeting of breast cancers (Stipsanelli & Valsamaki, 2005; Disis et al., 1994a, 1997b):

- Trastuzumab (Herceptin) that is bound to the extracellular domain of Her2/neu receptor
- Pertuzumab that is bound to a different epitope of Her2/neu receptor
- Bevacizumab that is bound to vascular endothelial growth factor receptors (VEGFRs).

Immunotherapy of breast cancer may cause side effects such as fever, chill, pain, weakness, nausea, vomiting, diarrhea, headache, and rash. These side effects generally become less severe after the first treatment. In addition, immunotherapy is a very expensive method for patients.

4. Targeted molecular imaging and therapy

The researchers are trying to improve the methods that can decrease the dose of drugs and transfer them just to the tumor cells with high efficiency and kill the cancer cells without affecting healthy cells. The recent improvements in biology of tumor cells, have introduced new methods in diagnosis and therapy of cancer named targeted molecular imaging and therapy (Sawyers, 2004). The knowledge of the diversities between tumor and normal tissues is the key to identify novel targets for new selective diagnosis and therapeutic strategies (Gasparini et al., 2005). The aim of these methods is to deliver a drug for therapy or a contrast agent for imaging just to the tumor site or cancer cells using different technologies. In these methods, not only the dose of drugs is decreased, but also the damage to the normal tissues is decreased. On the other hand, the probability of the diagnosis and therapy is increased too. In addition, the targeting methods in comparison with other methods have fewer side effects and the patients tolerate less physical and mental hurts. Tumor markers are used for targeting cancer cells in molecular imaging and therapy methods. Tumor marker is objectively measured and evaluated as an indicator of normal biological processes, pathogenic processes or pharmacologic responses to a therapeutic intervention (Meel et al., 2010).

4.1 Targeted molecular imaging

Recent advances in molecular and cellular biology have facilitated the discovery of novel molecular targets on tumor cells such as key molecules involved in proliferation, differentiation, cell death and apoptosis, angiogenesis, invasion and metastasis or associated with cancer cell stemness (William et al., 2008). Molecular imaging is defined as visualization, characterization and measurement of biological processes at the molecular and cellular levels in human beings and other living systems (Pysz et al., 2010). Today, molecular imaging is increasingly used in clinical oncology, because molecular imaging is a non-invasive diagnostic method that allows for more sensitive and specific monitoring of key cancer-related molecular targets in vivo and is expected to play an important role in future cancer diagnosis. Generally, molecular targets can be applied to (Meel et al., 2010; Neves & Brindle, 2006):

1. Detection: screening high-risk groups and large populations of asymptomatic individuals
2. Diagnosis of cancer in individuals with signs or symptoms
3. As a prognostic indicator
4. Localization of tumor and metastases

5. Staging the extent of disease
6. Monitor the clinical course of cancer patients
7. Determine the effectiveness of therapy
8. Early detection of recurrent or metastatic cancer

A molecular imaging agent typically consists of a signaling moiety (radionuclide in nuclear medicine) and a functional target. Specific targeting of cancer-associated targets with radiolabeled targeting agents (e.g. antibodies, peptides and non-immunoglobulin proteins) and the use of subsequent visualization systems like gamma camera, SPECT and PET are examples of molecular imaging methods in nuclear medicine.

4.2 Targeted molecular therapy

Major advances in molecular biology, cellular biology and genomics have substantially improved our understanding of cancers. Now, these advances are being translated into therapy. The term targeted therapy ideally connotes the ability to identify a known therapeutic target that is important in the biology of cancer cells and use a specific agent that can treat the disease by modifying the expression or activity of the target in the growth and progression of the cancer. With this approach, only patients with a likelihood of benefit are treated, so the therapeutic index will hopefully be improved. Selecting a biologically active target is usually the first step in molecular imaging research and leads to the design of a molecular imaging agent. Potential targets include proteins, DNA, RNA, carbohydrates and lipids. Several properties of these biomolecules as imaging targets need to be considered that are summarized in the following (Meel et al., 2010):

1. High specificity (i.e. binding specifically to a tumor-associated molecular target with minimal non-specific binding to non-target molecules).
2. High target binding affinity (low subnanomolar binding is typically desired).
3. Small size (enabling fast distribution to the tumor and quick clearance from the blood and other compartments).
4. High structural stability for labeling with signaling agents.
5. Available ligands that specifically target these biomolecules.

5. Targeted molecular agents of breast cancer

Molecular probes in nuclear medicine are the proof of principle for targeted molecular imaging and therapy. Molecular nuclear medicine holds the unique potential of being able to find, diagnose and treat diseases as well as to monitor treatment response. Several molecular targeting agents have been approved for clinical uses in nuclear medicine. Many others are under preclinical evaluation with high potential for clinical applications. The molecular targeting agents, that are common in nuclear medicine, are small molecules, oligonucleotides /PNAs, affibodys, peptides and antibodies.

5.1 Small molecules

Several radiolabeled small molecules have been applied for the detection and therapy of breast and prostate tumors and leukemia (Cornelissen & Vallis, 2010). For example, radiolabeled estrogens and estrogen receptor antagonists are bound to the estrogen receptor, a nuclear membrane receptor, which then translocate to the nucleus. 123I- tamoxifen, an estrogen receptor (ER) antagonist, has been used as a diagnostic tool to determine estrogen receptor status in patients with breast or head-and-neck cancer (Wiele et al., 2001). Other small-molecule radiopharmaceuticals include 125I-daunorubicin, 111In-folate, 123/131I metaiodo- benzyl-guanidine (MIBG), 125I-iododeoxyuridine and 111In-bleomycin (Jalilian et al., 2006, 2007). Small molecules such as tyrosine kinase inhibitors (TKIs) are less specific than therapeutic monoclonal antibodies (mAbs) (Huang & Armstrong,2004) and some of them can inhibit multiple targets simultaneously including cell receptors or signal transduction pathway proteins leading to a higher risk for toxicity (Xia et al., 2005).

5.2 Oligonucleotides/ PNAs/ MORF

The natural ability of oligonucleotides and the oligonucleotide mimetic peptide nucleic acids (PNAs) and phosphorodiamidate morpholinos (MORF) to anneal with RNA and DNA makes them the appealing vehicles to bring radionuclides in close proximity to the RNA/DNA. Both 125I and 111In have been used to radiolabel oligonucleotides and have been applied successfully to target over-expression of certain genes involved with cancer (Cornelissen & Vallis, 2010).

Aptamers are synthetically based DNA or RNA oligonucleotides that are highly stable structures and are considered to have low immunogenicity. They are selected for their ability to bind to a target of interest (Perkins & Missailidis, 2007). Hicke et al. demonstrated that the aptamers cleared quickly from the blood, reaching maximum tumor uptake within 10 min, but then decreasing to approximately 2% by 3 h. However, the rapid clearance from the blood and tissues resulted in highly favorable tumor/blood and kidney ratios but there was considerable additional clearance of the 99mTc through the liver and intestines (Hicke et al., 2006). However, using aptamers as the radiopharmaceuticals needs further improvements.

5.3 Affibody molecules

Affibody molecules are 58 amino-acid, three-helix bundle affinity proteins and are derived from the β-domain of the five-domain Ig-binding region protein A from *Staphylococcus aureus* (Orlova et al., 2007). They represent highly specific binders, selected by phage display from a library generated by randomization of 13 amino acids in helix 1 and 2, which are responsible for the Fc-binding site. Recently, affibody molecules have been investigated for tumor targeting purposes both for targeted imaging and therapy. The first generated and used affibody molecule for radionuclide imaging was Z_{HER2} with a binding affinity of 50 nM to HER2 protein (Capalaet al., 2009). Affibody molecules represent a promising novel class of targeting molecules that can be used as relatively small, high-affinity, cancer-specific ligands and that are well suited for tumor molecular imaging and therapy, providing a possible new route for imaging of tumor-specific receptors (Orlova et al., 2006). Since these structures are derived from a *Staphylococcal* protein, the potential immunogenicity of these molecules may be a concern (Sharkey & Goldenberg, 2008).

5.4 Peptides

During the past decade, proof of the principle that peptide receptors can be used successfully for in vivo targeting of human cancers, has been provided (Ferro-Flores et al., 2010). Peptides used for tumor targeting show some advantages over antibodies. Peptides are small and show rapid diffusion into the target tissues resulting in rapid pharmacokinetics (Ferro-Flores et al., 2010). Their fast blood clearance can lead to high tumor to background ratio shortly after administration of the radiopeptide. In addition, they can tolerate harsh chemical conditions and are easy to be purified and modified. The common peptides that are used in molecular imaging and therapy of breast cancer are somatostatin, bombesin, neuropeptide Y (NPY) and vasoactive intestinal peptide (VIP) (Ferro-Flores et al., 2010). The important disadvantage of peptides is rapid degrading from blood by endogenous peptidases and proteases (Ferro-Flores et al., 2010).

5.5 Antibodies

Antibodies are now increasingly recognized as important biological agents for the detection and treatment of cancer (Sharkey & Goldenberg, 2006). In the 1970s, polyclonal antibodies were already essential components of medical diagnosis as well as for therapy as antitoxins for the prevention of tetanus and other diseases (Goldsmith & Signore, 2010). The development of monoclonal antibody technology by Kohler and Milstein in the 1970s accelerated the exploitation of the chemo-specificity of antibodies for diagnostic and therapeutic purposes (Goldsmith & Signore, 2010). In the last two decades several different monoclonal antibodies have been approved by the Food and Drug Administration (FDA) for therapeutic purposes and some of these have also been radiolabeled for diagnostic and therapeutic purposes (Xiao et al., 2008). For imaging, it is highly desirable that targeting agents are rapidly excreted from the body. It is also essential that the targeting agent binds rapidly to its target, reducing the time between injection and imaging. The application of monoclonal antibodies for therapy and diagnosis is limited by generation of an immune response known as human anti-mouse antibody (HAMA) response (Salouti et al., 2011). One of the most successful approaches to overcome immunogenicity is "humanization" of rodent mAbs by genetic engineering (Waldmann&Morris, 2008). A simple approach to make an antibody to be more humanized is the replacement of the constant domains of the antibody with constant domains of a human antibody. The resulting chimeric antibody contains only the variable regions of murine origin and would therefore be expected to be less immunogenic in people. Many chimeric antibodies have been prepared and shown to retain the full antigen binding ability of the parent murine antibody as well as taking on the constant region effecter functions of the human antibody used (Waldmann&Morris, 2008). Humanization of rodent antibodies can be taken further to produce fully humanized antibodies in the form of reshaped, engineered human antibodies, in which much of the variable domain sequences are also replaced by human antibody sequence. In these approaches, the antigen binding loops are derived from the rodent antibody and much of the supporting framework is humanized (Waldmann&Morris, 2008). Targeting agents that have been approved for breast cancer include trastuzumab and pertuzumab directed against human epidermal growth factor receptor 2 (HER2) and bevacizumab, directed against vascular endothelial growth factor (VEGF) (Goldsmith & Signore, 2010). Several other targeting agents are currently under evaluation in preclinical and clinical trials (Carl & Roland, 2001).

5.5.1 Antibody derivatives

The use of mAbs has presented challenges in radionuclide imaging. Because of their large size (molecular weight of ~150 kDa), mAbs penetrate slowly and have long residence time in the blood circulation (days-weeks) due to active recycling by the neonatal Fc receptor, leading to limited tumor-to-normal organs ratio in biodistribution and low contrast images for the detection of biomarkers/tumors (Jonathan et al., 2000). Advances in protein engineering have led to a number of alternative constructs for imaging and therapy. These alternatives characterized by smaller size include:

- **Fragment antigen binding (Fab):** The area around the antibody hinge is more susceptible to proteolysis than the tightly folded domains and thus this is the point at which cleavage usually takes place. Proteolysis above the disulphide bonds in the hinge region with, for example papain, results in Fab fragments which are monovalent for antigen binding (~55 kDa).
- **Divalent fragment antigen binding ($F(ab')_2$):** If antibody proteolysis occurs below the hinge disulphide bonds, with enzymes such as pepsin, it results in a divalent $F(ab')_2$ fragment (~110 kDa).
- **Single chain fragment (scFv):** This antibody fragment consists only the variable heavy (VH) and the variable light (VL) chain of an antibody tethered together by a flexible linker, attaching the carboxyl terminus of the VL sequence to the amino terminus of the VH sequence (~25 kDa).
- **Nanobody:** Nanobodies are small antibody fragments (15 kDa) derived from the naturally occurring heavy-chain-only antibodies (Friedman. et al., 2009). These fragments have also been referred to VHH as they consist of a variable domain (VH) of the heavy chain (H) of antibodies (Meel et al., 2010).

When compared to intact IgGs, these antibody fragments have the advantages of faster biodistribution, rapid penetration into the tissues and improved tumor-to-normal organs ratio. These forms (e.g. $F(ab')_2$, Fab or other molecular constructs) achieve maximum tumor accretion more quickly with improved tumor/blood ratio that make earlier visualization, possible (Colcher et al., 1998). The use of fragments of antibodies has also been advocated as a possible means to reduce the immunogenicity of rodent antibodies in human beings. Antibody fragments generated by proteolysis or by genetic engineering, have been tested both in vitro and in vivo. As monovalent binding entities, antibody fragments suffer from relatively low avidity binding. Hence, to increase their binding avidity, they have also been engineered into multivalent constructs include:

- **Diabody:** "Diabody" is one of the engineered multivalent constructs. Diabodies can be produced to high levels in the form of stable dimmers (Wu & Yazaki, 2000; Hudson & Kortt, 1999; Lawrence et al., 1998). However, the stability of such dimeric species varies from one antibody to another.
- **Tribody:** In some cases, particularly with direct fusions of VH and VL, stable trimeric species are produced which have been termed "tribody" (Todorovskaet al., 2001). Some tribodies show improved avidity for antigens as expected from the increased number of binding sites, although this is not always the case (Todorovskaet al., 2001).

6. Target antigens

In recent years, there has been a significant improvement in the understanding of molecular events and critical pathways involved in breast cancer. The studies have confirmed the feasibility of using radiolabeled antibodies for imaging and therapy of primary and metastatic breast cancer and that a diverse array of molecules can serve as targets for localizing antibodies (Carlos et al., 2006). Theoretically, an ideal target for radionuclide detection and therapy of metastatic breast cancer would be tumor-specific, generously expressed on all the breast cancer cells, not expressed by normal tissues and not released into the blood circulation (Mohammadnejad et al., 2010). For antibody screening of breast cancer, it is essential that the antibody is well characterized with little cross-reactivity to other antigens. The antibodies show cross-reactivity with, e.g. leucocytes, potentially yielding false-positive images. The majority of breast cancer targeting antibody studies have used antibodies against MUC1, CEA, TAG-72 and L6 antigens (Carlos et al., 2006).

6.1 CEA

First described by Gold and Freedman in 1965, CEA was thought to be a specific marker for colon adenocarcinoma. However, subsequent studies demonstrated CEA expression in other human adenocarcinomas including the surface membrane of breast cancer cells (Jonathan et al., 2000). Expression of CEA has been reported in 10% to 95% of breast cancers (Hong et al., 2008, Denardo, 2005). Preliminary studies with 99mTc-labeled CEA antibody appeared to indicate a useful role for this agent in distinguishing between benign and malignant breast lesions in patients with indeterminate mammographic findings (Denardo, 2005). Therapy studies specifically in breast cancer have also been performed with T84.66 (Koppe et al., 2005). T84.66 is a well characterized murine IgG1 antibody with high specificity and affinity for a unique epitope of CEA molecules. A chimeric form of T84.66 (cT84.66) has been also used in clinical studies for the scintigraphic detection of breast cancer and in phase I/II therapy trials and scFv-based anti-CEA constructs are under study (Denardo, 2005). Another mAb that has been classified in this group is NP4. NP-4 belongs to the murine IgG1 subclass and is specific for CEA, reacting with a class III peptide epitope of CEA molecules (Richman & DeNardo, 2001).

6.2 MUC-1

MUC-1 mucins are large, complex glycoproteins that have a polypeptide core with multiple oligosaccharide side chains (Mukhopadhyay et al., 2011). The mature molecule is anchored within the cell surface by a characteristic transmembrane domain, but most of the mucins are expressed extracellular. This polar distribution is lost with neoplastic transformation and increased heterogenous MUC-1 synthesis is a common feature of breast cancer. This glycoprotein is aberrantly over expressed in adenocarcinomas including 80% of breast cancers (Salouti et al., 2011). Targeting, using antibodies directed against the MUC-1 antigen has been tested in patients with breast cancer using various antibodies. BrE-3 is an IgG1 antibody directed against the peptide epitope of the MUC-1 antigen that have been evaluated for RIT (Mohammadnejad et al, 2010). The studies of the application of BrE-3 mAbs in patients with breast cancer showed minimal cross reactivity with normal breast tissues (Howell et al., 1995; Blank et al., 1992). Because the majority of the patients rapidly showed HAMA response against the murine BrE-3 mAb, a humanized version of BrE-3 (hBrE-3) was developed (Kramer et al., 1993). Kramer and colleagues investigated the pharmacokinetics and biodistribution of 111In-MX-DTPA-labeled hBrE-3 in seven patients with metastatic breast cancer (Kramer et al., 1993). hBrE-3 was proved to have a lower immunogenicity compared to murine BrE-3 (only one patient developed a HAMA response) while tumor-targeting properties were preserved (Denardo, 2005). Monoclonal antibody 170H.82 (m170) is a murine IgG1 prepared using a synthetic asialo GM1 terminal disaccharide immunogen related to the Thomsen–Friedenreich disaccharide and selected by reactivity with MUC-1 expressing cancer cell membranes (Jonathan et al., 2000). The results of experimens showed that labeled m170 was effective for imaging of primary and metastatic breast cancer and was able to detect lesions as small as 1 cm in size using SPECT with an overall clinical accuracy of 92%. In particular, mAb 170H.82 has been studied in breast cancer patients, with reported a sensitivity and specificity for detecting locoregional soft tissue disease of 90% and 93%, respectively (Denardo, 2005). Because aberrant MUC-1 has provided effective target for breast cancer, gene-engineered antibody fragments (scFv) have been developed to MUC-1 antigen by phage display immunoglobulin gene libraries from mice immunized with MUC-1 peptide core and MCF-7 membranes. Numerous other monoclonal antibodies have been generated against MUC1 and have been used for breast cancer imaging such as HMFG-1 and HMFG-2, SM3, DF3, 12H12, BM2 (formerly called 2El 1), BM7, EBA-1, MA5 and PR81 (Richman & Denardo, 2001; Salouti et al., 2008). Although, not all of these antibodies necessarily react with the same MUC1 determinant, they have all shown the ability to target breast cancer either in animal xenografts or in patients. Thus, these antibodies have been shown to be suitable antibodies for radioimmunoscintigraphy and radioimmunotherapy studies in this cancer type.

6.3 TAG-72

Immunohistochemical and immunocytochemical techniques have demonstrated preferential expression of TAG-72 known as tumor-associated glycoprotein in breast, gastrointestinal and ovarian adenocarcinomas compared to normal tissues (Denardo, 2005). Antibodies against the TAG-72 antigen particularly B72.3 and chB72.3 were evaluated in patients after careful study in human xenograft mouse models (Lorraine et al., 1998). The TAG-72 target antigen reactive with B72.3 pancarcinoma antibody has been used to target and image breast cancer (Denardo, 2005). CC49, a newer antibody to a different epitope of TAG-72, is a murine IgG1 monoclonal antibody that was labeled with Lutitium-177 by Milenic et al. (Milenic et al., 1991). He found that Lutitium-177 was an attractive alternative radionuclide with a lower energy beta emission and longer half life than 90Y. The images demonstrated the activity uptake at the site of tumor as well as in bone marrow.

6.4 L6

L6 cell surface antigen is a 24-kDa surface protein containing 3 hydrophobic transmembrane regions that are followed by a hydrophilic region (Richman & Denardo, 2001). L6 antigen is related to a number of cell surface proteins with similar predicted membrane topology that have been implicated in cell growth. L6 antigen is highly expressed in 50% of breast cancer specimens. Two mAb of this family, L6 mAb and the chimeric version (ChL6) have been studied in clinical trials (Denardo et al., 1994). 131I-Chimeric L6 antibody demonstrated therapeutic promise for patients with breast cancer (John et al., 2009).

6.5 EGFR

Epidermal growth factor receptor (EGFR) is a family of transmembrane growth factor receptor tyrosine kinases involved in regulation of cell proliferation and survival of epithelial cells (Cleator & Heller, 2007). EGFR family includes four receptors: EGFR/ErbB1, HER2/ErbB2, HER3/ErbB3 and HER4/ErbB4. EGFR and HER2 are over expressed in approximately 40% and 25% of breast cancers, respectively and associated with aggressive clinical behavior and poor prognosis. Due to the important roles of EGFR and HER2 receptors in diagnosis and therapy of breast cancer patients, both receptors are discussed in details (Munagalaet al., 2011).

- **EGFR receptor**

EGFR (also known as ErbB1 or HER1) is a 170 kDa transmembrane protein with an intracellular tyrosine-kinase domain. Many epithelial cancers including tumors of the head and neck, breast, colon, lung, kidney, prostate, brain, bladder and pancreas overexpress EGFR. Such overexpression is associated with poor prognosis and this leads to several strategies to block this pathway and improve the outcome. Cetuximab is a chimeric IgG1 monoclonal antibody that competes with an endogenous ligand to bind to the extracellular domain of EGFR (Harris, 2004). On the basis of these findings and those of previous studies, Cetuximab received FDA approval in February 2004, for using in treatment of EGFR-positive metastatic colorectal cancer (Harris, 2004).

- **HER2/Neu receptor**

The HER2/Neu receptor is a member of the EGFR family and another important cancer-related receptor that is over expressed in several human tumors notably on a subset of breast cancer cells (Ross et al., 2004). Trastuzumab (commonly referred to Herceptin) was the first recombinant bivalent humanized mAb targeted against extracellular domain of HER2 reported in 1998, has been approved by FDA and is frequently used clinically in "naked antibody" therapy (Rasaneh et al., 2009). Trastuzumab binds with high affinity to HER2 and leads to internalisation of HER2 receptor and blockage of signal transduction. Unlike chemotherapy, trastuzumab do not have toxic effects such as nausea, vomiting, hair loss and bone marrow toxicity (Munagala, 2011). Pertuzumab, a recombinant humanized monoclonal antibody, binds to extracellular domain II of HER2 receptor and blocks its ability to dimerize with other HER family receptors (HER1, HER2, HER3, HER4) (Untch, 2010). Pertuzumab is the first in a new class of targeted agents known as HER dimerization inhibitors (HDIs). The drug showed promising activity with trastuzumab in the treatment of metastatic breast cancer in a phase II study (Baselga et al., 2007, 2010). The patients treated with trastuzumab have an increased risk of developing cardiac dysfunction (Widakowich et al., 2007). When trastuzumab was conjugated with a radioneclide, the dose of drug was decreased that led to decrease its cardiac toxicity (Harris, 2004). Radioactive anti-HER2/neu rhumAb are considered attractive agents for RIS and RIT of aggressive HER-2/neu-positive breast carcinomas (Munnink, 2009).

6.6 VEGF

Vascular-endothelial growth factor (VEGF) is a proangiogenic growth factor that regulates vascular proliferation and permeability and is an antiapoptotic factor for new blood vessels. VEGF acts via two receptors, VEGFR1 and VEGFR2, which are expressed on the vascular endothelium. VEGFR expression is commonly increased in response to hypoxia, oncogenes and cytokines and its expression is associated with poor prognosis. Bevacizumab (Avastin) is a humanised monoclonal antibody that inhibits angiogenic signaling. In February, 2004, bevacizumab received FDA approval for using in the first line treatment of metastatic colorectal cancer in combination with 5-fluorouracil-based chemotherapy (Munnink, 2009). FDA is still moving toward stripping the cancer drug bevacizumab of its indication for treating advanced breast cancer, but not other cancers (Munnink, 2009).

7. Radioimmunoscintigraphy

It is well known that mammography provides a high sensitivity at the cost of relatively low specificity. Therefore, breast cancer diagnosis requires an adjunctive test to mammography that can increase diagnostic specificity while maintaining a high positive predictive value. Although sestamibi imaging has been introduced as an adjunctive test to mammography, it fails to provide the necessary sensitivity, specificity and predictive values for nonpalpable lesions, thus resulting in a relatively high false-positive rate in patient population. Several strategies have been developed over the past two decades for earlier and more accurate diagnosis of disease and to evaluate response to therapy. One of the novel approaches for specific detection of cancers is the use of monoclonal antibodies conjugated with radionuclides so-called radioimmunoscintigraphy (is also called radioimmunodetection, radioimmunoimaging and radioimmunodiagnosis) (Salouti, et al., 2006). In this method, a radio-isotope labeled antibody is administered to a patient with cancer. Once localized to the tumor tissue, the radioisotope (and hence the sites of malignancy) can be detected with a nuclear medicine imaging system like gamma camera. The summery of history for RIS has been shown in table 1. The efficacy of this technique depends on antigen expression on tumor cells compared to normal tissues. Affinity, specificity, pharmacokinethics, properties of the radionuclide and imaging technique have influence on the efficacy of radioimmunoscintigraphy. The potential clinical applications of RIS are (1) evaluation of patients with suspected breast cancer, (2) locoregional staging of newly discovered breast cancer, (3) detection of distant metastases using whole body scintigraphy and (4) evaluation of tumor response to therapy (Berghammer et al., 2001).

1908	Paul Ehrlich is generally recognised as the inventor of the term "magic bullets", describing the potential of an antibody to specifically target tumor cells.	Ehrlich, 1906
1953	This approach was invented by Pressman and his associates who discovered that radioiodinated antisera could concentrate selectively in tumors when injected parenterally into animals bearing tumors.	Pressmanand Korngold, 1953
1957	Gamma camera as initially introduced in 1957 by Hal Anger was designed to detect gamma photons within an energy window between 30 and 300 keV.	Anger et al., 1957
1963	David Kuhl and Roy Edwards were the first to present tomographic images using the Anger camera by acquiring multiple planar images from different angles and back projecting data into a 3 dimensional space. The technology is called SPECT.	Kuhl & Edwards, 1963
1965	Gold and Freedman discovered carcinoembryonic antigen (CEA), the first well defined tumor-associated antigen and as a result of this finding purified polyclonal anti-CEA antibodies were shown to localise to CEA expressing tumors in vivo.	Gold & Freedman, 1965
1975	Discovery of the hybridoma technique by Kohler and Milstein was perhaps the single most important contribution to the development of radioimmunoscintigraphy. Using the hybridoma technique, mass production antibodies of predetermined specificity with high quality became possible.	Kohler & Milstein, 1975
1978	Goldenberg presented a trial using radiolabeled antibodies to detect breast cancer effectively.	Goldenberg et al., 1978
1983	Methodologic improvements included the combined use of optimized radionuclide tracers such as SPECT and antibody fragments such as Fab fragments to improve the quality of nuclear medicine images of metastatic cancer *in vivo*.	Larson *et al.*, 1983a, b
1986	As a further advancement of chimeric mAbs, in 1986, Jones *et al.* reported the production of humanized monoclonal antibodies.	Jones PT et al.1986
1998	Trastuzumab (Herceptin) was approved by FDA for using in patients with metastatic breast cancer.	Cobleigh et al, 1999
2004	Radioactive anti-HER-2/neu rhuMAb were considered attractive agents for radioimmunodiagnosis of aggressive HER-2/neu-positive breast carcinomas.	Olafsen et al, 2004

Table 1. The summery of history for radioimmunoscintigraphy.

7.1 Radionuclides for imaging

The most common radionuclides in nuclear medicine are ^{99m}Tc, ^{123}I, ^{67}Ga and ^{111}In. Lower energy γ-rays are readily absorbed in tissues and therefore less useful for external imaging. On the other hand, highest energy γ-rays cause to decrease the sensitivity of imaging system (Berghammeret al., 2001). Technetium-99m is so far the most commonly used radionuclide in nuclear medicine (Hamoudeh et al., 2008). This is due to the highly interesting physical properties of 99mTc which is advantageous for both effective imaging and patient safety perspectives. Its properties include short half-life (6 h), gamma energy at 140 keV with practically no alpha or beta emissions and latent chemical properties, facilitating thereby the labeling of several types of kits for versatile diagnostic applications and readily available and inexpensive (it is derived as a column elute from a 99Mo/99mTc generator) (Verhaar et al., 2000). It is most often used with smaller antibody forms such as Fab, scFv, diabodies and nanobodies. The gamma-ray emitting radionuclides are commonly used in gamma camera and single photon emission tomography (SPECT). Other groups of diagnostically used radionuclides are $ß^+$ emitters such as ^{11}C, ^{18}F, ^{13}N and ^{15}O (Hamoudeh et al., 2008). The positron emitting radionuclides are used in positron emission tomography (PET). The positive electron travels only a short distance through the tissues and interacts with a free or loosely bound negative electron. The outcome of this interaction is two photons, consisting each of 511 keV energy and being given off in opposite directions (Boswell & Brechbiel, 2007).

7.2 Imaging systems in nuclear medicine

Imaging systems in nclear medicine include gamma camera, single photon emission computed tomography (SPECT) and positron emission tomography (PET).

7.2.1 Gamma camera

Gamma camera is a one-headed, variable-angle diagnostic instrument that is used to image gamma radiation emitting radioisotopes, a technique known as scintigraphy. Gamma camera consists of a scintillation crystal, optically coupled to an array of photomultiplier tubes which converts the γ-rays into electric signals.

7.2.2 Single photon emission tomography

Single photon emission computed tomography (SPECT) is a sensitive nuclear imaging technique that provides a 3D spatial distribution of single-photon emitting radionuclide within the body (Gomes et al., 2010). Multiple 2D images, also called projections, are acquired from multiple angles around the patient and subsequently reconstructed using the reconstruction imaging methods to generate cross-sectional images of the internal distribution of the injected molecules (Wernick, & Aarsvold,2004). Because of the isotropic emission of γ-rays, a geometric collimation is needed to restrict the travelling direction of the emitted γ-rays from the body, through the use of lead collimators. In clinical systems, collimators typically have many parallel holes that produce no magnification. The photons that travel in other directions than those specified by the aperture of collimator are absorbed and do not contribute to the image, which reduces the detection efficiency and sensitivity of SPECT as compared to PET (Madsen, 2007). SPECT have several advantages including (1) whole body imaging, (2) quantitative molecular imaging and (3) can be combined with CT for preparing anatomical information. The disadvantages of this method are radiation exposure, low spatial resoulation (0.3-1 mm, 12-15 $mm^{3)}$ and long acquisition time (Pysz et al., 2010).

7.2.3 Positron emission tomography (PET)

Positron emission tomography is a nuclear medicine technique that produces high resolution tomographic imaging through the detection of high energy photon pairs emitted during positron decay (Costelloeet al., 2009). This method was initially developed in 1960s, but has largely been used as a research tool. However, PET can provide useful information for clinical practice. The images generated by PET represent the metabolic activity of the underlying tissues and can therefore distinguish benign from malignant lesions on the basis of differences in metabolic activity. Similarly, it can identify recurrent diseases in areas in which conventional scans are difficult to interpret because of prior treatment (Costelloeet al., 2009). PET represents the most advanced imaging technique, because it not only allows a three-dimensional image reconstruction, but also it can quantify the activity uptake (Fass, 2008). It combines the highest degree of sensitivity with a resolution of currently, 5-7 mm. The principal applied radionuclide for PET is Fluor-18 (18F) which is known for its ideal half-life to manage (1.83 h). The development of radiopharmaceutical [2-18F]-2-fluoro-2-deoxyglucose (18FDG) has been so far an important progress for PET imaging in oncology (Berghammer et al., 2001). 18FDG acts as a glucose analogue allowing for the visualization of glucose consumption, a metabolic process being massively enhanced in many malignancies (Einat & Moshe, 2010). PET has several advantages include (1) unlimited depth penetration; (2) whole body imaging possible, (4) quantitative molecular imaging and (5) can be combined with CT or MRI for anatomical information (Pysz et al., 2010). The disadvantage of PET is that it requires a conveniently located and expensive cyclotron and radiochemistry facilities to produce the short-half life isotopes and to incorporate these into suitable probe molecules (Fass, 2008).

8. Radioimmunotherapy

The first theory on the existence of proteins with specific binding capabilities to pathogenic organisms, thus acting as "magic bullet"', was postulated at the end of the 19th century by the german pathologist Paul Ehrlich (Enelich, 1906). He was the first to recognise antibodies for their ability to differentiate between normal cells and transformed malignant cells. He specifically introduced immunotherapy as a potential treatment modality for targeting and treating tumors. After it had been recognized in 1950 that proteins could be labeled with 131I without significantly altering their immunological specificity (Eisen & Keston, 1950), Pressman and Korngold tested the tumor-targeting potential of a 131I-labeled rabbit antiserum in rats bearing osteosarcoma and confirmed preferential antibody uptake in the tumor xenografts (Pressman & Korngold, 1953). The first clinical trial investigated the therapeutic efficacy of radiolabeled antibodies was performed in the 1950s by Beierwaltes, who treated fourteen patients with metastatic melanoma with 131I-labeled rabbit antibodies and reported a pathologically confirmed remission in one patient (Beierwaltes, 1974). In 1965, Gold and Freedman discovered carcinoembryonic antigen (CEA), the first well defined tumor-associated antigen. The purified polyclonal anti-CEA antibodies were shown to localize to CEA expressing tumors in vivo (Gold & Freedman, 1965). In the late 1970s, Goldenberg and colleagues successfully targeted colon cancer in patients using a polyclonal goat anti-CEA antiserum (Goldenberg et al., 1978). Nowadays, CEA has not only become one of the most extensively used tumor markers in clinical oncology, but also due to its pronounced expression in various carcinomas, it is one of the most targeted antigens in RIT. In 1975, Köhler and Milstein reformed the field of radioimmunotargeting as they introduced the hybridoma technology, a method that made it possible to produce large quantities of monoclonal antibodies with high purity and reproducibility (Kohler & Milstein, 1975). Since then, numerous antigen-antibody systems have been established and several of the antibodies have been taken to clinical trials. Radioimmunotherapy is a method of selectively delivering radionuclides with toxic emissions to cancer cells, while reducing the dose to normal tissues. Using mAbs labeled with radionuclides has two major advantages over the application of mAbs conjugated with either drugs or toxins. Firstly, tumor cells not expressing the target antigen can still be sterilized by the so-called crossfire phenomenon, i.e., radiation energy emitted by radionuclides bound to antibodies targeting adjacent tumor cells. Secondly, radionuclides are not subject to multidrug resistance. Although promising, RIT has been less effective for solid tumors, in part because they are less radiosensitive. However, early micrometatasis of breast cancer have been demonstrated to be radiosensitive (Koppe et al., 2005). On the other hand, an advantage of RIT is that it can target small metastatic lesions that are undetected by conventional scanning and would otherwise remain untreated. In addition, RIT is able to target multiple metastases throughout the body in a single treatment.

8.1 Radionuclides for treatment

The selection of a radionuclide for cancer treatments depends on several parameters including:

1. **Physical parameters**: The type of radiation emitted by the radionuclide, required energy necessary for therapy and half-life of the radionuclide are physical parameters that must be considered. The type of radiation and the content of its energy are important factors that determine what radionuclide is suitable for killing of single disseminated cells, small metastases or large cancer tissues. The physical half-life of the radionuclides should preferably be in the same order of magnitude as the biological half-life. A too long physical half-life increases the necessary amount of radionuclide to be delivered to the tumor cells to allow the reasonable amounts of decays before excretion. A shorter physical half-life, on the other hand, will not give enough time for the targeting process to take place. It seems reasonable to assume that the most suitable physical half-lives ranges from a few hours up to some days when targeting of disseminated cells is considered (Boswell & Brechbiel, 2007).
2. **Chemical parameters**: The chemical parameters are as follow: achievable specific activity, stability of the radionuclide/antibody complex after labeling and that the labeling procedure must not interfere with the immunological activity of the antibody.
3. **Biological parameters:** tumor type, size and location, antibody kinetics, antigen density and heterogeneity and antigenicity are the most important biological parameters.
4. **Other parameters:** radioisotope availability and its cost.

Three main categories of radionuclides have been investigated for their potential therapeutic characterisation in radioimmunotherapy including β-particle emitters, α-particle emitters and auger electron cascades.

1. β-particle emitters

So far, the vast majority of preclinical and clinical studies have been made to use β-emitting radionuclides such as ^{131}I, ^{90}Y, ^{186}Re and ^{188}Re. These radionuclides have a tissue range of about several millimeters. This can create a "cross fire" effect, so that antigen or receptor negative cells in a tumor can also be treated. High energy B-particles are not efficient for killing of single disseminated cells or small metastases. So, β-particle therapy is preferred for large tumors (Boswell & Brechbiel, 2007).

2. α-particle emitters

Radionuclides emitting α-particles such as 225Ac (half-life 10 days), 211At (half-life 7.2 h), 212Bi (half-life 60.55 min) and 213Bi (half-life 45.6 min) are options for treatment of small tumor nests or single disseminated tumor cells. Alfa particle emitting radionuclides are short ranged, high-energy helium nuclei with a high linear energy transfer (LET). As a consequence, α-emitters have a high relative biological effectiveness (RBE) which means, if nuclear localisation is possible, fewer radionuclides per cell are needed (Fass, 2009).

3. Auger electron cascades

Auger-electrons, discovered by Lise Meitner in 1922 and by Pierre Auger in 1923, are formed when the vacancy created in an inner shell is filled with an electron from a higher energy level after electron capture. Auger-electrons have high LET Like α-particles (Cornelissen & Vallis, 2010). Auger-electron emitters, like ^{125}I, deposit a concentrated amount of energy in even shorter distances than α-emitters. This means that these radionuclides need to be located in the vicinity of the tumor cell nucleus to be effective. For this reason, antibodies labeled with auger-emitting radionuclides need to target the entire tumor cell population for efficient therapy (Cornelissen & Vallis, 2010).

9. Improving the properties of antibody in radioimmunoscintigraphy and radioimmunotherapy

Several investigations using different radionuclides, engineered antibodies and methods to increase antibody accumulation and penetration are currently being evaluated and have so far shown promising results. The main properties of antibodies that have been manipulated to optimize efficacy are size, immunogenicity, affinity and avidity.

9.1 Size

Size is a factor that impacts the circulation time of antibodies. IgG antibodies are large proteins with a molecular weight of 150 kDa which limits the diffusion of the antibodies from the blood into the tumor, resulting in a heterogeneous intratumoral distribution. Furthermore, IgG antibodies are characterized by a long circulatory half-life in plasma for three to four days. Due to this slow clearance from the blood, tumor-to-background ratio is usually low. The primary concern for using radionuclide labeled IgG is that it remains in the blood for an extended period of time which continually exposes the highly sensitive red marrow to radiation resulting in dose-limiting myelosuppression. While intact mAbs are primarily catabolized by the liver and spleen, mAb fragments are mainly excreted via the kidneys, thereby increasing uptake in the kidneys and lead to increase consequently the kidney absorbed radiation dose. (Koppe et al., 2005). If radiometals are used as the radiolabel, they will accumulate in the hepatic parenchyma. The large size of an antibody impacts its ability to move through a tumor mass. The smaller forms of antibodies such as $F(ab')_2$ or Fab fragments and more recently, molecularly engineered antibody subfragments with more favorable pharmacokinetic properties, are removed more rapidly from the blood, thereby improving tumor/blood ratio. There have been reports of improved therapeutic responses using smaller-sized antibodies, but these smaller entities frequently are cleared from the blood by renal filtration and as a result many radionuclides (eg, radiometals) become trapped in a higher concentration in the kidneys than in the tumor. Changes in the molecular size/structure of the IgG can also alter the normal tissue distribution, shifting uptake from the liver to the kidneys (Sharkey & Goldenberg, 2009). Reducing the size of antibody below the filtration threshold of kidneys (70 kDa), increases renal excretion and therefore decreases toxicity to this organ. Hence, being smaller molecules, antibodies are more suited to RIT and RIS with short circulation time, lower absolute localisation to the tumor and rapid excretion by the kidneys (Yazaki et al., 2001).

9.2 Immunogenicity

The first mAbs being investigated for RIS and RIT were murine antibodies which can provoke an immune response in human beings. HAMA inactivate and eliminate murine antibodies after repeated administration. The formation of antibody-HAMA complexes also leads to the allergic-like HAMA response. In this way, therapeutic benefit of murine mAbs is limited by their side effect profile, short serum half-life and inability to trigger human immune effector functions. In order to reduce the immunogenicity of antibodies, chimeric antibodies were designed by combining constant domains of human antibodies with variable regions of murine antibodies (Carlssona et al., 2003). However, chimeric mAbs minimize the immunogenic content, trigger the immunologic efficiency and allow a prolonged serum half-life in comparison with murine mAbs. As a further advancement of chimeric mAbs, in 1986, Jones first reported the production of humanized monoclonal antibodies (Jones et al., 1986). Humanized antibodies are almost completely of human origin with only the complementarity determining regions (CDRs) being murine. To completely avoid the risk of immunogenicity, further developments have led to the production of fully human antibodies that contain 100% human proteins. For the development of fully human mAbs, phage display technology and genetically engineered mice are the key techniques that have been widely used to link genotype and phenotype. Immunosuppressive agents have been investigated to reduce HAMA. Low-dose cyclosporin, as used with a highly immunogenic antibody, was unable to significantly reduce HAMA following murine CC49 delivery. Thus, cyclosporin may have some efficacy in reducing immunogenicity of murine antibodies in patients, but does not appear to be sufficient to permit administration of multiple doses in all patients (Pagel, 2009).

9.3 Affinity and avidity

The antibody affinity is a measure of the strength of binding of an individual antibody binding site to a single antigenic site. This can be considered as the sum of all the non-covalent interactions between antibody and antigen involved in the binding reaction. However, antibody molecules usually have more than one binding site and many antigens contain more than one antigenic site and therefore multivalent binding may be possible. The strength with which a multivalent antibody binds to an antigen, is termed avidity. Although high affinity is a requirement for good tumor localization, there seems to be a point at which further increases in affinity do not increase uptake at the target site (Schlomet al., 1992; Colcher et al., 1988). Indeed, reduced tumor uptake and limitations on penetration of antibody into the tumor tissue can result from the increasing of antibody affinity (Dearling & Pedley, 2007).

10. Technical limitations of radioimmunoscintigraphy and radioimmunotherapy

Although this conceptually simple technique has been investigated and refined for almost 50 years, it still has inherent limitations. In the present part, the problems of imaging and therapy of breast cancer by radioimmunoscintigraphy and radioimmnotherapy methods are discussed.

10.1 Antibody

Monoclonal antibodies have inherent limitations for application in targeting methods of imaging and therapy that can be cited in followings:

- mAbs are large molecules and so have difficulty in penetrating to large tumor masses especially in the early stages of the malignancies (Sergides et al., 1999).
- mAbs are currently not entirely sensitive for malignant tissues. For example, mAb B72.3 recognizes TAG-72 and has been used extensively for the detection of several malignancies including breast, lung, ovary and colorectal (Granowska et al., 1991).

10.2 Antigen

Tumors produce a chaotic vascular system in which blood flow is slow and can be interrupted or even reversed. The ratio of tissue cells to vascular support is lower than most normal tissues. These effects create areas of tumor hypoxia which are relatively resistant to radiation therapy and therefore reduce the efficacy of RIT (Sergides et al., 1999). Some antigens of breast cancer are epithelial surface antigens lying on the inner surfaces of cells, thus being exposed to the circulation only by neoplastic architectural disruption. Other factors influencing the suitability of antigens for tumor targeting are internalization and shedding into the bloodstream. Unfortunately, the majority of identified antigens in human tumors represent tumor-associated antigens, not only present on the tumor tissues, but also detectable on normal tissues (Sergides et al., 1999).

10.3 Background radioactivity

A high background level of radiation due to the presence of radioactivity in normal tissues reduces the tumor/background ratio which reduces the success of diagnosis and therapy. Tumor/background ratio may be diminished by the following factors: (1) the relative long circulation time of nonlocalized murine immunoglobulin in human beings; (2) binding of radiolabeled antibodies to antigens, released by the tumor in the blood pool; (3) the presence of free radionuclides and the subsequent accumulation in kidneys, bladder and other tissues, (4) non-specific uptake antibody by binding Fc fragment of antibody to normal tissues; (5) phagocytosis of murine immunoglobulin especially in the liver; (6) the presence of immune complexes due to the reaction of labelled antibody with Fc cell surface receptors, if non-fragmented immunoglobulins are used and (7) unconjugation of radio-isotope from antibody in the patient body (Sergides et al., 1999).

11. Improving in radioimmunoscintigraphy and radioimmunotherapy techniques

A variety of methods have been developed to counter the inherent flaws in RIS and RIT techniques. The following section discusses the methods for overcoming these problems.

11.1 Pre-targeting

The pretargeting procedure was developed from the concept that the targeting antibody should be separated from the targeting radionuclide through the use of a bispecific antibody (Chang et al., 2002). An alternative approach to improve tumor:blood ratio for RIS is the use of pre-targeting strategies. The pre-targeting strategies have led to significant improvements in T/B ratio and better diagnostic imaging (Dearling & pedley, 2007). Also, pretargeting has been applied successfully for radioimmunoimaging, because the pretargeted antibody is nontoxic. High doses can be administered to saturate antigenic sites at the tumor. Pretargeting strategies for RIT have been applied to achieve higher intratumor concentration of isotope than achieved by conventional RIT (Kraeber-Bodere et al., 2009). The simplest form of pre-targeting is to use a second antibody reagent to clear blood background activity, hence improving the signal:noise ratio and the quality of the image. Immune complexes formed by a second antibody are rapidly removed from the circulation by the reticuloendothelial system, particularly in the liver. In the alternative approach, the administration of antibody and radiolabel are separated. Antibody is allowed to localize to the tumor and sufficient time is allowed for antibody clearance from the blood and non-target tissues (Dearling & pedley, 2007). Radioisotope is then injected separately in a form which can be readily captured by the tumor bound antibody. The approaches using streptavidin/biotin binding systems raised much interest, because the affinity of streptavidin for biotin is exceptionally high (Gruaz-Guyon et al., 2005). In this strategy, the high affinity of the avidin:biotin system is used to capture radiolabeled small molecules from the blood as a two-step imaging method. Antibody-avidin conjugate is injected and allowed to be localized to the tumor and cleared from the blood (Dearling & pedley, 2007). Radioactive avidin is then injected which localizes the tumor by taking advantage of the high affinity and specificity of avidin for biotin (Roland et al., 2010, Dearling & pedley, 2007).

11.2 Dose fractionation

Dose fractionation has been proposed as a method to improve the therapeutic effect of radioimmunotherapy (Dearling & pedley, 2007, Denardo et al., 2002). Fractionated radioimmunotherapy may improve therapeutic outcome by decreasing heterogeneity of the dose delivered to the tumor and by decreasing hematologic toxicity, thereby allowing an increased amount of radionuclide that can be administered (Linden et al,. 2005) . A variety of fractionation regimens have been developed and the studies have reported both against and in its favour (Goel et al., 2001; Buchsbaum et al., 1995; Pedley et al., 1993; Schlom et al.,1990; Beaumier et al., 1991). This technique has several advantages including more uniform distribution of mAb and radiation dose, patient-specific radionuclide and radiation dose, control toxicity by titration of an individual patient, reduced toxicity, increased tumor radiation and efficacy and prolongation of tumor response (Violet, 2008). This technique has some disadvantages including lower radiation dose rate, complex strategy to implement, treatment interruption, increased cost and potential delay in tumor regression (Dearling & pedley, 2007).

11.3 Delayed imaging

Kinetic differences in specific and non-specific uptake of radioactivity provide an opportunity to image at a time when the T/B ratio is optimal. Background radioactivity falls with time due to excretion and decay of the radioisotope. Tumor radioactivity also falls with time, but not as fast as the background. The optimum time for RIS is dependent on the selected antibody and radioisotope and detection method (Sergides et al., 1999).

11.4 Background subtraction

If the background is labeled using a non-specific antibody, the background signal can then be subtracted from the results of RIS (Sergides et al., 1999; Goldenberg et al., 1978). It should be remembered that this technique leads to increase the total dose of radioactivity in the patient body that leads to undesirable side effects.

11.5 Pre-scouting

In the latter application, RIS is performed as a scouting procedure prior to RIT to enable the confirmation of tumor targeting and the estimation of radiation dose delivered to both tumors and normal tissues. For this purpose, the radioimmunoconjugates used for RIS and RIT should demonstrate a similar biodistribution and therefore radionuclides with comparable chemical properties have to be chosen (Dearling & pedley, 2007). When using 131I for RIT, both 123I and 131I can be used for a RIS scouting procedure. When using 90Y for RIT, 111In can be used to represent this pure beta-emitter (Dearling & pedley, 2007). Finally, when aiming the therapeutic use of 186Re or 188Re, either these radionuclides themselves can be used for an imaging procedure or 99mTc (Pontus et al., 2004).

11.6 Increasing the dose delivery

The result of experiments indicated that increasing the dose of antibody will increase the amount of radioactivity in the tumor (Begent et al., 1987). On the other hand, this technique has side effects due to HAMA response against the dramatic rise in dose of administered antibody that limits the application of this technique (Dearling & pedley, 2007).

11.7 Combined imaging systems

The resolution of latest-generation of PET and SPECT cameras has been improved and the combination of these systems with an integrated CT (and also MRI) has led to a much better interpretation of the data (Dearling & pedley, 2007). In addition, the indirect combination of nuclear imaging and optical imaging systems can also serve shared purposes (Munnink et al, 2009).

11.8 Second antibody

The background counts can be reduced by removing radioactivity from the circulation. This can be achieved by the use of a second antibody active against the RIS antibody. In this technique, after the binding time of original antibody to tumor tissue, the second antibody administers to the patient (Sergides et al., 1999). The second antibody binds to the radioactive antibody that remains in the blood stream. The reticuloendothelial system uptakes antibody-antibody complex and leads to concentrate radioactivity in liver and spleen. This technique leads to increase in T/B ratio without adverse effects. The only disadvantage of this method is limitation in the detection of metastases at liver and spleen (Sergides et al., 1999).

11.9 Improving the internalization of the radiolabeled mAb

One significant factor that influences the absorbed radiation dose to the tumor is the fate of the radiolabel after internalization of the radiolabeled mAb into the tumor cells. In case of internalisation, the radionuclides will come closer to the critical radiation target, i.e. nuclear DNA. Internalization of the antibody depends on various factors including the antibody, the targeted antigen and the tumor cells. On the other hand, internalisation might be disadvantageous, if it leads to quick degradation of the targeting agent followed by diffusion and elimination of the radionuclide (Boswell et al., 2007). Most antibodies including those that target antigens located on the surface of the tumor cells such as anti-CEA antibodies, are eventually catabolized. Intracellular degradation of the targeting agent can be prevented by e.g. dextranation (Bue et al., 2000). Radiolabeling of antibodies with 90Y or 177Lu is performed by linking these radionuclides to chelators (DTPA or DOTA) which are chemical moieties that complex free metal ions. These chelators are conjugated to the antibodies and subsequently to the radiolabel. After catabolization of mAbs labeled with 90Y- or 177Lu-DTPA/-DOTA, the catabolic products are conjugated to, in most cases, lysine (e.g. 90Y- or 177Lu-DOTA-lysine). Whereas radioiodinated tyrosine is excreted by the cell, the 90Y- or 177Lu-DTPA/DOTA-lysine metabolites are trapped within the lysosomes, thereby increasing the tumor retention time of these radiolabels (Koppe et al., 2005). Cellular excretion can also be limited if the radionuclides are of metal type, e.g. indium or yttrium, and this is due to intracellular retention of metal containing catabolic products (Press et al., 1996).

11.10 Targeting agents

RIS may be improved by the production of superior targeting agents to deliver radioactivity to tumor sites. For example, instead of using intact antibodies to target tumors, fragments of antibodies retaining their antigenic specificity can be used (Sergides et al., 1999). Fragments of an antibody have several advantages including:

1. Shorter circulating half-life and faster execration by kidney that leads to decrease background signals.
2. Smaller molecular weight that leads to faster and more deeply diffuse into tumors.
3. Reduce non-specific antibody binding by Fc receptor on cells due to the loss of the Fc fragment
4. Reduce the HAMA response due to the loss of Fc fragment that is responsible for immune response to foreign proteins.

Further improvements in the structure of antibodies are being explored with antibody engineering technology. Single-chain antigen binding fragments (sF_7) consisting of variable heavy (V_H) or variable light (V_L) domains and recombinant sF_7 peptides which are V_H and V_L domains connected by peptide linkers are the productions of this technology. These productions has high affinity for antigen (Sergides et al., 1999).

11.11 Antibody affinity

The strength of the antibody:antigen interaction is measured through the binding affinity and is quantified through the association constant (K_a) (Boswell et al., 2007). Increasing Ka of antibody will be leads to an increase in uptake antibody in the tumor. However, they may be less able to penetrate deeply due to strongly bound at the tumor surface. The studies with iodine radiolabeled scFvs demonstrated that a threshold affinity between 10^{-7} and 10^{-8} M was required to observe detectable tumor uptake in mice 24 h post injection, whereas no gain in tumor accumulation was observed with affinities >10^{-9} M. Affinities >10^{-9} M were detrimental to rapid and uniform tumor penetration due to stable binding at the first pass of tumor antigens forming a binding site barrier (Adams et al., 2001).

11.12 Multivalency

Multivalency has been reported as an advantage in radioimmunotherapy (Dearling & pedley, 2007). Conversion of monovalent antibodies into multivalent format increases their functional affinity and decreases dissociation rates for cell-surface and optimizes biodistribution

(Dearling & pedley, 2007). In addition, it allows the creation of bispecific antibody molecules that can target two different antigens simultaneously (Sergey et al., 2008). During the last decade, several techniques in multivalency engineering have been developed. Each of these strategies proposed to link monovalent domains and to produce multivalent antibody, obviously has some advantages in some special cases, but none of them is universal. The advantages of tumor targeting with multivalent antibody derivatives have been investigated for scFv dimers, prepared as disulfide-linked dimers of scFv (Adams et al., 1995), non-covalent diabodies (Kortt et al., 2001) and some other bi(multi)valent variants of recombinant antibody fragments (Kubetzko et al.,2006; Shahied et al., 2004; Willuda et al., 2001). In most cases, dimeric/divalent antibodies showed significant improvement of their pharmacokinetics and biodistribution over monomers (Sergey et al., 2008).

11.13 CockTails

One problem of RIS is the existence of diversity of epitopes on surface tumor cells that reduces uptake radioactivity in tumor. An alternative approach to improve the uptake of radioactivity by the target is using cocktails of several radiolabelled antibodies that recognize different epitopes or antigens on the same tumor. However, some of the experiments indicated positive results by using cocktails, other experiments showed that the mAbs of cocktails competed to bind to epitopes with each other and reduce the efficacy of the mixture to less than that of one antibody used alone (sergey et al., 2008).

11.14 Increasing tumor uptake

By increasing the level of antigen expression, diagnosis and therapy based on targeting can be improved. For example, hyperthermia can increase the amount of presenting antigen in a tumor (Wilder et al., 1993). Furthermore, several cytokines such as interferon alpha and interleukin-6 have been found to upregulate the expression of cell surface antigens including histocompatibility antigens and tumor associated antigens such as carcinoembryonic antigen (CEA). In both *in vivo* and *in vitro* studies an improved antibody-uptake has been demonstrated as a result of the administration of vasoactive peptides and cytokines such as IL-2 or external beam radiation therapy may result in a specific increased vascular permeability at the tumor site and thus an increased antibody uptake (Guadagni, et al., 1990). Structural modification (e.g., PEGylation) and residue mutation are both useful strategies in reducing chemically or physically derived nontarget organ uptake of Abs, but these methods do not reduce the uptake due to receptor expression within nontarget organs. These are research areas of high interest (Boswell & Brechbiel, 2007).

11.15 Reducing kidney uptake

Elevated renal uptake and prolonged retention of radiolabeled antibody is a problem in the therapeutic application of such agents (Dearling & pedley, 2007). Because of the negative charge of the basement membrane of the glomeruli, positively charged catabolites of the radiopharmaceutical may be retained in the kidney, increasing the toxic absorbed dose to this radiosensitive organ (Dearling & pedley, 2007). The result of some studies demonstrated that lysine, histidine and arginine were effective in reducing the renal uptake of radiopharmaceutical and lysine was the most effective (Lin et al., 2007). In these studies it has been shown that renal retention can also be minimized by the administration of lysine, a cationic amino acid, whereas the uptake in all other organs as well as the tumor remains unaffected (Behr et al., 1995).

12. Conclusion

In recent years, significant developments in the application of targeted imaging and therapy have taken place in nuclear medicine. This chapter suggests that optimization of radioimmunoscintigraphy and radioimmunotherapy methods is still possible and emphasizes that these technologies are continuing to progress and are close to become routine modalities in the identification of breast cancer sites and its therapy. The development of effective imaging and therapy of breast cancer relies to a great extent on the development of effective carriers and target agents that can deliver radionuclids to the cancer cells. These agents should be able to carry a large load of radionuclids and selectively deliver them to the cancer cells with high accuracy to achieve effective cancer cells death without inducing nonspecific toxicity. This means that the use of new targeting agents such as peptides and affibodies can provide promising results. Liposomes, dendrimers, micelles and nanoparticles present large families of carriers that can be exploited for delivery of radionuclids and they can be further improved to diagnose and therapy of breast cancer in the future. The research in the field of targeted imaging and therapy will help us to avoid unnecessary costs and potentially allow these new methods to be available for the majority of patients who need them, leading to better quality and quantity of life.

13. References

Adam, F., Alberto, H., Piera, S., Cristina, C., Armando, G., & Fabio, M. (2000). Monoclonal antibodies and therapy of human cancers. *Biotechnology Advances,* Vol.18, pp. 385–401.

Adams, GP., McCartney, JE., Wolf, EJ., Eisenberg, J., & Huston, JS. (1995). Enhanced tumor specificity of 741F8-1(sFv')2, an anti-c-erbB-2 singlechain Fv dimer, mediated by stable radioiodine conjugation. *The Journal of Nuclear Medicine,* Vol.36, pp.2276–2281.

Adams, GP., Schier, R., McCall, AM., Simmons, HH., Horak, EM., & Alpaugh, RK. (2001). High affinity restricts the localization and tumor penetration of single-chain Fv antibody molecules. *Cancer Research,* Vol. 61, pp. 4750–5.

Balleyguier, C., Opolon, P., Mathieu, MC., Athanasiou, A., Garbay, JR., & Delaloge, S. (2008). New potential and applications of contrast-enhanced ultrasound of the breast: Own investigations and review of the literature. *European Journal of Radiology ,*

Baselga, J., & Cameron, D. (2007). Objective response rate in a phase II multicenter trial of pertuzumab (P), a HER2 dimerization inhibiting monoclonal antibody, in combination with trastuzumab (T) in patients (Pts) with HER2 positive metastatic breast cancer (MBC) which had progressed during trastuzumab therapy. *Journal of Clinical Oncology, American Society of Clinical Oncology (ASCO) Annual Meeting Proceedings,* Part I. Vol 25, No. 18S: 1004

Baselga, J., Gelmon, KA., Verma, S., Wardley, A., Conte, P., & Miles, D. (2010). Phase II trial of pertuzumab and trastuzumab in patients with human epidermal growth factor receptor 2-positive metastatic breast cancer that progressed during prior trastuzumab therapy. *Journal of clinical Oncology,* Vol. 28, pp.1138-44.

Beaumier, PL., Venkatesan, P., & Vanderheyden, JL. (1991). 186Re radioimmunotherapy of small cell lung carcinoma xenografts in nude mice. *Cancer Research, Vol.* 51, pp.676-681.

Begent, RHJ., Bagshawe, KD., & Pedley, RB. (1987). Use of second antibody in radioimmunotherapy. *Journal of the National Cancer Institute Monographs*, Vol. 3, pp. 59–61.

Behr, TM., Sharkey, RM., Juweid, ME., Blumenthal, RD., Dunn, RM., & Griffiths, GL. (1995). Reduction of the renal uptake of radiolabeled monoclonal antibody fragments by cationic amino acids and their derivatives, *Cancer Research*, 55(17):3825–34.

Behr, TM., Sharkey, RM., & Juweid, ME. (1997). Variables influencing tumor dosimetry in radioimmunotherapy of CEA-expressing cancers with anti-CEA and anti-mucin monoclonal antibodies. *The Journal of Nuclear Medicine*, vol. 38, pp. 409-418.

Berg, JR., Kalisher, L., & Osmond, JD. (1973). Technetium-99m- disphosphonate concentration in primary breast cancer. *Radiology*, Vol. 109, pp. 393-394.

Berg, WA., Gutierrez, L., NessAiver, MS., Carter, WB., Bhargavan, M., & Lewis, RS. (2004). Diagnostic accuracy of mammography, clinical examination, US, and MR imaging in preoperative assessment of breast cancer. *Radiology*, Vol. 233(3), pp.830-849.

Berghammer, P., Obwegeser, R., & Sinzinger, H. (2001). Nuclear medicine and breast cancer: a review of current strategies and novel therapies. *The Breast*, Vol. 10, pp. 184-197.

Blank, EW., Pant, KD., Chan, CM., Peterson, JA., & Ceriani, RL. (1992). A novel anti-breast epithelial mucin MoAb (BrE-3). *Cancer*, Vol. 5, pp. 38–44.

Boswell, C., Andrew, C., Brechbiel, & Martin, W. (2007).Development of radioimmunotherapeutic and diagnostic antibodies: an inside-out view. *Nuclear Medicine and Biology*, Vol. 34, pp. 757–778.

Brem, RF., Rapelyea, JA., & Zisman, G. (2005). Occult breast cancer: Scintimammography with high-resolution breast-specific gamma camera in women at high risk for breast cancer. *Radiology*, Vol. 237, pp. 274-80.

Buchsbaum, D., Khazaelli, MB., & Liu, T. (1995). Fractionated radioimmunotherapy of human colon carcinoma xenografts with 131I-labeled monoclonal antibody CC49. *Cancer Research*, Vol. 55, pp. 5881-5887.

Bue, P., Holmberg, AR., Marquez, M., Westlin, JE., Nilsson, S., & Malmstrom, PU. (2000). Intravesical administration of EGF-dextran conjugates in patients with superficial bladder cancer. *European Urology*, Vol. 38, pp. 584–589.

Capala, J., Kramer-Marek, G., Lee, S., Hassan, M., Kiesewetter, DO., Puri, A., Chernomordik, V., Gandjbakhche, A., Griffiths, G., & Blumentha, R. (2009). Molecular targeting of HER2 for diagnosis and therapy of breast cancer. *Cancer Research*, Vol. 69, Supplement 1

Carl, AK., Borrebaeck, & Roland, C. (2001). Human therapeutic antibodies. *Current Opinion in Pharmacology*, Vol. 1, pp. 404–408.

Carlos, M., Mery, MPH., Bilal, M., Shafi, MSE., & Gary, B. (2006). Molecular imaging and radioimmunoguided surgery. *Seminars in Pediatric Surgery* ,Vol. 15, pp. 259-266.

Carlssona, J., Aronssonb, EF., Hietalac, SO., Stigbrandd, T., & Tennvall, J. (2003). Tumor therapy with radionuclides: assessment of progress and problems. *Radiotherapy and Oncology*,Vol. 66, pp. 107–117.

Chang, CH., Sharkey, RM., Rossi, EA., Karacay, H., McBride, W., Hansen, HJ., Chatal, JF., Barbet, J., & Goldenberg, DM. (2002). Molecular advances in pretargeting radioimmunotherapy with bispecific antibodies. *Molecular Cancer Therapeutics*, Vol. 1(7), pp.553-563.

Cleator, S., Heller, W., & Coombes, RC. (2007). Triple-negative breast cancer: therapeutic options. *Lancet Oncology*, Vol. 8, pp. 235–44.

Cobleigh, M., Vogel, C., Tripathy, D., Robert, N., Scholl, S., & Fehrenbacher, L. (1999). Multinational study of the efficacy and safety of humanized anti-HER2 monoclonal antibody in women who have HER2-overexpressing metastatic breast cancer that has progressed after chemotherapy for metastatic disease. *Journal of clinical Oncology*, Vol. 17, pp. 2639–48.

Colcher, D., Minelli, MF., Roselli, M., Muraro, R., Simpson-Milenic, D., & Schlom, J. (1988). Radioimmunolocalisation of human carcinoma xenografts with B72.3 second generation monoclonal antibodies. *Cancer Research*, Vol. 48, pp. 4597-4603.

Cook, GJR. (2003). Oncological molecular imaging: nuclear medicine techniques. *British Journal of Radiology*, Vol. 76, pp. 152-158.

Cornelissen, B., & Vallis, KA. (2010). Targeting the Nucleus: An Overview of Auger-Electron Radionuclide Therapy. *Current Drug Discovery Technologies*,Vol. 7.

Costelloe, CM., Rohren, EM., Madewell, JE., Hamaoka, T., Theriault, RL., Tse-Kuan, Y., Lewis ,VO., & Jingfei, M. (2009). Imaging bone metastases in breast cancer: techniques and recommendations for diagnosis. *Lancet Oncology*, Vol. 10, pp. 606–14.

Dearling, JLJ., & Pedley, RB. (2007). Technological Advances in Radioimmunotherapy. *Clinical Oncology*, Vol. 19, pp. 457-469.

Denardo, GL., Schlom, J., Buchsbaum, DJ., Meredith, RF., Odonoghue, JA., Sgouros, G., Humm, JL., & DeNardo, SJ. (2002). Rationales, evidence, and design considerations for fractionated radioimmunotherapy. *Cancer*, Vol.94, pp.1332–1348.

Denardo, S J. (2005). Functional Imaging: Radioimmunodetection and Therapy of Breast Cancer. *Seminars in Nuclear Medicine*, Vol. 35, pp. 143-151.

Denardo, SJ., Mirick, GR., Kroger, LA., O'Grady, LF., Erickson, KL., Yuan, A., Lamborn, KR., Hellstrom, I., Hellstrom, KE., & Denardo, GL. (1994). The biologic window for chimeric L6 radioimmunotherapy. *Cancer*,Vol. 73, pp. 1023–32.

Disis, ML., Calenoff, E., & McLaughlin, G. (1994). Existent T-cell and antibody immunity to HER-2/*neu* protein in patients with breast cancer. *Cancer Research*, Vol. 54, pp.16–20.

Disis, ML., Pupa, SM., Gralow, JR., Dittadi, R., Menard, S., & Cheever, MA. (1997). High-titer HER-2/*neu* protein-specific antibody can be detected in patients with early-stage breast cancer. *Journal of clinical Oncology*, Vol. 15, pp. 3363–3367.

Ehrlich, P. (1906). Collected Studies on Immunology, *John Wiley*.

Einat, ES., & Moshe, I. (2010). PET in women with high risk for breast or ovarian cancer , *Lancet Oncology*, Vol. 11, pp. 899–905.

Eniu, A. (2007). Integrating biological agents into systemic therapy of breast cancer: Trastuzumab, lapatinib, bevacizumab. *J BUON*, Vol. 12, pp. 119-26.

Fass, L. (2008). Imaging and cancer: A review.*Molecular oncology*, Vol. 2, pp. 115–152.

Ferro-Flores, G., Ramírez, M., Melendez-Alafort, L., & Santos-Cuevas, CL. (2010). Peptides for *In Vivo* Target-Specific Cancer Imaging. *Mini-Reviews in Medicinal Chemistry*, Vol.10, pp. 87-97.

Frangioni, JV. (2008). New technologies for human cancer imaging. *Journal of clinical Oncology*, Vol. 26(24), pp. 4012-4021.

Friedman, M., et al. (2009). Engineering and characterization of a bispecific HER2xEGFR-binding affibody molecule. *Biotechnology and Applied Biochemistry*. Vol. 54, pp. 121–131.

Gaffer, SA., Pant, KD., & Shochat, D. (1981). Experimental studies of tumor radioimmunodetection using antibody mixtures against carcinoembryonic antigen (CEA) and colon-specific antigen. *cancer*, Vol. 27, pp. 101-5.

Gasparini, G.,Longo, R., Torino, F., & Morabito, A. (2005). Therapy of breast cancer with molecular targeting agents. *European Society for Medical Oncology*, Vol. 16, pp. 28-36.

Gianni, L., Llado, A., Bianchi, G., Cortes, J., Kellokumpu-Lehtinen, PL., & Cameron, DA. (2010). Open-label, phase II, multicenter, randomized study of the efficacy and safety of two dose levels of Pertuzumab, a human epidermal growth factor receptor 2 dimerization inhibitor, in patients with human epidermal growth factor receptor 2-negative metastatic breast cancer. *Journal of clinical Oncology*, Vol. 28, pp. 1131-7.

Glasspool, RM., & Evans, TRJ. (2000). Clinical imaging of cancer metastasis. *European Journal of Cancer*,Vol. 36, pp. 1661-1670.

Goel, A., Augustine, S., & Baranowska-Kortyewicz, J. (2001). Singledose versus fractionated radioimmunotherapy of human colon carcinoma xenografts using 131I-labeled multivalent CC49 single-chain Fvs. *clinical Cancer Research*, Vol. 7, pp. 175-184.

Goel, A., Augustine, S., Baranowska-Kortylewicz, J., & Colcher, D. (2001). Single-Dose versusFractionated Radioimmunotherapy of Human Colon Carcinoma Xenografts Using 131I-labeled Multivalent CC49 Single-chain Fvs1. *clinical Cancer Research*, Vol. 7, pp. 175-184.

Goel, A., Baranowska-Kortylewicz, J., Hinrichs, SH., Wisecarver, J., Pavlinkova, G., Augustine, S., Colcher, D., Booth, BJ., & Batra, SK. (2001). 99mTc-labeled divalent and tetravalent CC49 single-chain Fvs: Novel imaging agents for rapid *in vivo* localization of human colon carcinoma. *The Journal Of Nuclear Medicine, Vol.* 42, pp. 1519-1527.

Gold, P., & Freedman, SO. (1965). Specific carcinoembryonic antigens of the human digestive system. *The Journal of Experimental Medicine*, Vol. 122, pp. 467–481.

Goldenberg, DM., & Nabi, HA. (1999). Breast Cancer Imaging With Radiolabeled Antibodies. *Seminars in Nuclear Medicine*, Vol. XXIX, No 1, pp. 41-47.

Goldenberg, DM., Deland, F., & Kim, E. (1978). Use of radiolabeled antibodies to carcinoembryonic antigen for the detection and localization of diverse cancers by external photoscanning. *New England Journal of Medicine*, Vol. 298, pp. 1384–6.

Goldenberg, DM., Goldenberg, H., Sharkey, RM. (1990). In-vivo antibody imaging for the detection of human tumors. *Cancer Treatment Research*, Vol. 51, pp. 273–92.

Goldsmith, J., & Signore, A. (2010). An overview of the diagnostic and therapeutic use of monoclonal antibodies in medicine. *The Quarterly Journal of Nuclear Medicine And Molecular Imaging*, Vol. 54, pp. 574-81.

Gomes, CM., Abrunhosa, AJ., Ramos, P., & Pauwels, EKJ. (2010). Molecular imaging with SPECT as a tool for drug development. *Advanced Drug Delivery Reviews*. pp. 1-8.

Granowska, M., Mather, SJ., & Britton, KE. (1991). Diagnostic evaluation of 111In and 99mTc radiolabelled monoclonal antibodies in ovarian and colorectal cancer: correlations with surgery. *International journal of radiation applications and instrumentation Part B, Nuclear Medicine and Biology*, Vol . 18, pp. 413–24.

Gruaz-Guyon, A., Raguin, O., & Barbet, J. (2005). Recent advances in pretargeted radioimmunotherapy. *Current Medicinal Chemistry*, Vol. 12, pp. 319-338.

Guadagni, F., Witt, PL., & Robbins, PF. (1990). Regulation of carcinoembryonic antigen expression in different human colorectal tumor cells by interferon-gamma, *Cancer Research*, 50: 6248–6255.

Hamoudeh, M., Kamleh, MA., Diab, R., & Fessi, H. (2008). Radionuclides delivery systems for nuclear imaging and radiotherapy of cancer. *Advanced Drug Delivery Reviews*, Vol. 60, pp. 1329–1346.

Harris, M. (2004). Monoclonal antibodies as therapeutic agents for Cancer. *Monoclonal antibodies in cancer therapy*, Vol. 5, pp. 292–302.

Hassan, MS., Ansari, J., Spooner, D., & Hussain, SA. (2010). Chemotherapy for breast cancer (Review). *Oncology Reports*, Vol. 5, pp. 1121-31.

Hawrysz, DJ., & Sevick-Muraca, EM. (2000). Developments toward diagnostic breast cancer imaging using near-infrared optical measurements and fluorescent contrast agents. *Neoplasia*, Vol. 2(5), pp. 388-417.

Hicke, BJ., Stephens, AW., Gould, T., Chang, YF., Lynott, CK., Heil, J., Borkowski, S., Hilger, CS., Cook, G., Warren, S., & Schmidt, PG. (2006). Tumor targeting by an aptamer. *The Journal Of Nuclear Medicine*, Vol.47(4), pp. 668-678.

Hind, D., Ward, S., De Nigris, E., Simpson, E., Carroll, C., & Wyld, L. (2007). Hormonal therapies for early breast cancer: systematic review and economic evaluation. *Health Technol Assess*, Vol. 11, pp. 1-134.

Hong, H., Sun, J., & Cai, W. (2008). Radionuclide-Based Cancer Imaging Targeting the Carcinoembryonic Antigen. *Biomarker Insights*, Vol. 3, pp. 435–451.

Hou, D., Hoch, H., & Johnston, GS. (1984). A new 111In-bleomycin complex for tumor imaging: preparation, stability, and distribution in glioma-bearing mice. *Journal of Surgical Oncology*, Vol. 25, pp. 168-75.

Howell, LP., Denardo, SJ., Levy, N., Lund, J., &Denardo, GL. (1995). Immunohistochemical staining of metastatic ductal carcinomas of the breast by monoclonal antibodies used in imaging and therapy: a comparative study. *International Journal of Biological Markers*, Vol. 10, pp. 126–35.

Huang, S., Armstrong, EA.,Benavente, S. (2004). Dual-agent molecular targeting of the epidermal growth factor receptor (EGFR): Combining anti-EGFR antibody with tyrosine kinase inhibitor. *Cancer Research*, Vol.64, pp. 5355-5362.

Hudson, PJ., & Kortt. (1999). High avidity scFv multimers; diabodies and triabodies. *Immunological Methods*, Vol. 231, pp. 177-189.

Imai, K., & Takaoka, A. (2006). Comparing antibody and small-molecule therapies for cancer. *Nature*, Vol. 6, pp. 714-727.

Izumi,Y., Xu, L., di Tomaso, E., Fukumura, D., Jain, RK. (2002). Tumour biology: herceptin acts as an anti-angiogenic cocktail. *Nature*, Vol. 416, pp. 279–280.

Jalilian, AR., Aboudzadeh, R., Akhlaghi, M., Shirazi, B., Moradkhani,S.,&Salouti, M. (2007). Production and biological evaluation of [201Tl(III)]bleomycin. *Journal of Labelled Compounds and Radiopharmaceuticals*, Vol. 50, pp.556–557.

Jalilian, AR., Akhlaghi, M., ShiraziB., Aboudzadeh, R., Salouti, M., Babaii, MH. (2006). [201 Tl] (III)- Bleomycin for tumor imaging. *Radiochima Acta*, Vol. 94, pp. 453-459.

Jonathan, D., Cheng, PT., Rieger M Von., Mehren, G., Adams, P., Louis, m., & Ws, N. (2000). Recent advaces in immunotherapy and monoclonal antibody treatment of cancer. *Seminars in Oncology Nursing*, Vol. 16, pp. 2-12.

Jones, KL., & Buzdar, AU. (2004). A review of adjuvant hormonal therapy in breast cancer. *Endocrine-Related Cancer*, Vol. 11, pp. 391-406

Jones, PT., Dear, PH., Foote, J., Neuberger, MS., & Winter, G. (1986). Replacing the complementarity-determining regions in a human antibody with those from a mouse. *Nature,* Vol. 321, pp. 522-5.

Kepshire, DS., Davis, SC., Dehghani, H., Paulsen, KD., Pogue, BW. (2007). Subsurface diffuse optical tomography can localize absorber and fluorescent objects but recovered image sensitivity is nonlinear with depth. *Applied Optics,* Vol.46 (10), pp.1669-1678.

Keshtgar, M., Davidson, T., Pigott, K., Falzon, M., & Jones, A. (2010). Current status and advances in management of early breast cancer. *International Journal of Surgery,* Vol. 8, pp. 199-202.

Kohler, G., & Milstein, C. (1978). Continuous culture of fused cells secreting antibody for the detection and localization of diverse cancers by external photo scanning. *New England Journal of Medicine,* Vol. 298, pp. 1384-6.

Kohler, G., & Milstein, C. (1975). Continuous cultures of fused cells secreting antibody of predefined specificity. *Nature,* Vol. 256, pp. 495–497.

Kopans, DB. (1992). The positive predictive value of mammography. *American Journal of Roentgenology,* Vol. 158, pp. 521-526.

Koppe, MJ., Postema, EJ., & Aarts, F. (2005). Antibody-guided radiation therapy of cancer. *Cancer and Metastasis Reviews,* Vol.24, pp. 539–567.

Kortt, AA., Dolezal, O., Power, BE., & Hudson, PJ. (2001). Dimeric and trimeric antibodies: high avidity scFvs for cancer targeting. *Biomolecular Engineering,* Vol. 18, pp. 95–108.

Kraeber–Bodere, F., Goldenberg, DM., Chatal,JF., & Barbet,J. (2009). Pretargeted radioimmunotherapy in the treatment of metastatic medullary thyroid cancer. *Current Oncology,* Vol. 16(5), pp. 3–8.

Kramer, EL., Denardo, SJ., Liebes, L., Kroger, LA., Noz, ME., Mizrachi, H., Salako, QA., Furmanski, P., Glenn, SD., & Denardo, GL. (1993). Radioimmunolocalization of breast carcinoma using BrE-3 monoclonal antibody: phase I study. *The Journal Of Nuclear Medicine,* Vol. 34, pp. 1067–74.

Kubetzko, S., Balic, E., Waibel, R., Zangemeister-Wittke, U., & Pluckthun, A. (2006). PEGylation and multimerization of the anti-p185HER-2 single chain Fv fragment. D5:effects on tumor targeting. *The Journal of Biological Chemistry,* Vol. 281, pp. 35186–351201.

Larson, SM., Divgi, C., Scott, A., Daghighian, F., Macapilnac, H., & Welt, S. (1994). Current Status of Radioimmunodetection. *Nuclear Medicine and Biology,*Vol. 21, pp. 721-729.

Lawrence, LJ., Kortt, AA., Iliades, P., Tulloch, PA., & Hudson, PJ. (1998). Orientation of antigen binding sites in dimeric and trimeric single-chain Fv antibody fragments. *FEBS Letters,* Vol. 425(3), pp. 479-484.

Liberman, L. (2000). Percutanous imaging-guided core breast biopsy:state of the art the millennium . *American Journal of Roentgenology,* Vol. 174. pp. 1191-1199.

Lin, FI., & Iagaru, A. (2010). Current Concepts and Future Directions in Radioimmunotherapy. *Current Drug Discovery Technologies*

Lin, Y., Hung, G., Luo, T., Tsai, S., Sun, S., Hsia, C., Chen, S., & Lin,WY. (2007). Reducing renal uptake of 111In-DOTATOC: A comparison among various basic amino acids , *Annals of Nuclear Medicine,* Vol. 21, pp. 79–83.

Linden, O., Hindorf, C., Cavallin-Stahl, E., Wegener, WA., Goldenberg, DM., Horne, H., Ohisson, Tomas., Lars, S., Sven-Erik S., & Jan T. *(2005).* Dose Fractionated

Radioimmunotherapy in Non-Hodgkin's Lymphoma Using DOTA-Conjugated, ^{90}Y-Radiolabeled, Humanized Anti-CD22 Monoclonal Antibody, Epratuzumab. *Clinical Cancer Research,* Vol. *11, pp.* 5215-5220

Liu, X., Pop Laurentiu, M., & Vitetta, Es. (2008). Engineering therapeutic monoclonal antibodies. *Immunological Reviews,* Vol. 222, pp. 9–27

Lorraine, MF., Raya, SB., Lisa von M., Henry, DA., Ralph., S, Jay, H.,&David, A. (1998). Immunolymphoscintigraphy in Breast Cancer:valuation Using 131I-Labeled Monoclonal Antibody B72.3. *Nuclear Medicine and Biology,* Vol. 25, pp. 251–260.

Luini, A., Gatti, G., & Zurrida, S. (2007). The evolution of the conservative approach to breast cancer. *The Breast.*Vol. 16, pp. 120–129.

Madsen, MT. (2007). Recent advances in SPECT imaging. *The Journal of Nuclear Medicine,* Vol. 48 (4), pp. 661–673.

Meel , R., Gallagher, WM., Oliveira, S., O'Connor, AE., Schiffelers, R M., & Byrne, AT. (2010). Recent advances in molecular imaging biomarkers in cancer: application of bench to bedside technologies. *Drug Discovery Today,*Vol. 15.

Merkle, Van D. (2009). Blood Testing: Three Easy Steps. *Dynamic Chiropractic nutritional wellness,* Vol. 5, No. 2, pp.1-3.

Milenic, DE., Schlom, J., & Siler, K. (1991). Monoclonal antibody-based therapy of a human tumor xenograft with a 177-lutetium-labeled immunoconjugate. *Cancer Research,* Vol. 51, pp. 2889-2896.

Mohammadnejad, J., Rasaee, MJ., Babaei, MH., & Salouti, M.(2010). Radioimmunotherapy of MCF7 breast cancer cell line with 131I-PR81 monoclonal antibody against MUC1: Comparison of direct and indirect radioiodination methods, *Human Antibodies,* Vol. 19, pp. 15–25.

Mohammadnejad, MJ., Rasaee, J., Babaei, MH., Paknejadc. M., Zahir, MH., & Salouti, M. (2010). A new radiopharmaceutical compound (^{131}I-PR81) for radioimmunotherapy of breast cancer: Labeling of antibody and its quality control, *Human Antibodies,* Vol. 19, pp. 79–88.

Mukhopadhyay, P., & Chakraborty., S. (2011). Mucins in the pathogenesis of breast cancer: Implications in diagnosis, prognosis and therapy. *Biochimica et Biophysica Acta,*

Munagala, R., Aqil, F., & Gupta, RC. (2011). Promising molecular targeted therapies in breast cancer. *Indian Journal of Pharmacology,* Vol. 43, pp. 236-45.

Munninka, THO., Nagengasta, WB., Brouwersb, AH., Schr odera, CP., Hospersa, GA., Hoogec, MN., Lub-de, WE., Dieste, PJ., & Vries, EGE. (2009). Molecular imaging of breast cancer. *The Breast,* pp. 66–73

Murray, JL., Green, MC., & Hortobagyi, GN. (2000). Monoclonal antibody therapy for solid tumors. *Cancer treatment reviews,* Vol. 26, pp. 269–286.

Neves, AA., & Brindle, KM. (2006). Assessing responses to cancer therapy using molecular imaging. *Biochimica et Biophysica Acta,* Vol. 1766, pp. 242–261

Nguyen, BD., Roarke, MC., Karstaedt, PJ., Ingui, CJ., & Ram, PC. (2009). Practical Applications of Nuclear Medicine in Imaging Breast Cancer. *Current problems in diagnostic radiology,* Vol. 38, pp. 68-83.

Nystrom, L., Andersson, I., Bjurstam, N., Frisell, J., Nordenskjold, B., & Rutqvist, LE. (2002). Long-term effects of mammography screening: updated overview of the Swedish randomised trials. *Lancet,* Vol. 359(9310), pp. 909-919.

Olafsen, T., Tan, GJ., & Park, JM. (2004). Tumor targeting, biodistribution and micro-PET imaging of engineered anti-her2/Neu antibody fragments in xenograft-bearing mice. *The Journal Of Nuclear Medicine,,* Vol. 44, pp. 363-369.

Orlova, A., Magnusson, M., Eriksson, TL., Nilsson, M., Larsson, B., Hoiden-Guthenberg, I., Widstrom, C., Carlsson, J., Tolmachev,V., Stahl, S., & Nilsson, F Y. (2006). Tumor imaging using a picomolar affinity HER2 binding affibody molecule. *Cancer Research,* Vol. 66, pp. 4339–4348.

Orlova, A., Nilsson, FY., Wikman, M., Widstrom, C., Stahl, S., Carlsson, J,. & Tolmachev, V. (2006). Comparative *in vivo* evaluation of technetium and iodine labels on an anti-HER-2 affibody for single-photon imaging of HER-2 expression in tumors. *The Journal Of Nuclear Medicine,* Vol. 47(3), pp. 512-519.

Pagel, JM., Boferman, OC., Hazel, BB., & Ruby, F. (2009). Targeted radionuclide therapy of cancer. *Principles of Cancer Biotherapy,* 463 © Springer Science + Business Media B.V.

Pedley, RB., Boden, JA., Boden, R., Dale, R., & Begent, RH. (1993). Comparative radioimmunotherapy using intact or F(ab0)2 fragments of 131I anti-CEA antibody in a colonic xenograft model. *British Journal of Cancer,* Vol. 68, pp. 69-73.

Perkins, AC., & Missailidis, S. (2007). Radiolabelled aptamers for tumor imaging and therapy. *The Quarterly Journal Of Nuclear Medicine And Molecular Imaging,* Vol. 51(4), pp. 292-296.

Pontus, KE., Bforjessona, EJ., Postemab, R de B., Jan, C., Roosc, C., Rene L., Kalevi, JA., Kairemod, Guus, AMS., van Dongen. (2004). Radioimmunodetection and radioimmunotherapy of head and neck cancer.*Oral Oncology,* Vol. 40, pp. 761–772.

Press, OW., Shan, D., & Howell-Clark, J. (1996). Comparative metabolism and retention of iodine-125, yttrium-90, and indium-111 radioimmunoconjugates by cancer cells. *Cancer Research,* Vol. 56, pp. 2123–2129.

Pressman, D., & Korngold, L. (1953). The in-vivo localisation of anti-Wagner-osteogenic-sarcoma antibodies. *Cancer,* Vol. 6, pp. 619–623.

Pysz, MA., Gambhir, SS., Willmann, JK. (2010). Molecular imaging:currentstatusand emerging strategies, *Clinical Radiology,* Vol. 65, pp. 500-506.

Rasaneh, S., Rajabi, H., Babaei, MH., Johari Daha, F., & Salouti, M. (2009). Radiolabeling of trastuzumab with 177Lu via DOTA, a new radiopharmaceutical for radioimmunotherapy of breast cancer. *Nuclear Medicine and Biology,* Vol. 36, pp. 363–369.

Richman, CM., & Denardo, SJ., (2001). Systemic radiotherapy in metastatic breast cancer using 90Y-linked monoclonal MUC-1 antibodies. *Critical Reviews in Oncology: Hematology,* Vol. 38, pp. 25–35.

Roland, B., Walter, OW., Press, & Pagel, JM. (2010). Pretargeted Radioimmunotherapy for Hematologic and Other Malignancies, *Cancer Biotherapy & Radiopharmaceuticals.*Vol. 25(2).

Ross,RJ., & Thompson, JS. (1982), Nuclear magnetic resonance imaging and evaluation of human breast tissue: preliminary clinical trials . *Radiology,* Vol. 143, pp. 195-205.

Ross, JS., Fletcher, JA., Bloom, KJ., Linette, GP., Stec, J., Symmans, WF., Pusztai, L., & Hortobagyi, GN. (2004). Targeted therapy in breast cancer: the HER- 2/neu gene and protein. *Molecular and Cellular Proteomics,* Vol. 3, pp. 379–398.

Salouti, M., Babaei, MH., Rajabi, H., & Rasaee, MJ. (2011). Preparation and biological evaluation of 177Lu conjugated PR81 for radioimmunotherapy of breast cancer. *Nuclear Medicine and Biology,* pp. 1-7.

Salouti, M., Babaei, MH., Rajabi, H.,& Foroutan, H. (2011). Comparison of 99mTc-labeled PR81 and its F(ab0)2 fragments as radioimmunoscintigraphy agents for breast cancer imaging. *Annals of Nuclear Medicine,* Vol. 25, pp. 87–92.

Salouti, M., Rajabi, H., Babaei, MH., & Rasaee, MJ. (2008). Breast tumor targeting with 99mTc-HYNIC-PR81 complex as a new biologic radiopharmaceutical. *Nuclear Medicine and Biology,* Vol. 35, pp. 763–768.

Salouti, M., Rajabi, H., & Babaei, MH. (2006). A new monoclonal antibody radiopharmacetical for radioimmunoscintigraphyof breast cancer: direct labeling of antibody and its quality control. *DARU,* Vol. 14, pp. 51-56.

Sauer, G., Deissler, H., Strunz, K., Helms, G., Remmel, E., & Koretz, K. (2005). Ultrasound-guided large-core needle biopsies of breast lesions: analysis of 962 cases to determine the number of samples for reliable tumor classification. *British Journal of Cancer,* Vol. 92(2), pp. 231-235.

Sawyers, C. (2004). Targeted cancer therapy. *Nature,* Vol. 432, pp. 294-297.

Schillaci, O., & Buscombe, JR. (2004). Breast scintigraphy today: Indications and limitations. *European Journal of Nuclear Medicine and Molecular Imaging,* Vol. 31, pp. 35-45.

Schillaci, O., Danieli, R., & Filippi, L. (2007). Scintimammography with a hybrid SPECT/CT imaging system. *Anticancer Research,* Vol. 27, pp. 557-62.

Schlom, J., Eggensperger, D., & Colcher D. (1992). Therapeutic advantage of high-affinity anticarcinoma radioimmunoconjugates. *Cancer Research,* Vol. 52, pp. 1067-1072.

Schlom, J., Molinolo, A., & Simpson, JF. (1990). Advantage of dose fractionation in monoclonal antibody-directed radioimmunotherapy. *National Cancer Institute,* Vol. 82, pp. 763-771.

Schueller, G., Schueller-Weidekamm, C., & Helbich, TH. (2008). Accuracy of ultrasoundguided, large-core needle breast biopsy. *European Radiology,* Vol. 18(9), pp. 1761- 1773.

Sergey, MD., & Ekaterina, NL. (2008). Multivalency: the hallmark of antibodies used for optimization of tumor targeting by design. *BioEssays,* Vol. 30, pp.904–918.

Sergides, G., Austin, RCT., & Winslet, MC. (1999). Radioimmunodetection: technical problems and methods of improvement, *European Journal of Surgical Oncology,* Vol. 25, pp. 529–539.

Shahied, LS., Tang, Y., Alpaugh, RK., Somer, R., & Greenspon, D. (2004). Bispecific minibodies targeting HER2/neu and CD16 exhibit improved tumor lysis when placed in a divalent tumor antigen binding format. *Biological Chemistry,* Vol. 279, pp. 53907–53914.

Sharkey, RM., & Goldenberg, DM. (2006). Targeted Therapy of Cancer: New Prospects for Antibodies and Immunoconjugates. *A Cancer Journal for Clinicians,* Vol. 56, pp. 226-243.

Sharkey, RM., & Goldenberg, DM. (2008). Novel radioimmunopharmaceuticals for cancer imaging and therapy. *Current Opinion in Investigational Drugs* ,Vol. 9(12), pp. 1302-1316.

Slamon, D., Eiermann, W., & Robert, N. (2006). 2nd interim analysis phase III randomized trial comparing doxorubicin and cyclophosphamide followed by docetaxel (AC→T) with doxorubicin and cyclophosphamide followed by docetaxel and trastuzumab (AC→TH) with docetaxel, carboplatin and trastuzumab (TCH) in HER2 positive early breast cancer patients. *Proceeding of Breast Cancer Symposium,* San Antonio, December 14–17.

Slamon, DJ., Leyland-Jones, B., & Shak, S. (2001). Use of chemotherapy plus a monoclonal antibody against HER2 for metastatic breast cancer that overexpresses HER2. *New England Journal of Medicine, Vol .344, pp.* 783-792.

Stipsanelli, E., & Valsamaki, P. (2005). Monoclonal antibodies: old and new trends in breast cancer imaging and therapeutic approach. *Hellenic Society of Nuclear Medicine,* Vol. 8, pp. 103–108.

Todorovska, A., Roovers, RC., Dolezal, O., Kortt, AA., Hoogenboom, HR., & Hudson, PJ. (2001), Design and application of diabodies, triabodies and tetrabodies for cancer targeting. *Immunological Methods,* Vol. 248, pp. 47-66.

Untch, Michael. (2010). Targeted Therapy for Early and Locally Advanced Breast Cancer, *Breast Care (Basel),* Vol. 5(3), pp. 144–152.

Verhaar-Langereis, MJ., Zonnenberg, BA., de Klerk, JMH., & Blijham GH. (2000). Radioimmunodiagnosis and therapy. *cancer treatment reviews,* Vol. 26, pp. 3–10.

Violet, JA., Dearling, JLJ., Green, AJ., Begent, RHJ., & Pedley, RB. (2008). Fractionated 131I anti-CEA radioimmunotherapy: effects on xenograft tumor growth and haematological toxicity in mice. *British Journal of Cancer,* Vol. 99, pp. 632 - 638.

Waldmann, TA., & Morris, JC. (2006). Development of Antibodies and Chimeric Molecules for Cancer Immunotherapy.

Wernick, MN., & Aarsvold, JN., (2004). Emission Tomography: The Fundamentals of SPECT and PET, 1st ed, *Elsevier,* San Diego, CA.

Widakowich, C.,Gilberto, D., Castro, Jr., de Azambuja, E.,Dinh, P., &Awada, A. (2007). Review: Side Effects of Approved Molecular Targeted Therapies in Solid Cancers.*AlphaMed Press,* pp. 1083-7159.

Wiele, Van de C., Cocquyt, V., Vanden, BR. (2001). Iodinelabeled tamoxifen uptake in primary human breast carcinoma. *The Journal Of Nuclear Medicine,* Vol. 42, pp. 1818-20.

Wilder, RB., Langmuir, VK., & Medonca, HL. (1993). Local hyperthermia and SR 4233 enhance the antitumor effects of radioimmunotherapy in nude mice with human colonic adenocarcinoma xenografts. *Cancer Research,* Vol. 53, pp. 3022–3027.

William, C., Eckelman, Richard, CR., & Gary, JK. (2008). Targeted imaging: an important biomarker for understanding disease progression in the era of personalized medicine. *Drug Discovery Today,*Vol. 13, Numbers 17/18.

Willuda, J., Kubetzko, S., Waibel, R., Schubiger, PA., & Zangemeister-Wittke, U. (2001). Tumor targeting of mono-, di-, and tetravalent antip185(HER-2) miniantibodies multimerized by self-associating peptides. *Biological Chemistry,* Vol. 276, pp.14385–14392.

Wu, AM., & Yazaki. (2000). Designer genes: Recombinant antibody fragments for biological imaging. *Quarterly Journal of Nuclear Medicine,* Vol.44, pp. 268-283.

Xia, W., Gerard, CM., & Liu, L. (2005). Combining lapatininb (GW572016), a small molecule inhibitor of ErbB1 and ErbB2 tyrosine kinases, with therapeutic anti-ErbB2 antibodies enhances apoptosis of ErbB2-overexpressing breast cancer cells. *Oncogene,* Vol. 24, pp. 6213-6221.

Yazaki, PJ., Wu, AM., & Tsai, SW. (2001). Tumor targeting of radiometal labelled anti-CEA recombinant T84.66 diabody and t84.66 minibody: comparison to radioiodinated fragments. *Bioconjugate Chemistry,* Vol. 12, pp. 220-228.

Zonderland, HM. (2002). The role of ultrasound in the diagnosis of breast cancer. *Seminars in Ultrasound, CT and MRI,* Vol. 21, pp. 317-324.

8

Diagnosis of Dementia Using Nuclear Medicine Imaging Modalities

Merissa N. Zeman, Garrett M. Carpenter and Peter J. H. Scott
Department of Radiology, University of Michigan Medical School, Ann Arbor, MI, USA

1. Introduction

Dementia describes the loss of brain function that occurs with certain diseases, and which has the potential to affect memory, thinking, language, judgment, and behavior. Most types of dementia involve irreversible neurodegeneration, and Alzheimer's disease (AD) is the most common form. Beyond AD however, there are many other diseases that can lead to dementia including dementia with Lewy bodies (DLB), frontotemporal dementia (FTD), Parkinson's disease with dementia, corticobasal degeneration (CBD) and progressive supranuclear palsy (PSP). Dementia can also be the result of many small strokes and, in such cases, is called vascular dementia.

Whilst such clinically and neuropathologically overlapping dementia diseases can be predicted by clinical diagnosis, definitively differentiating them from one another has typically been attempted using high-risk diagnostic procedures (e.g. brain biopsy, Lumbar puncture) or, more commonly, during a *post-mortem* examination. This makes it difficult to a) differentiate dementias and treat each appropriately before patient death; b) manage the diseases early, before the onset of cognitive decline; c) select appropriate patients for assisting in dementia-related drug development; and d) track the impact of new dementia therapeutics in clinical trials. Therefore, new non-invasive diagnostic methods for managing dementia are in high demand and, reflecting this, many radiopharmaceuticals (drugs tagged with a radioactive isotope) have been developed over the last 2 decades that allow non-invasive examination of dementia pathophysiology in living human subjects using nuclear medicine imaging techniques. Such techniques include positron emission tomography (PET) and single photon emission computed tomography (SPECT) imaging, and have greatly enhanced diagnostic confidence across the entire dementia disease spectrum in recent years.

This chapter reviews radiopharmaceuticals commonly employed clinically in the management of dementia patients, suffering from the diseases outlined above, with nuclear medicine modalities. The chapter is divided by disease entity, and progress in imaging the pathophysiology of each disease is highlighted. In addition to those radiopharmaceuticals with approval for human use discussed herein, there are many experimental radiopharmaceuticals for dementia in pre-clinical development, which have not yet been translated into clinical use. Comprehensive review of such pre-clinical radiopharmaceuticals is outside the scope of this book, and pertinent examples are highlighted only when necessary to indicate key concepts involved in imaging dementia patients. The interested reader can obtain additional information on radiopharmaceuticals currently in development for dementia from many excellent and comprehensive review articles available in the literature (Brücke, et al., 2000; Herholz, 2003, 2011; Herholz, et al., 2007; Ishii, 2002; Jagust, 2004; Kadir and Nordberg, 2010; Nordberg, 2004, 2008; Pavese and Brooks, 2009; Sioka, et al., 2010; Vitali, et al., 2008).

2. Alzheimer's disease

2.1 Introduction

Alzheimer's disease (AD) is the most common form of dementia, affecting, for example, 5.3 million Americans, and this number is expected to rise as the baby boom generation comes of age. The cause of AD is presently not entirely understood but what is clear is that it results from a complex neurodegenerative cascade that includes misfolding and aggregation of proteins such as amyloid and tau, with concomitant decline of neurotransmitter systems. As set forth by the National Institute of Neurological and Communicative Diseases and Stroke-Alzheimer's Disease and Related Disorders Association (NINCDS-ADRDA) and the Diagnostic and Statistical Manual of Mental Disorders, fourth edition (DSM-IV-TR), a diagnosis of Alzheimer's disease (AD) requires two components: (1) clinical progressive dementia with episodic memory impairment and (2) hallmark neuropathological changes, including the presence of extracellular Aβ plaques and intraneuronal neurofibrillary tangles (NFTs) in the cortical brain (APA, 2000; McKhann, et al., 1984). Due to the difficulty of confirming histopathology *in vivo*, however, AD can only be definitively diagnosed *post-mortem*. Consequently, the prevailing criteria only allow a probabilistic diagnosis of AD based on clinical phenotype. Specifically, a patient must present with manifest dementia above a certain severity threshold, impairment of two or more cognitive domains, which must cause major interference with social function, and a daily regiment to receive a clinical diagnosis of AD (APA, 2000). After confirming the presence of dementia, a clinician must exclude other conditions that might account for cognitive decline (McKhann, et al., 1984). Since the criteria's enumeration in 1984, new data has emerged - specifically, with regards to the biological basis of AD. New clinical tests, (chiefly, MRI, CT and PET), coupled with the Mini-Mental State Examination (MMSE) and ECG, may foment a clinician's ability to differentiate between forms of dementia.

While clinical-neuropsychological testing remains one of the best tools in a clinician's armamentarium, the utility of such testing is limited in many respects. Evidence suggests that AD pathology (i.e. Aβ deposition in extracellular plaques and vascular walls, tau neurofibrillary tangles (NFTs), cerebral atrophy, synaptic reduction, and neuronal loss) may develop years to decades before the appearance of cognitive deterioration (Pike, et al., 2007; Price and Morris, 1999; Thal, et al., 2002). As dementia represents a late stage in the progression of this disease, early clinical diagnosis of AD is not possible with a great degree of accuracy. Clinical-neuropsychological testing has low sensitivity and specificity in early pre-dementia stages because, in part, a mere subset of individuals that is clinically diagnosed with mild cognitive impairment (MCI), an at-risk population, will progress to AD (Forsberg, et al., 2008; Petersen, et al., 2009; Pike, et al., 2007). Even within later stages, a clinical diagnosis of AD is only probable, not definitive. Only 70 to 90% of persons that match the aforementioned criteria have their diagnoses confirmed at autopsy (Jellinger, et al., 1990; Kukull, et al., 1990). A clinical differential diagnosis of dementia remains somewhat difficult, as many of the cognitive symptoms of AD overlap with those of other neurodegenerative disorders.

It is thus apparent that there is a great need to revise the way in which AD is conceptualized. Accurate and definitive diagnoses need to occur *ante-mortem*, in lieu of *post-mortem*, and preferably in the early pre-dementia (prodromal) stage. Dubois *et al.*, having moved beyond the NINCDS-ADRDA criteria for probable AD, introduced new standards for diagnosis (Dubois, et al., 2007). They include early and significant episodic memory impairment and at least one abnormal *in vivo* biomarker- particularly, medial temporal lobe atrophy, abnormal CSF biomarkers (increased total tau concentrations, increased phospho-tau concentrations, low $Aß_{1-42}$ concentrations, or a combination of all three), brain Aβ load, temporoparietal hypometabolism on [18F]FDG-PET, and/or specific binding pattern with particular PET ligands. Learning more about AD biomarkers, and how they fit into the accepted paradigm for this disease, will allow for decreased dependence on unreliable clinical diagnostic criteria. Non-invasive PET imaging can be particularly useful in this context. Probes are being developed that target specific AD biomarkers, allowing us to monitor AD pathophysiology *in vivo*. The main strategies for exploration of AD pathophysiology using PET imaging have been reviewed (Jagust, 2004; Nordberg, 2004, 2008), and are outlined in the following sections.

2.2 Imaging Alzheimer's disease with [^{18}F]FDG

[^{18}F]Fluoro-2-deoxy-D-glucose ([^{18}F]FDG) is the most commonly used radiopharmaceutical for clinical PET imaging to date. Patients receive an injection of [^{18}F]FDG, and then images are typically obtained 30 - 60 min later. As a radiolabeled analog of glucose, [^{18}F]FDG is typically employed as a marker of cell proliferation as it preferentially accumulates in cells with increased glucose consumption (e.g. tumors). Therefore, [^{18}F]FDG finds widespread application in oncology including diagnosis and staging of cancers, and monitoring tumor response to chemotherapy. However, glucose is also the main energy supply for the brain and, reflecting this, levels are closely coupled to neuronal function so that measurement of cerebral glucose metabolism can provide diagnostically relevant information about the neurodegenerative disorders described above. According to Herholz and colleagues (Herholz, et al., 2007), typical resting state cerebral metabolic rate for glucose is 40-60 μmol glucose/100 g/min for grey matter, and 15 μmol glucose/100 g/min for white matter, although this does drop off somewhat with age (Kuhl, et al., 1982). Observed regional differences include higher values in the striatum and parietal cortex. Other phylogenetically older brain structures (e.g. medial temporal cortex and cerebellum) have glucose metabolism rates between grey matter and white matter.

For at least two decades, significant efforts have been made to image patients at various stages of Alzheimer's disease (including high risk, asymptomatic patients; patients with mild cognitive impairment (MCI); and patients with fully developed Alzheimer's disease) with [^{18}F]FDG (e.g. Figure 1). In patients considered high risk for developing AD (for example because of family history and possession of the ApoE ε4 allele (Reiman, et al., 1996; Small, et al., 1995)), impairment of regional cerebral glucose metabolism has been observed decades before likely onset of dementia and certainly while the patients are still asymptomatic (Reiman, et al., 2004).

In 1997, Kuhl and colleagues reported the first example of using posterior cingulate glucose metabolism, determined from [^{18}F]FDG PET scans, to predict progression of disease in patients with MCI (Minoshima, et al., 1997). The results have been echoed by a number of subsequent longitudinal studies, which have confirmed the high predictive power of

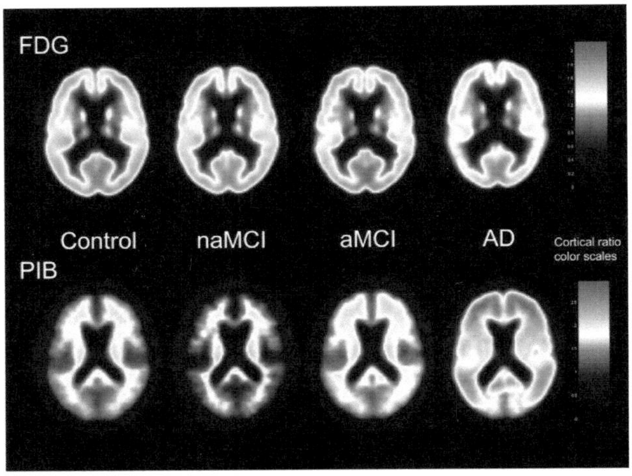

Fig. 1. ^{18}F-FDG and PiB group mean images for control, naMCI, aMCI, and AD subjects showing better visual separation of groups using PiB. Scaling shown to right using pons and cerebellar normalization, respectively. Regions with activity similar to these regions of normalization color in 1.0 color ranges (green), whereas regions with greater uptake show up in yellow and red. Color scaling is slightly different for 18F-FDG and PiB groups given different range of cortical ratios. *(Reprinted with permission from Loew VJ, Kemp BJ, Jack CR, et al. Comparison of 18F-FDG and PiB PET in Cognitive Impairment. J Nucl Med. 2009;50:878-886)*

[^{18}F]FDG PET. For example, Berent and colleagues reported 70% progression of disease in 3 years following an abnormal PET scan, but only 30% progression after a normal PET scan (Berent, et al., 1999). Anchisi and co-workers also showed that a normal FDG PET scan indicated low chance of progression of MCI into full AD within 1 year (Anchisi, et al., 2005). Generally speaking [^{18}F]FDG PET has >80% sensitivity and specificity for prediction of rapid progression. Moreover, a recent report by Drzezga and colleagues discovered that [^{18}F]FDG PET (92% sensitivity, 89% specificity) was superior to ApoE ε4 testing (75% sensitivity, 56% specificity) when used to predict disease progression (A. Drzezga, et al., 2005). Other aspects of [^{18}F]FDG PET scans have also proven pertinent to the assessment of MCI. For example, mesial temporal metabolic impairment (Heiss, et al., 1992), as well as hippocampal and antorhinal metabolic impairment (de Leon, et al., 2001), although the latter can be difficult to assess because of small size.

As MCI progresses and develops into Alzheimer's disease, numerous studies over the last two decades have shown that both cerebral blood flow and glucose metabolism are reduced in a number of areas of the brain. For example, impairment of glucose metabolism in the temporoparietal association cortices is typical in AD (on the order of 16-19% over 3 years (Smith, et al., 1992)), whilst no significant decline is apparent in the corresponding normal controls. These cortices are also prone to amyloid deposition during AD (Bartzokis, et al., 2007). Reduced glucose metabolism may also occur in the frontal association cortex, although more so as AD progresses. In contrast to the other dementia diseases discussed herein, the rate of glucose metabolism in other areas of the brain including the visual and motor cortex, basal ganglia and cerebellum is unaffected (Herholz, et al., 2007). This is in agreement with the clinical manifestation of AD, as primary motor and sensory function remain intact, whilst memory, associative thinking, planning of action and other higher sensory processing decline. Such clinical and imaging differences can be used as a means of differentiating AD from other related disorders.

More subtle differences between FDG PET scans of normal patients and AD patients are also apparent if more advanced image analysis is employed. Voxel-based analysis can detect differences in FDG PET that are not obvious upon visual interpretation of the scan. For example, comparison of FDG PET scans of AD patients versus normal controls reveals impaired glucose metabolism in the posterior cingulate gyrus as well as the precuneus (Minoshima, et al., 1997). This is not immediately obvious because metabolism in these areas is normally above average and the decrease in AD patients can obscure it into the background. The large amounts of FDG PET data obtained in AD patients now allow advanced analytical techniques to go one step further, and automatically detect the typical pattern of metabolic abnormalities associated with AD. This approach has been successfully used to distinguish AD patients for normal controls with >80% (and frequently >90%) accuracy, and such data have enabled the use of FDG PET in AD therapeutic trials (Heiss, et al., 1994).

2.3 Imaging amyloid-ß (Aß) plaque burden in Alzheimer's disease

As Aβ deposition is considered a hallmark neuropathological sign of AD and is thought to be one of the primary events in the pathogenesis of AD (the "amyloid cascade hypothesis"), Aβ PET imaging agents are at the forefront of this expanding field (Haass and Selkoe, 2007). In AD patients, Aβ deposits are composed of $A\beta_{1-40}$ and $A\beta_{1-42}$, peptides that are 40 and 42 amino acids in length, respectively, generated from the sequential proteolytic cleavage of amyloid precursor protein (APP) by β- and γ-secretases (Beyreuther and Masters, 1991; Martins, et al., 1991). Whilst $A\beta_{1-42}$ deposits have a higher propensity to oligomerize, both isoforms are found in fibrillar amyloid plaques (Tamaoka, et al., 1994), characteristic β-sheet-rich structures that represent the target for Aβ PET ligands.

The ability to image and measure Aβ load *in vitro* has considerable implications for the future study of AD. As Aβ deposition commences long before the onset of cognitive deficits, Aβ-targeting probes may support earlier diagnoses and interventions in the pre-dementia stage of this disease (Pike, et al., 2007; Price and Morris, 1999; Thal, et al., 2002). Aβ PET imaging additionally has some utility in accurately differentiating AD from Aβ-negative forms of dementia and, thus, in increasing the specificity of a clinical diagnosis. Objectively monitoring treatments and selecting candidates for particular drugs and clinical trials are other potential uses for this imaging technology (Rafii and Aisen, 2009); for example, patients with low cortical Aβ load, as measured by Aβ PET, are unlikely to qualify for anti-amyloid therapies.

Due to the large number of possible clinical applications, there has been a dramatic rise in the number of probes that target Aβ plaques over the last decade. The four Aβ PET imaging agents under active commercial development are [^{11}C]PIB, [^{18}F]flutemetamol, [^{18}F]florbetaben, and [^{18}F]florbetapir. Each imaging agent is currently undergoing FDA-approved Phase III clinical trials in the US, except [^{18}F]Florbetapir, which is awaiting FDA approval. Each Aβ PET imaging agent will be discussed individually in further detail below.

2.3.1 [^{11}C]Pittsburgh Compound B ([^{11}C]PiB)

The most well-characterized and studied radiopharmaceutical for Aβ pathology is [^{11}C]Pittsburgh Compound B ([^{11}C]PiB, (N-methyl-[^{11}C])2-(4'-methylamino-phenyl)-6-OH-

BTA), a 6-hydroxyl-substituted benzothiazole aniline; a team led by Mathis and Klunk developed this ^{11}C-labeled neutral derivative of Thioflavin-T amyloid dye at the University of Pittsburgh in 2002 (W. E. Klunk, et al., 2001; Mathis, et al., 2002). Pre-clinical studies of [^{11}C]PiB have demonstrated that this radiotracer has excellent brain penetration (approximately 7% injected dose per gram at 2 minutes post injection) and initial brain uptake, rapid clearance from normal brain tissue, high binding affinity to Aβ plaques (K_i=0.87±0.18 nM), and moderate lipophilicity (W. E. Klunk, et al., 2001; Mathis, et al., 2002; Mathis, et al., 2003). As a carbon-11 labeled ligand, [^{11}C]PiB has the advantage of delivering a lower radiation burden (whole-body effective dose conversion factor for a 70-kg adult= 4.74±0.8 μSv/MBq; typical administered dose= 489±61 MBq (13±1.65 mCi); effective dose= 2.37±0.53 mSv). Furthermore, [^{11}C]PiB is able to reach a maximum effect size more rapidly than ^{18}F-labeled radiopharmaceuticals, leading to shorter imaging times (50-70 minutes as the optimal time-window) (McNamee, et al., 2009; O'Keefe, et al., 2009; Scheinin, et al., 2007). Of particular interest, *in vitro* autoradiography studies have confirmed that [^{11}C]PiB binds to aggregated, fibrillar Aβ deposits in the cortex, striatum, and cerebral vessel walls, but not to amorphous, cerebellar Aβ deposits (Greenberg, et al., 2008; W. E. Klunk, et al., 2003; Lockhart, et al., 2007). At nanomolar concentrations, however, [^{11}C]PiB does not bind to free soluble amyloid, NFTs, or Lewy bodies (Fodero-Tavoletti, et al., 2007; W. E. Klunk, et al., 2003; Lockhart, et al., 2007).

In 2004, Klunk *et al.* published the results from their first in human proof-of-mechanism study (W. E. Klunk, et al., 2004). With 16 mild AD patients and 9 healthy controls, this study supported the use of [^{11}C]PiB uptake patterns for the reliable discrimination between the two diagnostic groups. AD patients had a twofold increase of [^{11}C]PiB uptake over healthy controls, as measured by regional and average neocortical standard uptake value ratios (SUVRs) with the cerebellum as the reference region, specifically in the frontal, temporal, parietal, and lateral temporal cortices, portions of the occipital cortex, and the striatum. This pattern of [^{11}C]PiB uptake is consistent with the distribution of Aβ plaques in previous *post-mortem* studies (Thal, et al., 2002). Three AD patients, however, had [^{11}C]PiB retention levels in the range typical for healthy controls. Contrastingly, all healthy controls, except one, showed little or no cortical [^{11}C]PiB binding. Non-specific binding was present in white matter areas, but at identical levels in healthy controls and AD patients. This study additionally cited a significant inverse correlation between [^{11}C]PiB uptake and cerebral metabolic rate, especially in the parietal cortex, but only when healthy controls and AD patients were pooled together. Despite this significant trend, [^{11}C]PiB uptake levels provided higher discriminatory power than cerebral metabolic rate in differentiating AD patients from healthy controls.

Since this groundbreaking study, the number of investigations using [^{11}C]PiB in humans, as well as research applications for this radiopharmaceutical, have greatly proliferated. Numerous studies have been dedicated to determining the relationship between [^{11}C]PiB retention and other AD biomarkers, as well as clinical features/parameters. For example, [^{11}C]PiB uptake negatively correlates with CSF $A\beta_{1-42}$ levels in AD patients and healthy controls (Fagan, et al., 2007; Forsberg, et al., 2010). Furthermore, tracer binding is directly proportional to CSF tau in MCI patients, but not AD patients, cerebral atrophy as measured by MRI in AD subjects (although NFTs correlate better), and temporoparietal hypometabolism as measured by [^{18}F]FDG-PET (Forsberg, et al., 2008; W. E. Klunk, et al., 2004; Storandt, et al., 2009). In addition, subjects with at least one Apolipoprotein E ε4 (ApoE ε4) allele, a genotype strongly associated with AD, are more likely to have a [^{11}C]PiB-positive scan than a negative one (A. Drzezga, et al., 2009; Storandt, et al., 2009).

While [^{11}C]PiB has primarily shown utility in differentiating AD patients from healthy controls, this tracer has also been assessed for the differential diagnosis of dementia. [^{11}C]PiB binding patterns allow for great separation between AD and Frontotemporal Lobar Degeneration (FTLD) patients, as those with the frontotemporal and semantic forms of the latter rarely have Aβ plaques *post-mortem* (A. Drzezga, et al., 2008; Engler, et al., 2008; Rabinovici, et al., 2007; Rowe, et al., 2007). Contrastingly, due to the presence of Aβ deposits in a large proportion of patients with Lewy body dementia (DLB) (only 15% of cases represent "pure" DLB with no Aβ pathology), it is harder to distinguish DLB from AD solely based on [^{11}C]PiB binding alone (McKeith, et al., 1996; Rowe, et al., 2007). In comparison to the distribution pattern typical of AD patients, DLB cortical [^{11}C]PiB uptake has been noted to be more variable and lower in a majority of cases (Rowe, et al., 2007). While [^{11}C]PiB cannot distinguish AD and DLB pathology with a high degree of accuracy, this technology could potentially be used to identify Aβ-negative and Aβ-positive DLB subsets. Whether this discrimination signifies differences in therapeutic options remains unknown at this time. In a study by *Rowe et al.*, the presence of Aβ deposition (high Aβ load) was associated with a more rapid onset of the full DLB phenotype (Rowe, et al., 2007). [^{11}C]PiB studies, thus, may be able to shed new insights into DLB pathophysiology. Healthy controls have been additional subjects of [^{11}C]PiB studies because 10-30% of cognitively normal elderly people have Aβ plaques at levels comparable to those of AD patients *post-mortem* (Aizenstein, et al., 2008; Price and Morris, 1999). Concomitantly, 10-30% of healthy controls with normal cognition show increased cortical [^{11}C]PiB binding (W. E. Klunk, et al., 2004; Mintun, et al., 2006; Morris, et al., 2009; Rowe, et al., 2007). To date, this technology does not allow discrimination between healthy controls with high Aβ load and AD patients. The meaning of these false-positive scans is unclear; while low specificity is possible, high [^{11}C]PiB uptake and thus Aβ load in cognitively normal people most likely represents either pre-clinical AD or "benign" pathology (Mintun, et al., 2006; Morris, et al., 2009; Rowe, et al., 2007).

There is evidence to suggest a prodromal stage of AD does exist, in which Aβ deposition begins in a small subset of adults as a primary event (Jack, et al., 2009; Pike, et al., 2007; Rowe, et al., 2007). As these individuals reach the MCI phase, the amount of Aβ accumulation approximates the levels seen in AD patients (Jack, et al., 2009; Pike, et al., 2007). Upon conversion to AD, Aβ load either plateaus or progresses slowly. Consequently, clinical cognitive decline (or severity of dementia) does not correlate with Aβ load, as measured *in vivo* by [^{11}C]PiB (Jack, et al., 2009; Rowe, et al., 2007). This time course for Aβ accumulation is further supported by a 2-year study in which a majority of 16 AD subjects did not show a significant change in [^{11}C]PiB uptake from baseline, despite decreases in clinical cognitive parameters and temporoparietal metabolism (as measured by [^{18}F]FDG-PET) (Engler, et al., 2006). The results from this study support the use of [^{11}C]PiB as a potential early biomarker for AD, but not as an indicator of disease severity. Other measures, such as [^{18}F]FDG-PET and tau PET imaging agents, which track later-developing biomarkers, correlate better with cognitive decline and thus can be used to assess neurodegeneration (Meyer, et al., 2011).

To further evidence [^{11}C]PiB's ability to act as an early biomarker for AD, radiotracer studies have been performed in MCI patients. [^{11}C]PiB distribution patterns in MCI patients are dichotomous, with one subset of MCI patients showing abundant "AD-like" neocortical binding ([^{11}C]PiB-positive) and the other subset showing low, non-specific binding ([^{11}C]PiB-negative) (Forsberg, et al., 2008; Okello, et al., 2009; Pike, et al., 2007; Rowe, et al., 2007). As only 40-60% of MCI patients progress to AD, longitudinal studies are needed to determine if this bimodal distribution pattern of [^{11}C]PiB uptake accurately predicts those who will convert to AD (Forsberg, et al., 2008; Kukull, et al., 1990; Okello, et al., 2009; Petersen, et al., 2009). In a study by Forsberg *et al.*, 7 out of 21 tested MCI patients converted to AD after 8.1±6.0 months (Forsberg, et al., 2008). Interestingly, there were detectable group differences between the 7 MCI converters and the 14 non-converters. MCI converters were shown to have lower levels of CSF $A\beta_{1-42}$ and MMSE test scores compared to non-converters. Additionally, MCI converters were more likely to be ApoE ε4 carriers (85%) than were non-converters (57%). Most importantly, MCI converters had high [^{11}C]PiB uptake in the frontal, parietal, and temporal cortices and the posterior cingulum, similar to levels in AD patients. Contrastingly, MCI non-converters had significantly lower cortical [^{11}C]PiB retention, indistinguishable from healthy controls. These promising results demonstrate the prognostic value of [^{11}C]PiB for predicting which MCI patients will progress to AD.

[^{11}C]PiB has now been used in a large number of subjects, consistently showing high sensitivity and specificity in detecting cerebral amyloid deposition *in vivo* with high intra- and inter-reader agreement (W. E. Klunk and Mathis, 2008). Due to the short physical half-life of carbon-11 (20.4 minutes), however, [^{11}C]PiB is limited in clinical availability. As a result, Aβ tracers that are radiolabeled with fluorine-18, a radioisotope with a considerably longer half-life (109.4 minutes) than carbon-11, have been developed. Fluorine-18 labeled Aβ PET tracers do not require on-site cyclotrons for their production, thus allowing for a more widespread distribution of this imaging technology.

2.3.2 [^{18}F]Flutemetamol (3'-[^{18}F]F-PiB or [^{18}F]GE067)

[^{18}F]Flutemetamol (3'-[^{18}F]F-6-OH-BTA1) is an ^{18}F-labeled thioflavin analog of [^{11}C]PiB licensed to GE Healthcare (Koole, et al., 2009). Due to its longer physical half-life in comparison to its parent molecule, [^{18}F]flutemetamol can potentially have a larger impact in clinical and research settings. Unlike other ^{18}F-labeled Aβ PET radiotracers, [^{18}F]flutemetamol has the advantage that there has been extensive work done on its parent molecule, [^{11}C]PiB, which can easily lend itself to the validation of [^{18}F]flutemetamol. Although [^{11}C]PiB and [^{18}F]flutemetamol exhibit similarities in structure, the two radiotracers have slightly different properties. Fortunately, pre-clinical studies of [^{18}F]flutemetamol have demonstrated favorable brain kinetics, good penetration of intact blood-brain barrier (BBB), and fairly rapid washout of non-specific binding (Nelissen, et al., 2009). [^{18}F]Flutemetamol has showed a good safety profile and biodistribution (Koole, et al., 2009). The average typical administered dose is 121 MBq (range=96-147 MBq; 2.59-3.98 mCi) (Koole, et al., 2009); It is important to note that [^{18}F]flutemetamol delivers an effective dose that is 1.7 times larger than that for [^{11}C]PiB (2.37 mSv versus 4.12 mSv) (O'Keefe, et al., 2009); this higher radiation burden is due to the relatively greater radiation dose associated with fluorine-18 (whole-body effective dose conversion factor= 33.6 μSv/MBq for [^{18}F]flutemetamol versus 4.74±0.8 μSv/MBq for [^{11}C]PiB). Nevertheless, there have been no adverse events reported for the use of this radiotracer and, therefore, it has been deemed safe for use in humans (Koole, et al., 2009).

Under the direction of Nelissen and co-workers, [^{18}F]flutemetamol entered Phase I clinical trials in 2009 (Nelissen, et al., 2009). Eight AD patients and 8 healthy controls were used in this proof-of-concept study. After 80 minutes post injection, most regions of the neocortex showed a large difference in SUVRs (with the cerebellum as the reference region) between AD patients and healthy controls, except in the medial temporal cortex, which is more prone to NFT buildup than amyloid deposition, and the occipital cortex. This spatial distribution of [^{18}F]flutemetamol uptake in AD patients closely resembles that typically seen in its parent molecule, [^{11}C]PiB. Interestingly however, non-specific binding in white matter was more pronounced, but not statistically significant, in healthy controls injected with [^{18}F]flutemetamol in comparison to when using [^{11}C]PiB (Fodero-Tavoletti, et al., 2009).

While this study showed that [^{18}F]flutemetamol PET imaging can be used to differentiate AD patients and healthy controls, 2 AD patients had particular regional SUVRs within the range seen in healthy controls. These results are comparable to previous [^{11}C]PiB studies, in which 10-20% of clinically diagnosed AD patients did not show high cortical tracer uptake (W. E. Klunk, et al., 2004). Conversely, one healthy control had cortical SUVRs in line with those seen in AD patients. One possible explanation is that high white matter binding led to increased cortical values. The proportion of [^{18}F]flutemetamol-positive healthy controls in this study, however, is comparable to the 10-30% of elderly healthy controls who have increased [^{11}C]PiB brain uptake at levels indistinguishable from AD patients.

Based on the positive Phase I results, [^{18}F]flutemetamol continued to be investigated in a clinical Phase II capacity (Vandenberghe, et al., 2010). Twenty-seven patients with clinically probable AD, 20 patients with amnestic MCI, 15 elderly healthy controls, and 10 younger healthy controls were used to determine the efficacy of blinded visual assessments of [^{18}F]flutemetamol scans as well as to directly measure [^{18}F]flutemetamol against its parent molecule [^{11}C]PiB in terms of its discriminatory power. Researchers found that mean SUVRs in the frontal cortex, lateral temporal cortex, parietal cortex, anterior/posterior cingulate, and striatum were significantly higher in AD patients than in the elderly healthy controls. These results are consistent with the Phase I clinical study for [^{18}F]flutemetamol. Based on blinded visual assessments of [^{18}F]flutemetamol scans, 25 of 27 scans from AD subjects and 1 of 15 scans from the elderly healthy controls were PET-positive, corresponding to a sensitivity of 93.1% and a specificity of 93.3% against the clinical standard of truth. For MCI patients, 9 of 20 subjects were assigned to the high tracer uptake category. The proportion of [^{18}F]flutemetamol-positive scans for MCI patients is comparable to that reported for [^{11}C]PiB (Forsberg, et al., 2008). Additionally, investigators found that the test-retest variability ranged from 1 to 4%, which is lower than that reported for [^{11}C]PiB. Most important to the validation of this radiotracer is that both visually and quantitatively, [^{18}F]flutemetamol uptake was highly concordant with that of [^{11}C]PiB for both AD and MCI patients. However, non-specific binding was greater with [^{18}F]flutemetamol. Regardless, as was seen in Phase I clinical studies, high white matter uptake did not lead to any misclassifications of the scans by the visual readers.

Before clinical application, flutemetamol PET imaging needs to be tested against histopathology findings at autopsy. Thus, GE Healthcare is currently organizing and recruiting for an ongoing [^{18}F]flutemetamol Phase III clinical study (Clinical Trial NCT01165554) that will include patients willing to undergo *post-mortem* studies. Results from this trial are pending (GEHC, Accessed 2011).

2.3.3 [^{18}F]Florbetaben ([^{18}F]BAY94-9172 or [^{18}F]AV-1/ZK)

[^{18}F]Florbetaben ([^{18}F]BAY94-9172, previously [^{18}F]AV-1/ZK, *trans*-4-(N-methyl-amino)-4′-[2-[2-(2-[^{18}F]fluoro-ethoxy)-ethoxy]-ethoxy]-stilbene) is a fluorinated polyethylene glycol

(PEG) stilbene derivative that was developed by Zhang *et al.* in 2005 through Avid Radiopharmaceuticals under the name [^{18}F]AV-1/ZK (Zhang, et al., 2005a). Due to their high binding affinities to Aβ aggregates, stilbene derivatives have been considered as potential Aβ-targeting probes for PET imaging (H. F. Kung, et al., 2001; Zhang, et al., 2005a; Zhang, et al., 2005b). Stilbene derivatives have similar structural characteristics as benzothiazoles (PiB derivatives) and thus compete for the same binding site on amyloid plaques (Zhang, et al., 2005b). [^{18}F]Florbetaben was chosen from a series of stilbenes for its appropriate lipophilicity, high binding affinity (K_i= 6.7±0.3 nM), good safety profile, high initial uptake and rapid washout in normal mouse brain (4 minutes post-injection), and being ^{18}F-radiolabeled (Barthel, et al., 2010; H. F. Kung, et al., 2001; Patt, et al., 2010). The typical administered dose for [^{18}F]florbetaben is 350 MBq (9.5 mCi), and the effective dose is 5.13 mSv using this dose (whole-body effective dose conversion factor= 14.67±1.39 μSv/MBq) (O'Keefe, et al., 2009). However, [^{18}F]florbetaben causes a much lower radiation burden than most other ^{18}F-labeled probes, such as [^{18}F]flutemetamol (Koole, et al., 2009). *In vivo* autoradiography of transgenic mouse brain and *in vitro* autoradiography of *post-mortem* human AD brain tissues have demonstrated specific [^{18}F]florbetaben binding to neuritic Aβ plaques and to cerebral amyloid angiopathy (Zhang, et al., 2005b); [^{18}F]florbetaben does not label Lewy bodies, Pick bodies, glial cytoplasmic inclusions, α-synuclein, NFTs, or other tau pathology to any appreciable extent (Zhang, et al., 2005b). Due to convincing pre-clinical data, [^{18}F]florbetaben entered clinical trials, under the license of Bayer Schering Pharma.

Rowe *et al.* performed the first-in-man proof of mechanism study in 2008, using 15 elderly healthy controls, 15 patients with probable AD, and 5 patients with frontotemporal lobe degeneration (FTLD) (Rowe, et al., 2008). AD patients showed extensive cortical [^{18}F]florbetaben uptake while healthy controls and FTLD patients only demonstrated non-specific binding in white matter, but at levels comparable to those of AD patients. Visual assessment of [^{18}F]florbetaben scans correctly differentiated AD patients from both healthy controls and FTLD patients in all but two cases, leading to a sensitivity and specificity of 100% and 90%, respectively. Results for this study are comparable with previous [^{11}C]PiB studies, in terms of radiotracer distribution. However, the amount of tracer uptake is slightly higher for [^{11}C]PiB. At 90-120 minutes post-injection, the mean neocortical SUVR, with the cerebellum as the reference region, for [^{18}F]florbetaben was 57% greater in AD patients than in healthy controls; but in comparison, [^{11}C]PiB binding is, on average, 70% higher in AD patients than in healthy controls (Rowe, et al., 2007). Nevertheless, [^{18}F]florbetaben PET imaging was shown to be highly sensitive and specific in discriminating between AD patients, healthy controls, and FTLD patients, at a level similar to [^{11}C]PiB.

Subsequent studies have confirmed [^{18}F]florbetaben's high discriminatory power, low inter- and intrareader variability, and clinical utility (Barthel, et al., 2010). As an optimal imaging agent, [^{18}F]florbetaben reaches maximum effect size fairly quickly (90 minutes post-injection) and maintains this contrast for up to 4 hours post-injection (Barthel, et al., 2010; Rowe, et al., 2007). This implies a certain flexibility of the imaging time window, which is advantageous in the clinical arena. [^{18}F]Florbetaben has also been useful in better clarifying the relationship between Aβ load and other AD biomarkers. For example, regional radiotracer uptake, particularly in the lateral temporal cortex, is slightly, but significantly inversely proportional to MMSE and word-list memory scores when AD patients and healthy controls are pooled together (Barthel, et al., 2011; Rowe, et al., 2007). Moreover, there is a higher frequency of ε4 allele(s) of apolipoprotein E (APOE ε4), a strong risk factor for the development of AD, in AD patients with [^{18}F]florbetaben-positive scans than in those with [^{18}F]florbetaben-negative scans (Barthel, et al., 2011). These results are comparable to findings using [^{11}C]PiB.

Barthel *et al.* reported the largest study to date, using 81 patients with probable AD and 69 healthy controls in the primary analysis (Barthel, et al., 2011). This Phase II study confirmed the diagnostic accuracy and efficacy of [^{18}F]florbetaben in a larger cohort of subjects. Neocortical tracer uptake was significantly higher for AD patients compared with healthy controls in frontal, temporal, parietal and occipital cortices, and anterior / posterior cingulate. On a regional level, the posterior cingulate presented the greatest separation between AD patients and healthy controls and, thus, allowed for the differentiation between the two diagnostic groups. These results are consistent with previous [^{11}C]PiB studies that have shown that tracer uptake in the posterior cingulate is a good and early indicator of probable AD (Ziolko, et al., 2006). Visual assessment of [^{18}F]florbetaben scans have a sensitivity of 80% and specificity of 91% for distinguishing AD patients from healthy controls. Upon statistical adjustment, due to the fact that somewhat unreliable clinical diagnoses (70-90% accuracy) were used as the standard of truth, the sensitivity increased to 96% while the specificity was determined to be 97%.

While Phase II clinical trial showed promising results, [^{18}F]florbetaben imaging needs to be compared to *post-mortem* studies to validate this technique. As of November 30, 2009, [^{18}F]florbetaben has entered Phase III FDA-approved clinical studies in the US (Bayer, Accessed 2011). Using approximately 232 individuals, this trial (Clinical Trial NCT01020838) will assess the efficacy of [^{18}F]florbetaben PET imaging for detection of cerebral Aß against the golden standard of *post-mortem* histopathology. The trial is not expected to be completed until April 2014.

2.3.4 [^{18}F]Florbetapir ([^{18}F]AV-45 or Amyvid)

[^{18}F]Florbetapir ([^{18}F]AV-45, (E)-2-(2-(2-(2-[^{18}F]fluoroethoxy)ethoxy)ethoxy,)-5-(4-methylaminostyryl)pyridine, Amyvid) was recently developed by Avid Radiopharmaceuticals. As a fluoropegylated stilbene derivative, [^{18}F]Florbetapir is similar in structure to [^{18}F]florbetaben, but the stilbene backbone has been replaced with a styrylpyridine core (Zhang, et al., 2007; Zhang, et al., 2005a). [^{18}F]Florbetapir was chosen from a small number of ^{18}F-labeled styrylpyridine analogs due to its optimum *in vivo* kinetics and high selectivity for Aβ plaques (Zhang, et al., 2007). Pre-clinical characterization of [^{18}F]florbetapir demonstrated that this radiotracer has excellent binding affinity (K_d=3.72±0.30 nM) to Aβ aggregates, moderate lipophilicity, high initial brain uptake (7.33±1.54% injected dose per gram at 2 min post-injection) and rapid washout kinetics (1.88±0.14% injected dose per gram remaining in the brain 60 minutes post injection) in normal mice and primate brain (Choi, et al., 2009). Additionally, as supported by *in vitro* autoradiography of *post-mortem* human brain tissue sections and *ex vivo* autoradiography of transgenic mouse brain, [^{18}F]florbetapir selectively labels fibrillar Aβ plaques, but not tau NFTs (Choi, et al., 2009; Choi, et al., 2011). Non-specific binding is low or non-existent. This spatial distribution of [^{18}F]florbetapir uptake is similar to the pattern observed for [^{18}F]florbetaben (Zhang, et al., 2005b).

Favorably, [^{18}F]florbetapir also exhibits fast brain kinetics comparable to that of [^{11}C]PiB (McNamee, et al., 2009). The signal-to-noise ratio for this radiotracer asymptotes at 50-60 minutes post injection and remains stable until at least 90 minutes post-injection (Wong, et al., 2010); contrastingly, both [^{18}F]flutemetamol and [^{18}F]florbetaben reach maximum effect size at 85-90 minutes post injection (Barthel, et al., 2010; Nelissen, et al., 2009). This property of [^{18}F]florbetapir creates a large time-frame to obtain a 10 minute image and allows for shorter imaging times, if necessary. Moreover, [^{18}F]florbetapir has a good safety profile and biodistribution. The typical administered dose is 382.0±14 MBq (10.3±0.38 mCi), and the effective dose is 6.66±0.38 mSv using an administered dose of 370 MBq (whole-body effective dose conversion factor = 18.0±1.01 μSv/MBq) (Lin, et al., 2010). As expected, [^{18}F]florbetapir delivers a higher radiation burden than [^{11}C]PiB, but still within the normal range for ^{18}F-labeled radiopharmaceuticals (O'Keefe, et al., 2009); and thus it remains suitable for clinical imaging applications.

Clinical studies of [^{18}F]florbetapir have consistently shown its high discriminatory power in being able to differentiate between AD patients, patients with amyloid positive and amyloid negative MCI, and healthy controls (e.g. Figure 2) (Lister-James, et al., 2011). For example, in a study of 15 elderly healthy controls and 11 AD patients, [^{18}F]florbetapir uptake was significantly higher in AD patients than in healthy controls, especially in cortical target areas, such as the frontal and temporal cortices and the precuneus (Wong, et al., 2010). Variable tracer uptake was seen in the occipital cortex, in which Aβ deposition is thought to occur inconsistently. Contrastingly, healthy controls had tracer accumulation predominantly in white matter areas, as non-specific binding. It was noted, however, that two elderly healthy controls presented with increased tracer accumulation, indistinguishable from AD patients, and two other healthy controls had borderline levels of tracer uptake, especially in the precuneus. This finding is consistent with previous [^{11}C]PiB studies, in which 10-30% of

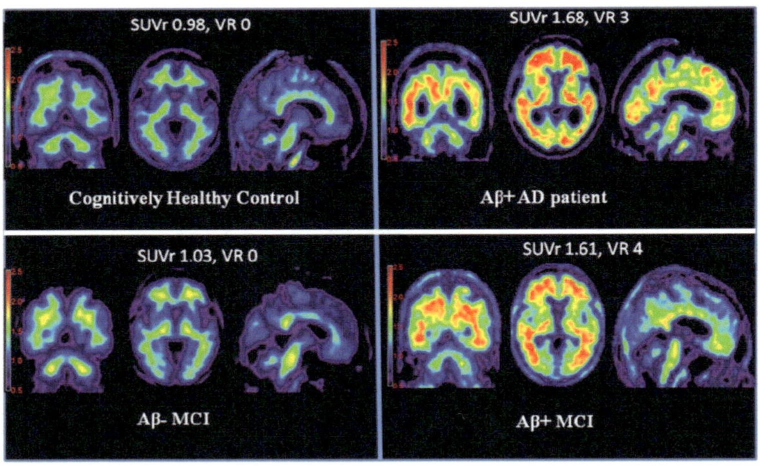

Fig. 2. Florbetapir F-18 PET imaging (coronal, axial, and sagittal views). Top left, healthy control (SUVR = 0.98; visual read score = 0); top right: patient with clinically diagnosed AD and interpreted as Aß+ (SUVR = 1.68; visual read score = 3); bottom left, patient with mild cognitive impairment and interpreted as Aß- (SUVR = 1.03; visual read score = 0); bottom right, patient with mild cognitive impairment and interpreted as Aß+ (SUVR = 1.61; visual read score = 4). *(Reprinted with permission from Lister-James J, Pontecorvo MJ, Clark C, et al. Florbetapir F-18: A histopathologically validated beta-amyloid positron emission tomography imaging agent. Semin. Nucl. Med. 2011;50:300-304)*

cognitively intact healthy subjects have increased tracer uptake (W. E. Klunk, et al., 2004; Mintun, et al., 2006; Morris, et al., 2009; Rowe, et al., 2007).

Lin and co-workers presented similar results for [^{18}F]florbetapir in a clinical study, using 6 healthy controls and 3 AD patients (Lin, et al., 2010). Tracer uptake was particularly high in the frontal, parietal, and occipital cortices of AD patients; healthy controls showed substantial non-specific binding in subcortical white matter. Consequently, simple semi-quantitative measures (SUVRs with the cerebellum as the reference region) could be used to discriminate between AD patients and healthy controls. Of importance, one AD patient showed little uptake of the radiotracer, similar to the binding pattern of healthy controls. This negative scan may be due to a lack of tracer sensitivity, but more likely is indicative of a low Aβ load in this clinically diagnosed AD patient.

In 2011, Clark *et al.* published the results from the first study of its kind, comparing the efficacy of an Aβ PET imaging agent against the golden standard of neuropathology confirmation at autopsy (Clark, et al., 2011b). This study included individuals near end of life who consented to donating their brain after death. Thirty-six subjects with clinically diagnosed AD were included in the autopsy cohort (but only 29 were included in the primary analysis) while 74 young healthy controls were in the non-autopsy cohort. All 74 young healthy controls were found to have a [^{18}F]florbetapir-negative scan. For the primary analysis autopsy cohort, visual assessment scores of [^{18}F]florbetapir scans and average neocortical and regional SUVRs (cerebellum as reference region) correlated well with *post-mortem* amyloid pathology (as measured by immunohistochemistry and silver stain neuritic plaque score).

Interestingly, only 15 participants met pathological criteria for AD in the primary analysis autopsy cohort. Of these 15 participants, 14 had [^{18}F]florbetapir PET scans visually assessed as positive, giving a sensitivity of 93%. Fourteen participants in the primary analysis autopsy cohort had histologically-confirmed low levels of Aβ aggregation at *post-mortem* and thus did not meet the criteria for AD. All 14 participants had [^{18}F]florbetapir-negative scans, leading to a specificity of 100%. This study also cited good interreader agreement among the three nuclear medicine physicians who visually rated the [^{18}F]florbetapir PET images ($0.68 \leq \kappa \leq 0.98$). While these Phase III results are very promising, Clark cautioned that this study does not explicitly highlight the specific clinical applications of this imaging agent. Currently, only a [^{18}F]florbetapir-negative scan is considered clinically useful, as it can help rule out the presence of pathologically significant levels of Aβ in the brain and thus AD pathology. [^{18}F]Florbetapir cannot, however, diagnose AD because cerebral amyloid deposition is not specific to this diagnosis. Due to encouraging results from its Phase III clinical study, Avid Radiopharmaceuticals (now a sub-company under Eli Lilly and Company) filed for FDA approval of [^{18}F]florbetapir in late 2010 (Sullivan, 2011). In a vote of 13-3, the Peripheral and Central Nervous System Drugs Advisory Committee did not recommend approval of [^{18}F]florbetapir in January 2011, citing high inter-reader variability and the lack of a single clinically applicable binary reading method as outstanding issues (Sullivan, 2011). The advisory committee did, however, subsequently vote 16-0 in favor of approval if Avid were to implement reader-training programs (Sullivan, 2011). Such implementation is currently in progress.

The committee's decision was partially based on the results presented in the study by Clark and co-workers (Clark, et al., 2011b). Upon independently analyzing the critical individual reader score data, the FDA found substantial inter-reader variability among independent, extensively trained readers of [^{18}F]florbetapir PET scans for individuals in the autopsy cohort (Carome and Wolfe, 2011); in particular, sensitivities ranged from 55% to 90%, while specificities were between 80% and 100%. The FDA determined that the readers probably had different thresholds for positive and negative scans on their visual assessment scale; and thus, education initiatives are needed to introduce a consistent binary reading method (Clark, et al., 2011a). In March 2011 the FDA echoed the advisory committee's recommendation in their official response on [^{18}F]florbetapir, requesting that Avid Radiopharmaceuticals work to implement a reader-training program that will lead to better inter-reader reliability. When this issue has been adequately addressed, it is expected that FDA approval will be gained for [^{18}F]florbetapir.

2.4 Imaging tau neurofibrillary tangle burden in Alzheimer's disease

2.4.1 Introduction to tauopathies

Besides amyloid-β, tau is the other hallmark protein that plays a primary role in the pathogenesis of Alzheimer's disease. Tau microtubule-associated protein is essential for maintaining proper neuronal function, but in some individuals this protein can accumulate intraneuronally due to abnormal changes in the regulation of the protein. This process is believed to be the cause of a wide spectrum of different types of dementias known collectively as neurodegenerative tauopathies. In addition to Alzheimer's disease, other common tauopathies in humans include Frontotemporal dementia (FTD), Pick's disease, progressive Supranuclear Palsy (PSP), and Parkinson's disease (Ludolph, et al., 2009), and, unfortunately, many of these diseases are currently not curable.

As addressed above, there is currently no effective way to definitively diagnose AD (or other tauopathy) patients before the disease has done irreversible damage. As is the case with amyloid-β plaques, risky brain biopsies can be used to determine the presence of tau, but *post-mortem* examination of the brain is needed to definitively diagnose these types of disease. While many clinical diagnostic techniques can be used, they require patients to be in moderate to late stages of the disease, a time when treatment is much less effective. New diagnostic techniques, however, are being explored to enable earlier and more definitive diagnosis of AD with PET imaging. While numerous probes have targeted amyloid-β plaques, the most promising possibility is to develop a tau-specific PET biomarker that would improve diagnostic confidence, enable detection of early stages of AD, and allow doctors to monitor the progress of future treatments.

Microtubules are the cytoskeletal components that allow nutrients to be transported far distances along the length of axons. Axoplasmic transport in neurons is an essential process, necessary to maintain proper neuron function. Microtubules however are somewhat unstable and must be stabilized by tau proteins in order to function properly. In normally functioning human brains, tau binds to microtubules to promote stability and polymerization in order to enable axoplasmic flow and preserve overall neuronal functioning. Six tau isoforms exist in the adult human brain, each with an alternative exon splicing sequence. Three of these isoforms, known as 3R-tau are made up of three carboxy-terminal tandem repeat sequences and the other three isoforms, known as 4R-tau consist of four carboxy-terminal tandem repeat sequences. In adult humans the ratio of 3R-tau to 4R-tau is approximately 1:1 (V. M. Y. Lee, et al., 2001). The purpose of these different isoforms is not completely understood. It is known, however, that only the shortest form of 3R-tau is expressed in the fetus, while all six isoforms are expressed in adult brains. One study suggests that the 4R-tau isoform is more effective in promoting microtubule binding than the 3R-tau isoform. The exact mechanism by which tau is regulated in the brain is also largely unknown; however, recent studies suggest that phosphorylation levels of tau play an important role in tau regulation. Increased phosphorylation of tau likely decreases the ability of the protein to bind to microtubules. For this reason, it is believed that protein kinases and phosphatases play a role in tau regulation. The malfunction of this phosphorylation regulation mechanism is thought to be a major cause of tauopathies. In normally functioning brains, tau proteins contain approximately 2-3 moles of phosphate per mole of tau protein (Iqbal, et al., 2005).

In the case of AD, tau proteins are hyperphosphorylated, which causes a decrease in the ability of the tau to bind to microtubules, leading to microtubule dysfunction and neuronal death. Hyperphosphorylated tau is observed in the plaques of AD patients upon *post-mortem* examination. The mechanism by which this hyperphosphorylated tau is converted into a plaque is currently unknown. One theory for this process is that hyperphosphorylation of the tau causes it to lose binding affinity with microtubules, causing the aggregation of tau into insoluble intraneuronal brain deposits. In all neurodegenerative tauopathies, deposits and tangles of tau proteins are observed in the brain. In AD, tau accumulates in the brain in different structures known as neurofibrillary tangles (NFTs). These NFTs are composed of different structures of tau consisting of paired helical filaments (PHFs) and straight filaments. Tau aggregates are very insoluble in neurons and ultimately cause neuronal death by interfering with the essential axoplasmic flow of nutrients to different cell structures. As so little is known about the cause of Alzheimer's disease and other tauopathies, it is important to develop a better method for studying tau.

2.4.2 PET imaging of tau neurofibrillary tangle burden

Non-invasive functional molecular imaging techniques such as PET imaging have the potential to become the future diagnostic standard for Alzheimer's disease and related tauopathies as they would allow for earlier and more definitive diagnosis of such diseases, and provide an effective method for monitoring possible treatments. One such approach being aggressively explored is the development of tau specific radiopharmaceuticals that would allow for the non-invasive quantification of tau NFTs in the brain. Developing appropriate biomarkers for detecting tau has proven challenging as they must cross the blood brain barrier (BBB), bind selectively to tau, demonstrate safe biodistribution, and exhibit low non-specific binding. Nevertheless, several tau-targeting radiopharmaceuticals, radiolabeled with fluorine-18 or carbon-11, are in various stages of clinical and pre-clinical development. Experimental radiopharmaceuticals including BF-158, FDDNP and T808 are possible candidates for PET imaging of tau, and are outlined below for proof-of-concept purposes.

2.4.2.1 [^{18}F]FDDNP

2-(1-[6-[(2-[^{18}F]fluoroethyl)(methyl)amino]-2-naphthyl]ethylidene)malononitrile ([^{18}F]FDDNP) is a recently developed radiopharmaceutical designed to elucidate brain plaques and NFTs (Small, et al., 2006). Unlike [^{11}C]PiB, [^{18}F]FDDNP can bind to both amyloid-ß plaques as well as tau NFTs, and it has been used in this capacity to quantify NFT and plaque build-up in AD (Small, et al., 2006). Currently [^{18}F]FDDNP is the only biomarker of its kind being studied in human clinical trials, and such trials demonstrated the ability of [^{18}F]FDDNP PET to distinguish healthy control patients from patients with mild cognitive impairment, and from patients with AD. Initial studies have shown that patients with AD have significantly more [^{18}F]FDDNP binding in the temporal, parietal, and frontal regions of the brain than the corresponding healthy controls. The non-specificity of [^{18}F]FDDNP, however, appears to have limited its application to date, as the study of this probe has not progressed past these initial clinical studies.

2.4.2.2 Quinoline and benzamidizole PET biomarkers

Investigations into the possibility of using radiolabeled quinoline and benzamidizole derivatives for PET imaging of tau NFTs have been reported recently by Okamura and colleagues (N. Okamura, et al., 2005). Initial experiments, with [^{11}C]BF-126, [^{11}C]BF-158, and [^{11}C]BF-170, demonstrated that these compounds have a high affinity for tau NFTs. Furthermore, these compounds appear to bind specifically to tau, without extensive non-specific binding to amyloid plaques. Through the use of *in vitro* staining of AD brain slices, [^{11}C]BF-158 was shown to be the most promising compound for PET imaging of tau NFTs. These radiopharmaceuticals only interact with tau formations in the brains of AD patients. This could prove beneficial for distinguishing early AD from other types of tauopathies. For example, these radiopharmaceuticals do not bind strongly to the tau structures present in the brain slices of patients with Pick's disease and PSP. Although these radiopharmaceuticals have not yet been translated into human clinical trials, the promising pre-clinical data suggest they possess the appropriate properties to make them realistic radiopharmaceuticals for future testing.

2.4.2.3 [^{18}F]T794, [^{18}F]T807 and [^{18}F]T808

Recently, Kolb and colleagues reported development of PET radiopharmaceuticals with high binding affinity and selectivity for tau tangles (Szardenings, et al., 2011), and three lead compounds were identified: [^{18}F]T794, [^{18}F]T807 and [^{18}F]T808. Initial autoradiographical and rodent microPET studies suggest these compounds have the desired binding affinity for tau and good selectivity for tau over amyloid, to fill the void in clinical tau PET imaging. Translation into the clinic is underway, although human imaging studies with these compounds have also yet to be reported.

2.5 Imaging the cholinergic system

The abnormal aggregation of amyloid and tau proteins in AD pathophysiology is accompanied by concomitant decline of neurotransmitter systems, primarily the cholinergic system (Bierer, et al., 1995; Bohnen, et al., 2005; Contestabile, 2011; Francis, et al., 1999; Terry and Buccafusco, 2003). Thus, from a diagnostic perspective, there is interest in being able to image the cholinergic system with PET. To date, efforts have focused upon developing radiolabeled analogs of acetylcholine that are substrates for acetylcholinesterase. Acetylcholinesterase (AChE) is the enzyme responsible for the degradation of acetylcholine, leading to the termination of cholinergic neurotransmission. AChE deficits in *post-mortem* AD brain samples have been observed, suggesting that cholinergic decline is part of the complex neurodegenerative cascade that occurs in AD. Therefore, radiopharmaceuticals suitable for quantifying AChE *in vivo* have potential for tracking the progression of the cholinergic aspect of this cascade in AD patients. The synthetic acetylcholinesterase substrate, 1-[^{11}C]methylpiperidin-4-yl propionate ([^{11}C]PMP) (Shao, et al., 2003; Snyder, et al., 1998), is currently in routine clinical use as a radiopharmaceutical for the study of AChE function in AD patients, and results from such studies have been encouraging (K. A. Frey, et al., 1997; Iyo, et al., 1997; Koeppe, et al., 1997; Kuhl, et al., 1996). For example, statistically significant decreases in the cortical hydrolysis rate of [^{11}C]PMP in AD brains, versus age-matched controls, have been detected, and correlations identified (Bohnen, et al., 2005; Iyo, et al., 1997; Kilbourn, et al., 1996; Kuhl, et al., 1996). Similar results have also been obtained using [^{11}C]-*N*-methyl-4-piperidyl-acetate ([^{11}C]AMP) (Namba, et al., 1994).

2.6 Measurement of neuroinflammation

Microglial activation is the body's natural response to brain injury and associated neuroinflammation. In addition, microglial activation is also thought to play a significant role in the immune response to AD-related neuronal degeneration and, in AD patients, activated microglia can be found at sites associated with the deposition of aggregated Aβ (Kadir and Nordberg, 2010). There is consequently significant interest in developing radiopharmaceuticals that allow exploration of microglial activation using PET imaging, and the most common are ligands that target the peripheral benzodiazepine receptor including [^{11}C]PK11195 and [^{11}C]PBR28. Cagnin and co-workers reported increased levels of [^{11}C]PK11195 in the entorhinal, temporoparietal, and cingulate cortices in patients with mild AD (when compared to normal controls) (A. Cagnin, et al., 2001). In related work, Edison and colleagues imaged AD patients with both [^{11}C]PK11195 and [^{11}C]PiB. They found a negative correlation between cortical microglial activation and cognition in AD patients, but there was no observable correlation between [^{11}C]PK11195 uptake and [^{11}C]PiB binding (Edison, et al., 2008).

3. Parkinsonian dementias

3.1 Introduction

Parkinson's disease (PD) is a progressive degenerative neurological disease, characterized by asymmetric onset of resting tremors, rigidity, and bradykinesia in the limbs, leading ultimately to unstable posture. The disease is less common in adults under 60, but not unheard of, and it does become more common with increasing age. Progression of symptoms in PD typically occurs over 10–30 years, but progression can be accelerated in certain individuals, especially those with the so-called Parkinson's-plus syndrome.

The hallmark pathology of Parkinson's disease is loss of dopaminergic neurons in the substantia nigra pars compacta (SNc), leading to striatal dopamine deficiency, and classical symptoms of PD are thought to develop when 80% of striatal dopamine and 50% of the SNc neurons are lost. In addition to dopamine loss, concomitant formation of Lewy bodies also occurs in PD. Lewy bodies are composed primarily of synuclein and appearance of such intraneuronal Lewy body inclusions occurs initially in the lower brainstem and medulla oblongata, followed by midbrain and nigral involvement and, eventually, limbic and association cortical areas. Despite this, Pavese and Brooks indicate that even with the prevalence of Lewy bodies, decline of the dopaminergic system is still the primary factor in PD. Other related Parkinsonian syndromes are known however, and dementia occurs in most of them. For example, Dementia with Lewy bodies (DLB) is a common neurodegenerative dementia that is also associated with the development of α-synuclein positive Lewy body neuronal inclusions in the cortex, substantia nigra and brainstem. Patients with DLB, suffer from progressive cognitive decline including memory loss, visual hallucinations, cognitive circadian fluctuations and sleep disorders. Reflecting the seriousness of these conditions, enormous research has been undertaken to develop numerous radiopharmaceuticals (Figure 3) that can be used to differentiate these conditions and monitor their progression. Progress in this area to date has also been recently reviewed (Pavese and Brooks, 2009; Sioka, et al., 2010).

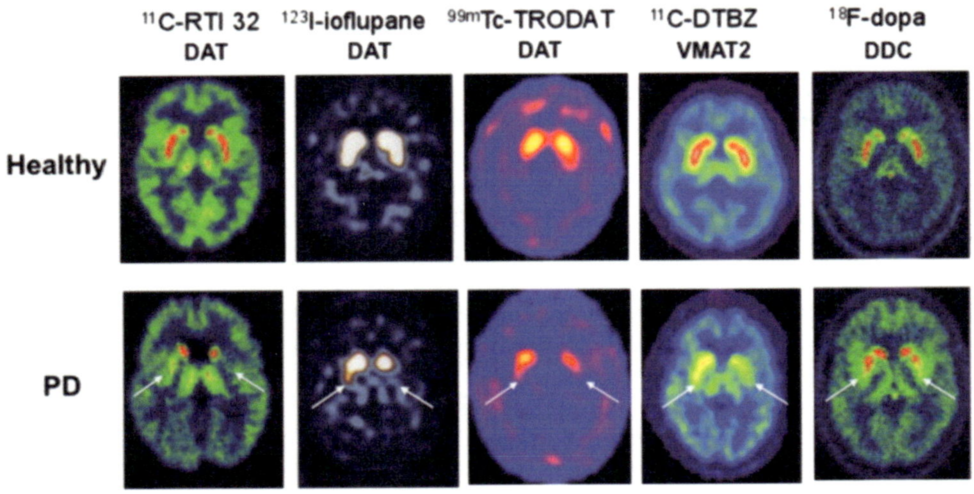

Fig. 3. Imaging dopamine terminal function in healthy controls and early Parkinson's disease. (Reprinted with permission from Pavese N and Brooks DJ, Imaging neurodegeneration in Parkinson's disease. Biochim. Biophys. Acta. 2009;1792:722-729)

3.2 Measurement of striatal aromatic amino acid decarboxylase activity

[^{18}F]DOPA is a radiopharmaceutical used for neuroimaging and for evaluation and quantification of presynaptic dopaminergic integrity. For example, analyzing the uptake of [^{18}F]DOPA in the striatal nuclei provides valuable information on both the density of the axonal terminal plexus and the activity of striatal aromatic amino acid decarboxylase (AADC), an enzyme that converts [^{18}F]DOPA to [^{18}F]dopamine (Pavese and Brooks, 2009). Therefore [^{18}F]DOPA uptake in the striatum of patients with PD is dependent upon the number of remaining dopaminergic cells, and can be used to track progression of the disease. It is worth noting, however, that early degeneration can be underestimated due to compensatory upregulation of AADC in remaining terminals (Ribeiro, et al., 2002).

Significant research has been undertaken to investigate the uptake of [^{18}F]DOPA in the putamen region of the brain, and noticeable [^{18}F]DOPA reductions have been shown to correlate with the clinical severity of rigidity and bradykinesia in PD patients (Brooks, et al., 1990; Broussolle, et al., 1999; Vingerhoets, et al., 1997). However, there is no correlation with the degree of tremors, and Pavese and Brooks highlight that this lack of correlation is suggestive of non-nigrostriatal and/or non-dopaminergic origins of the tremors associated with PD (Pavese and Brooks, 2009). In patients with hemiparkinsonism (i.e. Parkinsonian symptoms on one half of the body only), a corresponding reduction in dorsal posterior putamen uptake of [^{18}F]DOPA on the opposite side of the body has been observed (Morrish, et al., 1995). As the disease progresses to become bilateral, so to does the reduction of [^{18}F]DOPA uptake, and losses are detected in the ventral and anterior putamen and dorsal caudate. In the end stages of the disease, reduced [^{18}F]DOPA uptake in the ventral head of the caudate is also apparent. Such findings also correspond well to *post-mortem* data

(Fearnley and Lees, 1991; Kish, et al., 1988). Beyond these obvious areas of reduced [18F]DOPA uptake, if voxel analysis of the PET scans is performed, then less obvious reductions in [18F]DOPA uptake can also be detected across the entire brain (Kaasinen, et al., 2001; Rakshi, et al., 1999; Whone, et al., 2003).

3.3 Measurement of the Vesicular Monoamine Transporter (VMAT) 2

In neurodegenerative diseases there are typically characteristic losses of particular types of neurons in the human brain. As outlined above, progressive losses of dopaminergic neurons is the hallmark of Parkinson's disease. Reflecting this, a number of strategies have been developed for *in vivo* imaging of such neuronal losses. One such approach involves targeting the vesicular monoamine transporter type 2 (VMAT2) using radioligands such as (+)-α-[11C]dihydrotetrabenazine ([11C]DTBZ: (2*R*,3*R*,11b*R*)-(1,3,4,6,7,11b-hexahydro-9-[11C]methoxy-10-methoxy)-3-(2-methylpropyl)-2-hydroxy-2H-benzo[a]quinolizine) (K. A. Frey, et al., 2001). The VMAT2 is not specific for any monoamine, but is a common protein capable of transporting dopamine, norepinephrine, serotonin and histamine (Eiden and Weihe, 2011). Despite this non-specificity, the utility of VMAT2 imaging in neurodegenerative disease is still possible due to the compartmentalization of neuronal types in the human brain (K. A. Frey, et al., 2001). For example, dopaminergic nerve terminals predominate in the basal ganglia, and so enable specificity for examining losses of such terminals in PD patients (Figure 3). The VMAT2 is found in presynaptic vesicles, and transports monoamines from the cell cytosol into the storage vesicle, from where they can be released into the synapse (Wimalasena, 2011).

Lee and colleagues conducted a comparison between [11C]DTBZ, [18F]DOPA and [11C]methylphenidate (a radiopharmaceutical targeting the dopamine transporter (DAT)) (C. S. Lee, et al., 2000). Reflecting the upregulation of aromatic amino acid decarboxylase, and concomitant down regulation of the DAT, that occurs to increase dopamine turnover and reduce its reuptake in Parkinson's disease patients, this study found that [18F]DOPA Ki was reduced less than the [11C]DTBZ binding potential in the PD striatum, and [11C]DTBZ binding was reduced when compared to [11C]methylphenidate binding. The authors suggest that [11C]DTBZ PET is the most reliable method for quantifying dopaminergic terminal density although, per Pavese and Brooks (Pavese and Brooks, 2009), this needs to be validated and the effect of dopaminergic drugs upon [11C]DTBZ uptake determined.

Reflecting the drive to convert short lived carbon-11 labeled radiopharmaceuticals ($t_{1/2}$ = 20 min) into longer lived fluorine-18 labeled analogs ($t_{1/2}$ = 110 min) to facilitate distribution to satellite PET centers that do not own a cyclotron, [18F]FP-TBZ ([18F]AV-133) has also been developed to image the VMAT2, and is licensed to Avid Radiopharmaceuticals (H. F. Kung, et al., 2008). In studies by Frey and colleagues, AV-133 PET of normal and PD patients were compared (K. A. Frey, et al., 2008). Findings were similar to [11C]DTBZ, and AV-133 PET provided excellent images of the VMAT2. All PD patients had severe reduction of AV-133 accumulation in the striatum, most severe in the PP contralateral to worst PD symptoms. Similar findings were confirmed in further studies by Okamura and co-workers in 2010 (N. Okamura, et al., 2010), and very clear images showing the differences in AV-133 PET between PD patients and healthy controls were obtained (Figure 4).

3.4 Measurement of dopamine transporter binding

The presynaptic dopamine transporter (DAT) is found in dendrites and axons of dopaminergic neurons and is responsible for uptake of dopamine. Therefore, measurement

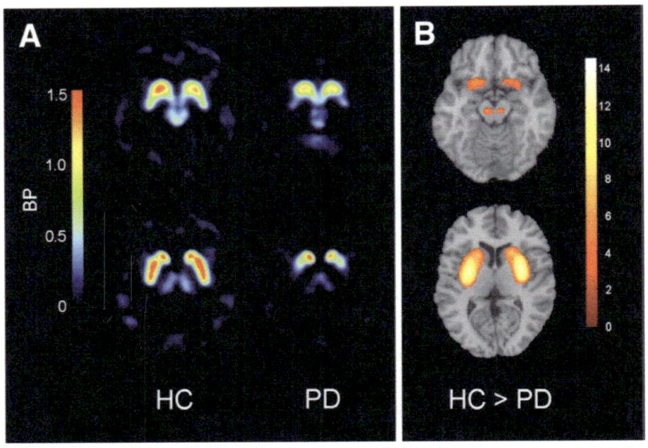

Fig. 4. (A) Representative images of 18F-AV-133 PET BP in HC and PD patient. (B) Areas of reduction in BP of PD patients, compared with HCs, in SPM analysis. Color bars represent t values. $P < 0.05$, corrected for multiple comparisons. *(Reprinted with permission from Okamura N, Villemagne VL, Drago J, et al. In vivo measurement of vesicular monoamine transporter type 2 density in Parkinson disease with ^{18}F-AV-133. J Nucl Med. 2010;51:223-228)*

of the DAT can be used as an indicator of the integrity of nigrostriatal projections. Reflecting this, a number of radiopharmaceuticals have been developed that allow for the analysis of DAT activity by PET and SPECT imaging (see the review by Pavese and Brooks for additional information (Pavese and Brooks, 2009)). These include phenyltropane derivatives such as ^{123}I-ß-CIT (Brucke, et al., 1997; Seibyl, et al., 1995), ^{123}I-FP-CIT ([^{123}I]ioflupane; DaTSCAN) (Castrejón, et al., 2005; Hauser and Grosset, 2011), and [^{99m}Tc]trodat (M. P. Kung, et al., 1997), that lead to distinctive images such as those shown in Figure 3. For example, [^{123}I]ioflupane, a radiolabeled analog of cocaine, is approved for clinical use in Europe and the United States, and marketed as DaTSCAN. Nuclear medicine physicians use [^{123}I]ioflupane to diagnose Parkinson's disease (PD), and to differentiate PD from other related neurological disorders that present with similar clinical symptoms (e.g. dementia with Lewy bodies (Antonini, 2007; Castrejón, et al., 2005)). [^{123}I]Ioflupane has a high binding affinity for presynaptic dopamine transporters (DAT). Thus, a SPECT scan conducted using [^{123}I]ioflupane provides physicians with a quantitative measure and the spatial distribution of DAT in the brain. A marked reduction in DAT in the striatal region of the brain is indicative of PD (Figure 3), allowing physicians to diagnose or differentiate a patient's neurological condition with improved diagnostic confidence when compared to diagnosing from clinical symptoms alone.

A review of the two major clinical trials of [^{123}I]ioflupane was recently published by Hauser and Grosset (Hauser and Grosset, 2011). The first study compared baseline scans in patients with early suspected Parkinsonism to the consensus clinical diagnosis established 3 years later (Marshall, et al., 2009). The study found 78-79% positive agreement (abnormal baseline scan and positive diagnosis of PD at 3 yrs, n = 71) and 97% negative agreement (normal baseline scan and negative for PD at 3 yrs, n = 28). The second study was a trial of [^{123}I]ioflupane in patients with established diagnoses of PD or essential tremor (ET), and obtained similar results (Benamer, et al., 2000). This study found 92-97% positive agreement (abnormal baseline scan and positive diagnosis of PD at 3 yrs, n = 158) and 74-96% negative agreement (normal baseline scan and clinical diagnosis of ET, n = 27). Castrejón and colleagues have also demonstrated that [^{123}I]ioflupane SPECT can distinguish between PD and other Parkinsonian disorders that do not have associated degeneration of the nigrostriatal pathway, such as ET (Castrejón, et al., 2005). Despite these positive findings, it is important to note that an abnormal [^{123}I]ioflupane SPECT scan does not necessarily indicate a diagnosis of PD. Similarly, a normal scan is not entirely indicative of ET (Hauser and Grosset, 2011). In each case, multiple other conditions must be considered and eliminated. For example, abnormal striatal uptake of [^{123}I]ioflupane would be expected in all degenerative Parkinsonian syndromes associated with a loss of nigrostriatal dopamine neurons including PD, progressive supranuclear palsy (PSP), multisystem atrophy (MSA), and corticobasal degeneration (CBD). [^{123}I]Ioflupane SPECT cannot differentiate these related disorders and so, in such cases, it might be necessary to run other tests (FDG PET, PiB PET etc.) to further distinguish such diseases.

3.5 Measurement of neuroinflammation in PD

As discussed above in the context of AD, microglial activation is the body's natural response to brain injury and associated neuroinflammation. Reflecting this, [^{11}C]PK11195 and [^{11}C]PBR28 have been developed to image microglial activation, and recent studies have explored the use of [^{11}C]PK11195 PET in PD patients. Such studies report significant increases in [^{11}C]PK11195 uptake in striatal and extrastriatal regions of PD patients when compared to healthy control subjects (Gerhard, et al., 2006; Ouchi, et al., 2005; Pavese and Brooks, 2009). These findings, which have been correlated with reduced striatal DAT binding (Ouchi, et al., 2005), suggest that significant microglial activation (and associated neuroinflammation) could contribute to dopaminergic neuron loss in PD. This represents an avenue of research that has yet to be extensively explored.

3.6 Imaging of dementia with Lewy bodies

Dementia with Lewy bodies (DLB) is a common Parkinsonian neurodegenerative dementia that is characterized by the development of α-synuclein positive Lewy body neuronal inclusions in the cortex, substantia nigra and brainstem. Patients with DLB, suffer from progressive cognitive decline including memory loss, visual hallucinations, cognitive circadian fluctuations and sleep disorders. In FDG PET of DLB patients, unique hypometabolism in the medial and lateral occipital lobes is observed, and is the feature that distinguishes DLB from AD (Ishii, 2002). DLB can also be distinguished from AD using [^{18}F]DOPA PET. Dopamine deficiencies, similar to PD, have been observed in DLB patients, but not in AD patients (Hu, et al., 2000).

4. Frontotemporal lobe degeneration

4.1 Introduction

Frontotemporal lobe degeneration (FTLD) is a cause of degenerative dementias that recent research suggests, in individuals younger than 65, is as common as AD. Frontotemporal dementia (FTD) is the most common example of such diseases, for which clinical and pathological criteria were proposed in 1994 by Brun and colleagues (Brun, et al., 1994). The disease is characterized by behavioral and personality changes that result from the frontotemporal involvement and include apathy, disinhibition, and often sever impairment of language production. In related conditions, such as semantic dementia and progressive non-fluent aphasia, language impairment can be the major symptom, and dementia the lesser symptom. In contrast to other dementias however, there is no (or less prominent) memory impairment associated with FTLD. Therefore, clinical differentiation from other diseases such as AD is usually relatively straightforward. The main difficulty associated with managing FTLD is that it is not typically diagnosed in its early stages because mild symptoms often go unnoticed, or are difficult to verify. To address this issue, FDG PET has been investigated as a possibility for diagnosing and staging the FTLD-related conditions by identifying areas of reduced glucose metabolism that are characteristic of these conditions.

4.2 FDG PET for imaging frontotemporal dementia

Reduced glucose metabolism in the frontal (mostly the frontal cortex) and anterior temporal regions is the characteristic hallmark observed in FDG PET scans of FTD patients. Such impairment is not always symmetric, and thought to be related to the aphasia and semantic memory deficits common in such patients. This (mostly) frontal impairment allows distinction of FTD from AD. For example, Foster and co-workers were recently able to distinguish FTD from AD with 86% specificity and 97.6% sensitivity, beyond clinical features alone (Foster, et al., 2007). Frontal metabolic decline, however, is not limited to FTD and can be apparent in certain cases of AD. In such cases where there is FTD / AD overlap in the FDG PET scans, it is recommended to conduct additional scans exploring microglial activation or amyloid deposits (see Section 2). For example, microglial activation characteristic of FTD has been investigated (A. Cagnin, et al., 2004). Alternatively, an amyloid positive scan would strongly suggest AD, whilst an amyloid negative scan would indicate FTD (Figure 5) (Kadir and Nordberg, 2010).

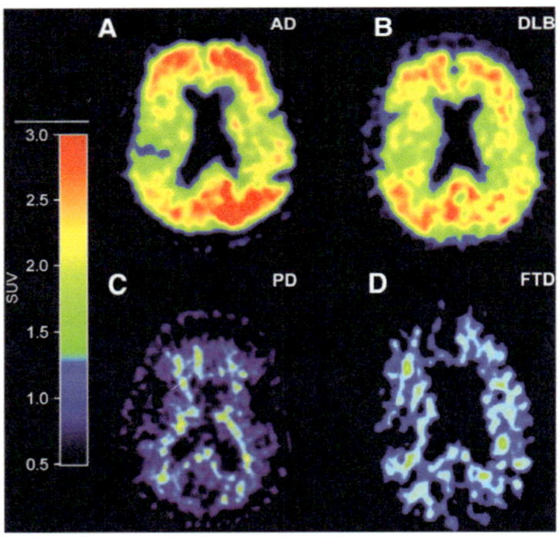

Fig. 5. High PIB retention was observed in patient with AD (A) and patient with DLB (B). In contrast, low PIB retention was observed in patient with PD (not demented) (C) and in patient with FTD (D). *(Parts A and B reprinted with permission from Ahmadul K and Nordberg A, Target-specific PET probes for neurodegenerative disorders related to dementia. J Nucl Med. 2010;51:1418-1430; Part C reprinted with permission from A. Johansson, et al. [11C]-PIB imaging in patients with Parkinson's disease: preliminary results. Parkinsonism Relat. Disord. 2008;14:345-347; Part D courtesy of Professor Henry Engler, Uppsala PET Center, Academical Hospital, Uppsala, Sweden).*

Other diseases (e.g. progressive supranuclear palsy, spino-cerebellar atrophy) or lifestyle choices (e.g. cocaine abuse) can also lead to frontal metabolic impairment. Consequently, other areas of reduced cerebral glucose metabolism should be considered when making a diagnosis as, despite its name, there are more widespread hemispheric defects in glucose metabolism that occur in FTD. For example, reduced glucose metabolism in the orbital gyrus, anterior cingulate gyrus, frontal cortices, anterior temporal cortices, hippocampus, subcortical structures, parietal region, sensorimotor cortex, and the cerebellar cortex, discussed by Ishii (Ishii, 2002), are consistent with the pathological features and *post-mortem* findings of FTD.

5. Imaging of other dementias

5.1 Corticobasal degeneration

Corticobasal degeneration (CBD) is a progressive dementia in which patients have cognitive decline, significant dementia and unique motor symptoms such as akineto-rigid syndrome (Ishii, 2002). In FDG PET of CBD patients, there is a decrease in absolute glucose metabolism in several regions of the brain, and distinct asymmetry in glucose metabolism patterns that is characteristic of the condition. For example, Hirono and colleagues showed that CBD patients had greater glucose metabolic asymmetries in the lateral frontal, lateral temporal, central and lateral parietooccipital regions than did the corresponding healthy controls (Hirono, et al., 2001). In the same study it was reported that the most significant pathologic changes in CBD appear in the pre- and post-central gyri, and parietal association cortices. Moreover, the associated metabolic asymmetries in the pre- and post-central gyri, as well as the thalamus, were larger in CBD than AD allowing differentiation of these conditions using FDG PET.

5.2 Progressive supranuclear palsy

Progressive supranuclear palsy (PSP) is a condition associated with Parkinsonism and dementia. Pathological changes are most common in the basal ganglia and brain stem, and features of this neurodegenerative condition include behavioral derangement and cognitive decline (Ishii, 2002). In FDG PET of PSP patients, glucose metabolism is reduced in the lateral and medial frontal lobes, caudate nucleus and midbrain, when compared to normal controls (Blin, et al., 1990; Hosaka, et al., 2002).

5.3 Vascular dementia

When dementia results from many small strokes, it is known as vascular dementia. In contrast to other dementias, it is relatively straightforward to diagnose vascular dementia from clinical symptoms, and with MRI or CT. Typically therefore nuclear medicine imaging is not needed for patients with pure vascular dementia (Ishii, 2002). On occasion however, vascular dementia can be associated with AD pathology. In such cases, FDG PET can be employed to distinguish vascular dementia from the reduced glucose metabolism profile associated with AD (see Section 2.2).

6. Conclusion

In conclusion, the sophisticated array of radiopharmaceuticals that have been developed for imaging dementia using PET and SPECT scans is highlighted. Using such imaging techniques alone, or in combination with each other (and/or MRI, CT etc.), allows physicians to differentiate between related, and frequently clinically overlapping, disease entities with a high degree of diagnostic confidence. However, whilst [^{18}F]FDG is readily available, the more specialized radiopharmaceuticals described herein are still limited to sites typically possessing a cyclotron and advanced radiochemistry laboratories. In order for patients and physicians alike to benefit from these radiopharmaceuticals, global access has to be provided. The new partnerships growing between big pharma, small radiopharmaceutical companies, and larger companies possessing global radiopharmaceutical distribution networks, as well as the appearance of mobile scanner technology, should greatly facilitate access to nuclear medicine imaging in the next decade.

7. Acknowledgement

This article was made available as Open Access with the generous support of the University of Michigan COPE Fund (http://lib.umich.edu/cope).

8. References

Aizenstein, H. J., et al. (2008). Frequent amyloid deposition without significant cognitive impairment among the elderly. *Arch. Neurol.*, Vol. 65, No. 11, (Nov. 2008), pp. 1509-1517, ISSN 00039942.

Anchisi, D., et al. (2005). Heterogeneity of brain glucose metabolism in mild cognitive impairment and clinical progression to Alzheimer disease. *Arch. Neurol.*, Vol. 62, No. 11, (Nov. 2005), pp. 1728-1733, ISSN 00039942.

Antonini, A. (2007). The role of 123I-ioflupane SPECT dopamine transporter imaging in the diagnosis and treatment of patients with dementia with Lewy bodies. *Neuropsychiatr. Dis. Treat.*, Vol. 3, No. 3, (Jun. 2007), pp. 287-292, ISSN 1176-6328.

APA (2000). *Diagnostic and statistical manual of mental disorders (IV-TR), 4th edition* Americam Psychiatric Association, ISBN 978-0890420256, Washington, D.C.

Barthel, H., et al. (2011). Cerebral amyloid-ß PET with florbetaben (18F) in patients with Alzheimer's disease and healthy controls: a multicentre phase 2 diagnostic study. *Lancet Neurol.*, Vol. 10, No. 5, (May 2011), pp. 424-435, ISSN 1474-4422.

Barthel, H., et al. (2010). Individualized quantification of brain ß-amyloid burden: results of a proof of mechanism phase 0 florbetaben PET trial in patients with Alzheimer's disease and healthy controls. *Eur. J. Nucl. Med. Mol. Imaging*, Vol. 49, No. Suppl. 1, (May 2011), pp. 33P, ISSN 1619-7070.

Bartzokis, G., et al. (2007). Human brain myelination and amyloid beta deposition in Alzheimer's disease. *Alzheimer's and Dement.*, Vol. 3, No. 2, (Apr. 2007), pp. 122-125, ISSN 1552-5260.

Bayer (Accessed 2011). *Phase III study of florbetaben (BAY94-9172) PET imaging for detection/exclusion of cerebral ß-amyloid compared to histopathology-NCT01020838.* http://clinicaltrials.gov/ct2/show/NCT01020838 *(accessed May 20, 2011)*

Benamer, H. T. S., et al. (2000). Accurate differentiation of parkinsonism and essential tremor using visual assessment of [123 I]-FP-CIT SPECT imaging: the [123 I]-FP-CIT SPECT study group. *Mov. Disord.*, Vol. 15, No. 3, (May 2000), pp. 503-510, ISSN 0885-3185.

Berent, S., et al. (1999). Neuropsychological function and cerebral glucose utilization in isolated memory impairment and Alzheimer's disease. *J. Psychiatr. Res.*, Vol. 33, No. 1, (Feb. 1999), pp. 7-16, ISSN 0022-3956.

Beyreuther, K. and Masters, C. L. (1991). Amyloid precursor protein (APP) and beta A4 amyloid in the etiology of Alzheimer's disease: precursor-product relationships in the derangement of neuronal function. *Brain Pathol.*, Vol. 1, No. 4, (Jul. 1991), pp. 241-251, ISSN 1750-3639.

Bierer, L. M., et al. (1995). Neurochemical correlates of dementia severity in Alzheimer's disease: relative importance of the cholinergic deficits. *J. Neurochem.*, Vol. 64, No. 2, (Feb. 1995), pp. 749-760, ISSN 0022-3042.

Blin, J., et al. (1990). Positron emission tomography study in progressive supranuclear palsy. Brain hypometabolic pattern and clinicometabolic correlations. *Arch. Neurol.*, Vol. 47, No. 7, (Jul. 1990), pp. 747-752, ISSN 00039942.

Bohnen, N. I., et al. (2005). Cognitive correlates of alterations in acetylcholinesterase in Alzheimer's disease *Neurosci. Lett.*, Vol. 380, No. 1-2, (May 2005), pp. 127-132, ISSN 0304-3940.

Brooks, D. J., et al. (1990). The relationship between locomotor disability, autonomic dysfunction, and the integrity of the striatal dopaminergic system in patients with multiple system atrophy, pure autonomic failure and Parkinson's disease studied by PET. *Brain*, Vol. 113, No. 5, (Oct. 1990), pp. 1539-1552, ISSN 0006-8950.

Broussolle, E., et al. (1999). The relation of putamen and caudate nucleus 18F-dopa uptake to motor and cognitive performances in Parkinson's disease. *J. Neurol. Sci.*, Vol. 166, No. 2, (Jul. 1999), pp. 141-151, ISSN 0022-510X.

Brucke, T., et al. (1997). Measurement of dopaminergic degeneration in Parkinson's disease with [123I]beta-CIT and SPECT. Correlation with clinical findings and comparison with multiple system atrophy and progressive supranuclear palsy. *J. Neural Transm.*, Vol. 50, No. Suppl., pp. 9-24, ISSN 0300-9564.

Brücke, T., et al. (2000). SPECT and PET imaging of the dopaminergic system in Parkinson's disease. *J. Neurol.*, Vol. 247, No. Suppl. 4, (Sep. 2000), pp. 2-7, ISSN 0340-5354

Brun, A., et al. (1994). Clinical and neuropathological criteria for frontotemporal dementia. *J. Neurol. Neurosurg. Psychiatry*, Vol. 57, No. 4, (Apr. 1994), pp. 416-418, ISSN 0022-3050.

Cagnin, A., et al. (2001). In-vivo measurement of activated microglia in dementia. *Lancet*, Vol. 358, No. 9280, (Aug. 2001), pp. 461-467, ISSN 0140-6736.

Cagnin, A., et al. (2004). In vivo detection of microglial activation in frontotemporal dementia. *Ann. Neurol.*, Vol. 56, No. 6, (Dec. 2004), pp. 894-897, ISSN 0364-5134.

Carome, M. and Wolfe, S. (2011). Florbetapir-PET imaging and postmortem β-amyloid pathology. *J. Am. Med. Assoc.*, Vol. 305, No. 18, (May 2011), pp. 1857, ISSN 0098-7484.

Castrejón, A. S., et al. (2005). 123-I Ioflupane (Datscan) presynaptic nigrostriatal imaging in patients with movement disorders. *Braz. Arch. Biol. Technol.*, Vol. 48, No. Special Issue, (Oct. 2005), pp. 115-125, ISSN 1516-8913.

Choi, S. R., et al. (2009). Preclinical properties of 18F-AV-45: a PET agent for Aβ plaques in the brain. *J. Nucl. Med.*, Vol. 50, No. 11, (Nov. 2009), pp. 1887-1894, ISSN 0161-5505.

Choi, S. R., et al. (2011). Correlation of Amyloid PET Ligand Florbetapir F 18 Binding with Aß Aggregation and Neuritic Plaque Deposition in Postmortem Brain Tissue. *Alz. Dis. Assoc. Dis.*, Vol. 25, No. ASAP On-line, (Mar. 2011), pp. doi: 10.1097/WAD.1090b1013e31821300bc, ISSN 0893-0341.

Clark, C. M., et al. (2011a). Florbetapir-PET imaging and postmortem β-amyloid pathology. *J. Am. Med. Assoc.*, Vol. 305, No. 3, (Jan. 2011), pp. 1857-1858, ISSN 0098-7484.

Clark, C. M., et al. (2011b). Use of Florbetapir-PET for Imaging ß-Amyloid Pathology. *J. Am. Med. Assoc.*, Vol. 305, No. 3, (Jan. 2011), pp. 275-283, ISSN 0098-7484.

Contestabile, A. (2011). The history of the cholinergic hypothesis. *Behav. Brain Res.*, Vol. 221, No. 2, (Aug 2011), pp. ISSN 0166-4328.

de Leon, M. J., et al. (2001). Prediction of cognitive decline in normal elderly subjects with 2-F-18-fluoro-2-deoxy-D-glucose posi- tron-emission tomography (FDG PET). *Proc. Natl. Acad. Sci. USA*, Vol. 98, No. 19, (Sep. 2001), pp. 10966-10971, ISSN 0027-8424.

Drzezga, A., et al. (2008). Imaging of amyloid plaques and cerebral glucose metabolism in semantic dementia and Alzheimer's disease. *Neuroimage*, Vol. 39, No. 2, (Jan. 2008), pp. 619-633, ISSN 1053-8119.

Drzezga, A., et al. (2009). Effect of APOE genotype on amyloid plaque load and gray matter volume in Alzheimer disease. *Neurology*, Vol. 72, No. 17, (Apr. 2009), pp. 1487-1494, ISSN 0028-3878.

Drzezga, A., et al. (2005). Prediction of individual clinical outcome in MCI by means of genetic assessment and (18)F-FDG PET. *J. Nucl. Med.*, Vol. 46, No. 10, (Oct. 2005), pp. 1625-1632, ISSN 0161-5505.

Dubois, B., et al. (2007). Research criteria for the diagnosis of Alzheimer's disease: revising the NINCDS-ADRDA criteria. *Lancet Neurol.*, Vol. 6, No. 8, (Aug. 2007), pp. 734-746, ISSN 1474-4422.

Edison, P., et al. (2008). Microglia, amyloid, and cognition in Alzheimer's disease: an [11C](R)PK11195-PET and [11C]PIB-PET study. *Neurobiol. Dis.*, Vol. 32, No. 3, (Dec. 2008), pp. 412-419, ISSN 0969-9961.

Eiden, L. E. and Weihe, E. (2011). VMAT2: a dynamic regulator of brain monoaminergic neuronal function interacting with drugs of abuse. *Ann. NY Acad. Sci.*, Vol. 1216, No. Addiction Reviews, (Jan 2011), pp. 86-98, ISSN: 0077-8923.

Engler, H., et al. (2006). Two year follow-up of amyloid deposition in patients with Alzheimer's disease. *Brain*, Vol. 129, No. 11, (Nov. 2006), pp. 2856-2866, ISSN 0006-8950.

Engler, H., et al. (2008). In vivo amyloid imaging with PET in frontotemporal dementia. *Eur. J. Nucl. Med. Mol. Imaging*, Vol. 35, No. 1, (Jan. 2008), pp. 100-106, ISSN 1619-7070.

Fagan, A. M., et al. (2007). Cerebrospinal fluid tau/β-amyloid 42 ratio as a predictor of cognitive decline in non-demented older adults. *Neurology*, Vol. 64, No. 3, (Mar. 2007), pp. 343-349, ISSN 0028-3878.

Fearnley, J. M. and Lees, A. J. (1991). Ageing and Parkinson's disease: substantia nigra regional selectivity. *Brain*, Vol. 114, No. 5, (Oct. 1991), pp. 2283-2301, ISSN 0006-8950.

Fodero-Tavoletti, M. T., et al. (2009). Characterization of PiB binding to white matter in Alzheimer disease and other dementias. *J. Nucl. Med.*, Vol. 50, No. 2, (Feb. 2009), pp. 198-204, ISSN 0161-5505.

Fodero-Tavoletti, M. T., et al. (2007). In vitro characterization of Pittsburgh compound-B to Lewy bodies. *J. Neurosci.*, Vol. 27, No. 39, (Sep. 2007), pp. 10365-10371, ISSN 0270-6474.

Forsberg, A., et al. (2010). High PIB retention in Alzheimer's disease is an early event with complex relationship with CSF biomarkers and functional parameters. *Curr. Alz. Res.*, Vol. 7, No. 1, (Feb. 2010), pp. 56-66, ISSN 1567-2050.

Forsberg, A., et al. (2008). PET imaging of amyloid deposition in patients with mild cognitive impairment. *Neurobiol. Aging*, Vol. 29, No. 10, (Oct. 2008), pp. 1456-1465, ISSN 0197-4580.

Foster, N. L., et al. (2007). FDG-PETimproves accuracy in distinguishing frontotemporal dementia and Alzheimer's disease. *Brain*, Vol. 130, No. 10, (Oct. 2007), pp. 2616-2635, ISSN 0006-8950.

Francis, P. T., et al. (1999). The cholinergic hypothesis of Alzheimer's disease: a review of progress. *J. Neurol. Neurosurg. Psychiatry* Vol. 66, No. 2, (Feb. 1999), pp. 137-147, ISSN 0022-3050.

Frey, K. A., et al. (2008). Imaging VMAT2 in Parkinson disease with [F-18]AV-133. *J. Nucl. Med.*, Vol. 49, No. Suppl. 1, (May 2008), pp. 5P, ISSN 0161-5505.

Frey, K. A., et al. (2001). Imaging the Vesicular Monoamine Transporter. *Adv. Neurol.*, Vol. 86, No. pp. 237-247, ISSN 0091-3952.

Frey, K. A., et al. (1997). PET quantification of cortical acetylcholinesterase inhibition in monkey and human. *J. Nucl. Med.*, Vol. 38, No. Suppl. 1, (May 1997), pp. 146P, ISSN 0161-5505.

GEHC (Accessed 2011). *GE Healthcare. Positron Emission Tomography (PET) imaging of brain amyloid compared to post-mortem levels-NCT01165554.* http://clinicaltrials.gov/ct2/show/NCT01165554 *(accessed May 20, 2011)*

Gerhard, A., et al. (2006). In vivo imaging of microglial activation with [11C](R)- PK11195 PET in idiopathic Parkinson's disease. *Neurobiol. Dis.*, Vol. 21, No. 2, (Feb. 2006), pp. 404-412, ISSN 0969-9961.

Greenberg, S. M., et al. (2008). Detection of isolated cerebrovascular β-amyloid with Pittsburgh Compound B. *Ann. Neurol.*, Vol. 64, No. 5, (Nov. 2008), pp. 587-591, ISSN 0364-5134.

Haass, C. and Selkoe, D. J. (2007). Soluble protein oligomers in neurodegeneration: lessons from the Alzheimer' s amyloid β-peptide. *Nat. Rev. Mol. Cell Biol.*, Vol. 82, No. 2, (Feb. 2007), pp. 239-259, ISSN 1471-0072.

Hauser, R. A. and Grosset, D. G. (2011). [^{123}I]FP-CIT (DaTscan) SPECT brain imaging in patients with suspected Parkinsonian syndromes. *J. Neuroimaging*, Vol. No. ASAP On-line, pp. DOI: 10.1111/j.1552-6569.2011.00583.x., ISSN 1051-2284.

Heiss, W. D., et al. (1994). Long- term effects of phosphatidylserine, pyritinol, and cognitive training in Alzheimer's disease. A neuropsychological, EEG, and PET investigation. . *Dementia*, Vol. 5, No. 2, (Mar-Apr. 2004), pp. 88-98, ISSN 1471-3012.

Heiss, W. D., et al. (1992). PET correlates of normal and impaired memory functions. *Cerebrovasc. Brain Metab. Rev.*, Vol. 4, No. 1, (Spring 1992), pp. 1-27, ISSN 1040-8827.

Herholz, K. (2003). PET studies in dementia. *Ann. Nucl. Med.*, Vol. 17, No. 2, (Apr. 2003), pp. 79-89, ISSN 0914-7187.

Herholz, K. (2011). Molecular imaging in Alzheimer's disease. *Eur. Neurol. Rev.*, Vol. 6, No. 1, (Mar. 2011), pp. 16-20, ISSN 1758-3837.

Herholz, K., et al. (2007). Positron emission tomography imaging in dementia. *Br. J. Radiol.*, Vol. 80, No. Special Issue 2, (Dec. 2007), pp. S160-167, ISSN 0007-1285.

Hirono, N., et al. (2001). Neuroral substrates for semantic memory: A positron emission tomography study in Alzheimer's disease. *Dement. Geriatr. Cogn. Disord.*, Vol. 12, No. 1, (Jan-Feb 2001), pp. 15-21, ISSN 1420-8008

Hosaka, K., et al. (2002). Voxel-based comparison of regional cerebral glucose metabolism between PSP and corticobasal degeneration. *J. Neurol. Sci.*, Vol. 199, No. 1, (Jul. 2002), pp. 67-71, ISSN 0022-510X.

Hu, X. S., et al. (2000). 18F-fluorodopa PET study of striatal dopamine uptake in the diagnosis of dementia with lewy bodies. *Neurology*, Vol. 55, No. 10, (Nov. 2000), pp. 1575-1577, ISSN 0028-3878.

Iqbal, K., et al. (2005). Tau Pathology in Alzheimer disease and other tauopathies. *Biochim. Biophys. Acta*, Vol. 1739, No. 2-3, (Jan. 2005), pp. 198-210, ISSN 0006-3002.

Ishii, K. (2002). Clinical application of positron emission tomography for diagnosis of dementia. *Ann. Nucl. Med.*, Vol. 16, No. 8, (Dec. 2002), pp. 515-525, ISSN 0914-7187.

Iyo, M., et al. (1997). Measurement of acetylcholinesterase by positron emission tomography in the brains of healthy controls and patients with Alzheimer's disease. *Lancet*, Vol. 349, No. 9068, (Jun. 1997), pp. 1805-1809, ISSN 0140-6736.

Jack, C. R., et al. (2009). Alzheimer's Diseae Neuroimaging Initiative. Serial PIB and MRI in normal, mild cognitive impairment and Alzheimer's disease: implications for sequence of pathological events in Alzheimer's disease. *Brain*, Vol. 132, No. 5, (May 2009), pp. 1355-1365, ISSN 0006-8950.

Jagust, W. (2004). Molecular neuroimaging in Alzheimer's disease. *NeuroRX*, Vol. 1, No. 2, (Apr. 2004), pp. 206-212, ISSN 1545-5343.

Jellinger, K., et al. (1990). Clinicopathological analysis of dementia disorders in the elderly. *J. Neurol. Sci.*, Vol. 95, No. 3, (Mar. 1995), pp. 239-258, ISSN 0022-510X.

Kaasinen, V., et al. (2001). Increased frontal [(18)F]fluorodopa uptake in early Parkinson's disease: sex differences in the prefrontal cortex. *Brain*, Vol. 124, No. 6, (Jun. 2001), pp. 1125-1130, ISSN 0006-8950.

Kadir, A. and Nordberg, A. (2010). Target-specific PET probes for neurodegenerative disorders related to dementia. *J. Nucl. Med.*, Vol. 51, No. 9, (Sep. 2010), pp. 1418-1430, ISSN 0161-5505.

Kilbourn, M. R., et al. (1996). In vivo studies of acetylcholinesterase activity using a labeled substrate, N[11C]methylpiperdin-4-yl propionate ([11C]PMP). *Synapse*, Vol. 22, No. 2, (Feb. 1996), pp. 123-131, ISSN 0887-4476.

Kish, S. J., et al. (1988). Uneven pattern of dopamine loss in the striatum of patients with idiopathic Parkinson's disease. Pathophysiologic and clinical implications. *New Engl. J. Med.*, Vol. 318, No. 14, (Apr. 1998), pp. 876-880, ISSN 0028-4793.

Klunk, W. E., et al. (2004). Imaging brain amyloid in Alzheimer's disease with Pittsburgh compound-B. *Ann. Neurol.*, Vol. 55, No. 3, (Mar. 2004), pp. 306-319, ISSN 0364-5134.

Klunk, W. E. and Mathis, C. A. (2008). The future of amyloid-beta imaging: a tale of radionuclides and tracer proliferation. *Curr. Opin. Neurol.*, Vol. 21, No. 6, (Dec. 2008), pp. 683-687, ISSN 1350-7540.

Klunk, W. E., et al. (2001). Uncharged thioflavin-T derivatives bind to amyloid-beta protein with high affinity and readily enter the brain. *Life Sci.*, Vol. 69, No. 13, (Aug. 2001), pp. 1471-1484, ISSN 0024-3205.

Klunk, W. E., et al. (2003). The binding of 2-(4'-methylaminophenyl)benzothiazole to postmortem brain homogenates is dominated by the amyloid component. *J. Neurosci.*, Vol. 23, No. 6, (Mar. 2003), pp. 2086-2092, ISSN 0270-6474.

Koeppe, R. A., et al. (1997). Kinetic analysis alternatives for assessing AChE activitiy with N-[C-11]methylpiperidinyl propionate (PMP): to constrain or not to constrain? *J. Nucl. Med.*, Vol. 38, No. Suppl. 1, (May 1997), pp. 198P, ISSN 0161-5505.

Koole, M., et al. (2009). Whole-Body Biodistribution and Radiation Dosimetry of 18F-GE067: A Radioligand for In Vivo Brain Amyloid Imaging. *J. Nucl. Med.*, Vol. 50, No. 5, (May 2009), pp. 818-822, ISSN 0161-5505.

Kuhl, D. E., et al. (1996). Mapping acetylcholinesterase in human brain using PET and N-[C-11]methylpiperidinyl propionate. *J. Nucl. Med.*, Vol. 37, No. Suppl. 1, (May 1996), pp. 21P, ISSN 0161-5505.

Kuhl, D. E., et al. (1982). Effects of human aging on patterns of local cerebral glucose utilization determined by the [18F]fluorodeoxyglucose method. *J. Cerebr. Blood Flow Metab.*, Vol. 2, No. 2, pp. 163–171, ISSN 0271-678X.

Kukull, W. A., et al. (1990). The validity of 3 clinical diagnostic criteria for Alzheimer's disease. *Neurology*, Vol. 40, No. 9, (Sep. 1990), pp. 1364-1369, ISSN 0028-3878.

Kung, H. F., et al. (2008). Radiolabeled dihydrotetrabenazine derivatives and their use as imaging agents, US 2008/0050312 A1, 45 pp. Vol. No. pp.

Kung, H. F., et al. (2001). Novel stilbenes as probes for amyloid plaques. *J. Am. Chem. Soc.*, Vol. 123, No. 50, (Dec. 2001), pp. 12740-12741, ISSN 0002-7863.

Kung, M. P., et al. (1997). [99mTc]TRODAT-1: a novel technetium-99m complex as a dopamine transporter imaging agent. *Eur. J. Nucl. Med.*, Vol. 24, No. 4, (Apr. 1997), pp. 372-380, ISSN 0340-6997.

Lee, C. S., et al. (2000). In vivo positron emission tomographic evidence for compensatory changes in presynaptic dopamine nerve terminals in Parkinson's disease. *Ann. Neurol.*, Vol. 47, No. 4, (Apr. 2000), pp. 493-503, ISSN 0364-5134.

Lee, V. M. Y., et al. (2001). Neurodegenerative Tauopathies. *Ann. Rev. Neurosci.*, Vol. 24, No. pp. 1121-1159, ISSN 0147-006X

Lin, K. J., et al. (2010). Whole-body biodistribution and brain PET imaging with [18F]AV-45, a novel amyloid imaging agent- a pilot study. *Nucl. Med. Biol.*, Vol. 37, No. 4, (May 2010), pp. 497-508, ISSN 0047-0740.

Lister-James, J., et al. (2011). Florbetapir F-18: a histopathologically validated beta-amyloid positron emission tomography imaging agent. *Semin. Nucl. Med.*, Vol. 41, No. 4, (Jul. 2011), pp. 300-304, ISSN 0001-2998.

Lockhart, A., et al. (2007). PIB is a non-specific imaging marker of amyloid-beta (Abeta) peptide-related cerebral amyloidosis. *Brain*, Vol. 130, No. 10, (Oct. 2007), pp. 2607-2615, ISSN 0006-8950.

Ludolph, A. C., et al. (2009). Tauopathies with parkinsonism: clinical spectrum, neuropathologic basis, biological markers, and treatment options. *Eur. J. Neurol.*, Vol. 16, No. 3, (Mar. 2009), pp. 297-309, ISSN 1351-5101.

Marshall, V. L., et al. (2009). Parkinson's disease is overdiagnosed clinically at baseline in diagnostically uncertain cases: a 3-year European multicenter study with repeat [123 I]-FP-CIT SPECT. *Mov. Disord.*, Vol. 24, No. 4, (Mar. 2009), pp. 500-508, ISSN 0885-3185.

Martins, R. N., et al. (1991). The molecular pathology of amyloid deposition in Alzheimer's disease. *Mol. Neurobiol.*, Vol. 5, No. 2-4, (Jun. 1991), pp. 389-398, ISSN 0893-7648.

Mathis, C. A., et al. (2002). A lipophilic thioflavin-T derivative for positron emission tomography (PET) imaging of amyloid in brain. *Bioorg. Med. Chem. Lett.*, Vol. 12, No. 3, (Feb. 2002), pp. 295-298, ISSN 0960-894X.

Mathis, C. A., et al. (2003). Synthesis and Evaluation of 11C-Labeled 6-Substituted 2-Arylbenzothiazoles as Amyloid Imaging Agents. *J. Med. Chem.*, Vol. 46, No. 13, (Jun. 2003), pp. 2740-2754, ISSN 0022-2623.

McKeith, I. G., et al. (1996). Consensus guidelines for the clinical and pathologic diagnosis of dementia with Lewy bodies (DLB): report of the Consortium on DLB International Workshop. *Neurology*, Vol. 47, No. 5, (Nov. 1996), pp. 1113-1124, ISSN 0028-3878.

McKhann, G., et al. (1984). Clinical diagnosis of Alzheimer's disease—report of the NINCDS–ADRDA work group under the auspices of Department of Health and Human Services Task Force on Alzheimer's disease. *Neurology*, Vol. 34, No. 7, (Jul. 1984), pp. 939-944, ISSN 0028-3878.

McNamee, R. L., et al. (2009). Consideration of optimal time window for Pittsburgh Compound B PET summed uptake measurements. *J. Nucl. Med.*, Vol. 50, No. 3, (Mar. 2009), pp. 348-355, ISSN 0161-5505.

Meyer, P. T., et al. (2011). Dual-biomarker imaging of regional cerebral amyloid load and neuronal activity in dementia with PET and 11C-labeled Pittsburgh Compound B. *J. Nucl. Med.*, Vol. 52, No. 3, (Mar. 2011), pp. 393-400, ISSN 0161-5505.

Minoshima, S., et al. (1997). Metabolic reduction in the posterior cingulate cortex in very early Alzheimer's disease. *Ann. Neurol.*, Vol. 42, No. 1, (Jul. 1997), pp. 85-94, ISSN 0364-5134.

Mintun, M. A., et al. (2006). [11C]PIB in a nondemented population. *Neurology*, Vol. 67, No. 3, (Aug. 2006), pp. 446-452, ISSN 0028-3878.

Morris, J. C., et al. (2009). Pittsburgh Compound B imaging and prediction of progression from cognitive normality to symptomatic Alzheimer disease. *Arch. Neurol.*, Vol. 66, No. 12, (Dec. 2009), pp. 1469-1475, ISSN 00039942.

Morrish, P. K., et al. (1995). Clinical and [18F] dopa PET findings in early Parkinson's disease. *J. Neurol. Neurosurg. Psychiatry*, Vol. 59, No. 6, (Dec. 1995), pp. 597-600, ISSN 0022-3050.

Namba, H., et al. (1994). In vivo measurement of acetylcholinesterase activity in the brain with a radioactive acetylcholine analog. *Brain Res.*, Vol. 667, No. 2, (Dec. 1994), pp. 278-282, ISSN 0006-8993.

Nelissen, N., et al. (2009). Phase 1 study of the Pittsburgh compound B derivative 18F-Flutemetamol in healthy volunteers and patients with probably Alzheimer disease. *J. Nucl. Med.*, Vol. 50, No. 8, (Aug. 2009), pp. 1251-1259, ISSN 0161-5505.

Nordberg, A. (2004). PET imaging of amyloid in Alzheimer's disease. *Lancet Neurol.*, Vol. 3, No. 9, (Sep. 2004), pp. 519-527, ISSN 1474-4422.

Nordberg, A. (2008). Amyloid imaging in Alzheimer's disease. *Neuropsychologia*, Vol. 46, No. 6, (May 2008), pp. 1636-1641, ISSN 0028-3932.

O' Keefe, G. J., et al. (2009). Radiation dosimetry of β-amyloid tracers 11C-PiB and 18F-BAY94-9172. *J. Nucl. Med.*, Vol. 50, No. 2, (Feb. 2009), pp. 309-315, ISSN 0161-5505.

Okamura, N., et al. (2005). Quinoline and Benzimidazole Derivatives: Candidate Probes for In Vivo Imaging of Tau Pathology in Alzheimer's Disease. *J. Neurosci.*, Vol. 25, No. 47, (Nov. 2005), pp. 10857-10862, ISSN 0270-6474.

Okamura, N., et al. (2010). In vivo measurement of vesicular monoamine transporter type 2 density in Parkinson disease with 18F-AV-133. *J. Nucl. Med.*, Vol. 51, No. 2, (Feb. 2010), pp. 223-228, ISSN 0161-5505.

Okello, A., et al. (2009). Conversion of amyloid positive and negative MCI to AD over 3 years. *Neurology*, Vol. 3, No. 10, (Sep. 2009), pp. 754-760, ISSN 0028-3878.

Ouchi, Y., et al. (2005). Microglial activation and dopamine terminal loss in early Parkinson's disease. *Ann. Neurol.*, Vol. 57, No. 2, (Feb. 2005), pp. 168-175, ISSN 0364-5134.

Patt, M., et al. (2010). Metabolite analysis of [18F]Florbetaben (BAY 94-9172) in human subjects: a substudy within a proof of mechanism clinical trial. *J. Radioanal. Nucl. Chem.*, Vol. 284, No. 3, (Mar. 2010), pp. 557-562, ISSN 0236-5731.

Pavese, N. and Brooks, D. J. (2009). Imaging neurodegeneration in Parkinson's disease. *Biochim. Biophys. Acta*, Vol. 1792, No. 7, (Jul. 2009), pp. 722-729, ISSN 0006-3002.

Petersen, R. C., et al. (2009). Mild cognitive impairment: ten years later. *Arch. Neurol.*, Vol. 66, No. 12, (Dec. 2009), pp. 1447-1455, ISSN 00039942.

Pike, K. E., et al. (2007). β-amyloid imaging and memory in non-demented individuals: evidence for preclinical Alzheimer' s disease. *Brain*, Vol. 130, No. 11, (Nov. 2007), pp. 2837-2844, ISSN 0006-8950.

Price, J. L. and Morris, J. C. (1999). Tangles and plaques in nondemented aging and "preclinical" Alzheimer's disease. *Ann. Neurol.*, Vol. 45, No. 3, (Mar. 1999), pp. 358-368, ISSN 0364-5134.

Rabinovici, G. D., et al. (2007). 11C-PIB PET imaging in Alzheimer disease and frontotemporal lobar degeneration. *Neurology*, Vol. 68, No. 15, (Apr. 2007), pp. 1205-1212, ISSN 0028-3878.

Rafii, M. S. and Aisen, P. S. (2009). Recent developments in Alzheimer's disease therapeutics. *BMC Med.*, Vol. 7, No. (Feb 2009), pp. 7, ISSN 1741-7015.

Rakshi, J. S., et al. (1999). Frontal, midbrain and striatal dopaminergic function in early and advanced Parkinson's disease. A 3D [18F]Dopa-PET study. *Brain*, Vol. 122, No. 9, (Sep. 1999), pp. 1637-1650, ISSN 0006-8950.

Reiman, E. M., et al. (1996). Preclinical evidence of Alzheimer's disease in persons homozygous for the epsilon 4 allele for apolipoprotein E. *New Engl. J. Med.*, Vol. 334, No. 12, (Mar. 1996), pp. 752-758, ISSN 0028-4793.

Reiman, E. M., et al. (2004). Functional brain abnormalities in young adults at genetic risk for late-onset Alzheimer's dementia. *Prod. Natl. Acad. Sci. USA*, Vol. 101, No. 1, (Jan. 2004), pp. 284-289, ISSN 0027-8424.

Ribeiro, M. J., et al. (2002). Dopaminergic function and dopamine transporter binding assessed with positron emission tomography in Parkinson disease. *Arch. Neurol.*, Vol. 59, No. 4, (Apr. 2002), pp. 580-586, ISSN 00039942.

Rowe, C. C., et al. (2008). Imaging of amyloid β in Alzheimer' s disease with 18F-BAY94-9172, a novel PET tracer: proof of mechanism. *Lancet Neurol.*, Vol. 7, No. 2, (Feb. 2008), pp. 129-135, ISSN 1474-4422.

Rowe, C. C., et al. (2007). Imaging beta-amyloid burden in aging and dementia. *Neurology*, Vol. 68, No. 20, (May 2007), pp. 1718-1725, ISSN 0028-3878.

Scheinin, N. M., et al. (2007). Biodistribution and radiation dosimetry of the amyloid imaging agent 11C-PIB in humans. *J. Nucl. Med.*, Vol. 48, No. 1, (Jan. 2007), pp. 128-133, ISSN 0161-5505.

Seibyl, J. P., et al. (1995). Decreased single- photon emission computed tomographic [123I]beta-CIT striatal uptake correlates with symptom severity in Parkinson's disease. *Ann. Neurol.*, Vol. 38, No. 4, (Oct. 1995), pp. 589-598, ISSN 0364-5134.

Shao, X., et al. (2003). *N*-methylpiperidinemethyl, *N*-methylpyrrolidyl and *N*-methylpyrrolidinemethyl esters as PET radiotracers for acetylcholinesterase activity *Nucl. Med. Biol.*, Vol. 30, No. 3, (Apr. 2003), pp. 293-302, ISSN 0047-0740.

Sioka, C., et al. (2010). Recent advances in PET imaging for evaluation of Parkinson's disease. *Eur. J. Nucl. Med. Mol. Imaging*, Vol. 37, No. 8, (Aug. 2010), pp. 1594-1603, ISSN 1619-7070.

Small, G. W., et al. (2006). PET of Brain Amyloid and Tau in Mild Cognitive Impairment. *New Engl. J. Med.*, Vol. 355, No. 25, (Dec. 2006), pp. 2652-2663, ISSN 0028-4793.

Small, G. W., et al. (1995). Apolipoprotein E type 4 allele and cerebral glucose metabolism in relatives at risk for familial Alzheimer disease. *J. Am. Med. Assoc.*, Vol. 273, No. 12, (Mar. 1995), pp. 942-947, ISSN 0098-7484.

Smith, G. S., et al. (1992). Topography of cross-sectional and longitudinal glucose metabolic deficits in Alzheimer's disease. Pathophysiologic implications. *Arch. Neurol.*, Vol. 49, No. 11, (Nov. 1992), pp. 1142-1150, ISSN 00039942.

Snyder, S. E., et al. (1998). Synthesis of 1-[11C]methylpiperidin-4-yl propionate ([11C]PMP) for in vivo measurements of acetylcholinesterase activity,. *Nucl. Med. Biol.*, Vol. 25, No. 8, (Nov. 1998), pp. 751-754, ISSN 0047-0740.

Storandt, M., et al. (2009). Cognitive decline and brain volume loss as signatures of cerebral amyloid-β peptide deposition identified with Pittsburgh Compound B. *Arch. Neurol.*, Vol. 66, No. 12, (Dec. 2009), pp. 1476-1481, ISSN 00039942.

Sullivan, M. G. (2011). FDA panel on amyloid imaging agent: not yet. *Family Practice News*, Vol. 41, No. 3, (Feb. 2011), pp. 15, ISSN 0300-7073.

Szardenings, K., et al. (2011). Novel, small molecule [F18]-PET tracers for imaging of tau in human AD brains. *J. Nucl. Med.*, Vol. 52, No. Suppl. 1, (May 2011), pp. 25P, ISSN 0161-5505.

Tamaoka, A., et al. (1994). Biochemical evidence for the long-tail form (A beta 1-42/43) of amyloid beta protein as a seed molecule in cerebral deposits of Alzheimer's diseae. *Biochem. Biophys. Res. Commun.*, Vol. 205, No. 1, (Nov. 1994), pp. 834-842, ISSN 0006-291X.

Terry, A. V. and Buccafusco, J. J. (2003). The Cholinergic Hypothesis of Age and Alzheimer's Disease-Related Cognitive Deficits: Recent Challenges and Their Implications for Novel Drug Development *J. Pharm. Expt. Ther.*, Vol. 306, No. 3, (Sep. 2003), pp. 821-827, ISSN 0022-3565.

Thal, D. R., et al. (2002). Phases of A-beta deposition in the human brain and its relevance for the development of AD. *Neurology*, Vol. 58, No. 12, (Jun. 2002), pp. 1791-1800, ISSN 0028-3878.

Vandenberghe, R., et al. (2010). 18F-Flutemetamol Amyloid Imaging in Alzheimer Disease and Mild Cognitive Impairment A Phase 2 Trial. *Ann. Neurol.*, Vol. 68, No. 3, (Sep. 2010), pp. 319-329, ISSN 0364-5134.

Vingerhoets, F. J. G., et al. (1997). Which clinical sign of Parkinson's disease best reflects the nigrostriatal lesion? *Ann. Neurol.*, Vol. 41, No. 1, (Jan. 1997), pp. 58-64, ISSN 0364-5134.

Vitali, P., et al. (2008). Neuroimaging in Dementia. *Semin. Nucl. Med.*, Vol. 28, No. 4, (Oct. 2008), pp. 467-483, ISSN 0001-2998.

Whone, A. L., et al. (2003). Plasticity of the nigropallidal pathway in Parkinson's disease. *Ann. Neurol.*, Vol. 53, No. 2, (Feb. 2003), pp. 206-213, ISSN 0364-5134.

Wimalasena, K. (2011). Vesicular monoamine transporters: Structure-function, pharmacology, and medicinal chemistry. *Med. Res. Rev.*, Vol. 31, No. 4, (Jul. 2011), pp. 483-519, ISSN 0198-6325.

Wong, D. F., et al. (2010). In Vivo Imaging of Amyloid Deposition in Alzheimer Disease Using the Radioligand 18F-AV-45 (Florbetapir F 18). *J. Nucl. Med.*, Vol. 51, No. 6, (Jun. 2010), pp. 913-920, ISSN 0161-5505.

Zhang, W., et al. (2007). 18F-labeled styrylpyridines as PET agents for amyloid plaque imaging. *Nucl. Med. Biol.*, Vol. 34, No. 1, (Jan. 2007), pp. 89-97, ISSN 0047-0740.

Zhang, W., et al. (2005a). F-18 polyethyleneglycol stilbenes as PET imaging agents targeting Aβ aggregates in the brain. *Nucl. Med. Biol.*, Vol. 32, No. 8, (Nov. 2005), pp. 799-809, ISSN 0047-0740.

Zhang, W., et al. (2005b). F-18 stilbenes as PET imaging agents for detecting beta-amyloid plaques in the brain. *J. Med. Chem.*, Vol. 48, No. 19, (Sep. 2005), pp. 5980-5988, ISSN 0022-2623.

Ziolko, S. K., et al. (2006). Evaluation of voxel-based methods for the statistical analysis of PIB PET amyloid imaging studies in Alzheimer's disease. *Neuroimage*, Vol. 33, No. 1, (Oct. 2006), pp. 94-102, ISSN 1053-8119.

9

Post-Therapeutic I-131 Whole Body Scan in Patients with Differentiated Thyroid Cancer

Ho-Chun Song and Ari Chong
Chonnam National University Medical School, Republic of Korea

1. Introduction

Therapy with radioiodine (I-131) has been used for patients with well-differentiated thyroid cancer such as papillary and follicular thyroid carcinoma to ablate normal thyroid tissue or to treat metastatic lesions. The improvement of survival rates and decrease of recurrence rates after I-131 therapy has been documented by retrospective studies (Mazzaferri & Jhiang, 1994; Samaan et al., 1992). Even those patients categorized as low risk also had significantly lower recurrence and death rates after they received I-131 (Dietlein et al., 2005). Diagnostic I-123 or I-131 whole body scan (DxWBS) can be performed to detect persistent disease before radioiodine therapy. The post-therapeutic I-131 whole body scan (RxWBS) can be done after administration of therapeutic dose of I-131.

1.1 Rationale of RxWBS

The purpose of RxWBS is for detection and localization or exclusion of functioning thyroid remnants, persistent or recurrent local disease or distant metastasis in patients receiving I-131 therapy (Luster et al., 2008). There are several reports regarding the higher detection ability of RxWBS than DxWBS. Therefore, the disease stage also can be changed after RxWBS. Fatourechi et al. reported that 13% of 117 patients of thyroid papillary cancer demonstrated abnormal foci on RxWBS, which were not seen on DxWBS (111 MBq (3 mCi), I-131) (Fatourechi et al., 2000). They also reported that RxWBS changed management strategy in 9% of 81 patients. Souza Rosario et al. reported that RxWBS on first ablation changed the disease stage in 8.3% of the patients and therapeutic approach in another 15% among total 106 patients (Souza Rosario et al., 2004). They also reported that RxWBS provided clinically relevant information for 26% of patients with 1 previous ablation. In their report, even when excluding cases whose lesions were known before scanning, the therapeutic approach was influenced by RxWBS in 15.6% of the patients.

There are also several reports regarding comparison of I-123 DxWBS and RxWBS. In the retrospective study by Donahue et al., they reported that RxWBS could find more lesions in 18% of 108 patients and clinical upstaging occurred in 10% of patients compared with DxWBS (I-123) (Donahue et al., 2008). In a study by Alzahrani et al., they showed 209 pairs of 238 pairs of RxWBS and DxWBS (I-123) were concordant (87.8% concordance rate) (Alzahrani et al., 2001). They also revealed that there were 29 discordant pairs, 13 RxWBS (5.5%) demonstrated additional foci of uptake at sites that were already positive on DxWBS

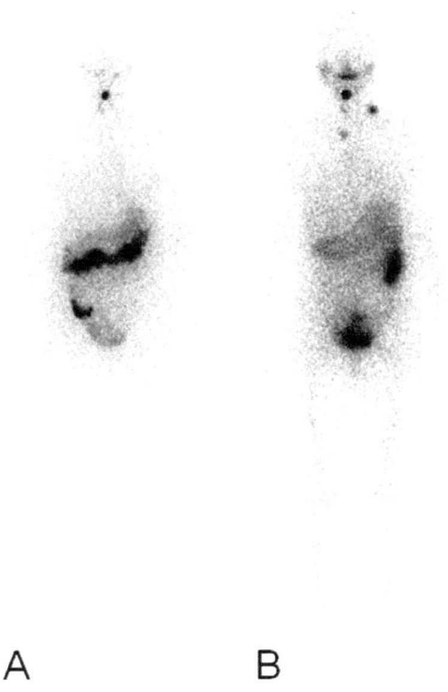

Fig. 1. Detection of metastatic lymph nodes on RxWBS, not on DxWBS. A 53-year-old woman with papillary thyroid cancer who underwent total thyroidectomy with left lateral neck dissection. A. I-123 DxWBS reveals a focal uptake in the anterior neck, suggesting remnant thyroid tissues in the thyroid bed. B. On RxWBS obtained 2 days after administration of 6.66 GBq (180 mCi) I-131, several focal hot uptake are noted in her left lateral neck and right highest mediastinal area. Neck ultrasonography revealed (image not shown) lesions suspicious of metastatic lymph nodes.

(I-123). Distant metastasis of thyroid cancer is not extremely rare. There have been studies reported the distant metastasis was found in 7-23% (Casara et al., 1991; Cooper et al., 2009; Mazzaferri, 1986; Samaan et al., 1985; Schlumberger et al., 1986). Iwano et al. reported that the concordance rates between DxWBS (I-123) and RxWBS were high for thyroid bed and bone metastases (89% and 86%, respectively), while they were low for lymph node and lung metastases on RxWBS (61% and 39%, respectively) (Iwano et al., 2009).

There are several reasons of performing RxWBS.

a. Metastasis is not extremely rare in thyroid cancer.
b. Presence of distant metastasis can change treatment strategies.
c. RxWBS has better detection performances of detecting remnant or metastatic lesions than DxWBS.
d. Performing scan after therapy does not require additional radiation exposure, like other radiologic evaluation.

2. Protocols of RxWBS

2.1 Imaging protocol

2.1.1 Gamma camera or SPECT

The efficacy of a system for imaging I-131 is dependent on the thickness of the crystal of camera and the collimator (Mazzaferri, 1986). I-131 whole body scan was usually done

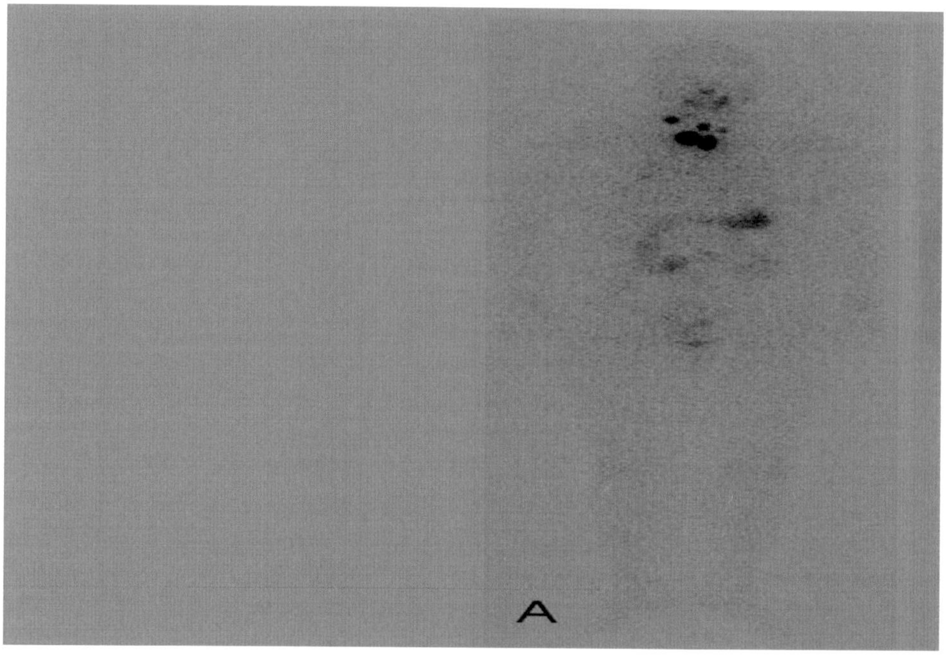

Fig. 2. Multiple pulmonary metastases detected on RxWBS which were invisible on DxWBS. A 54-year-old woman who underwent total thyroidectomy for papillary thyroid cancer. A, I-123 DxWBS shows several hot uptake in the anterior neck and upper mediastinum. B, On RxWBS obtained 3 days after the administration of 7.4 GBq (200 mCi) I-131, multiple metastatic lesions are newly detected in both the lung fields.

using a large field of view gamma camera with a medium-energy, parallel-hole collimator, and the photo peak was 364 KeV with a 20% window. Continuous acquisition mode can be used with a scanning ratio of 9 - 13 cm/s with a 512 x 512 or 1,024 × 256 matrix. Anterior and posterior views of the whole body can be obtained simultaneously. Spot views of suspected sites of metastasis can be done additionally using a 256 × 256 matrix for a total of 500,000 counts. Additional image such as scanning after drinking a glass of water to wash out physiologic uptake in the esophagus is sometimes needed (Figure 3).

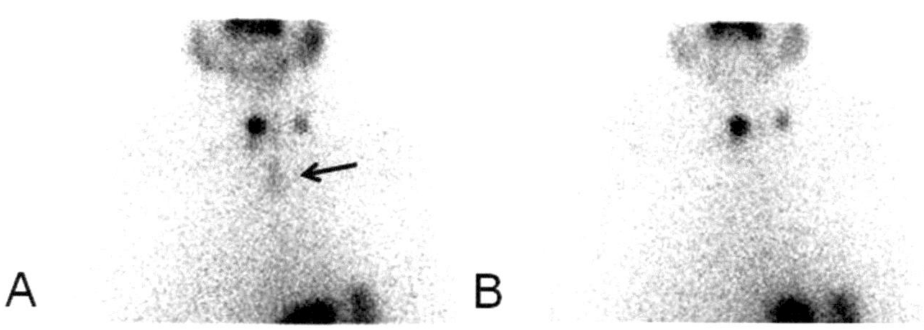

Fig. 3. Physiologic retention of I-131 in the esophagus. The physiologic I-131 retention (arrow) in the esophagus on RxWBS obtained after administration of 3.7 GBq (100 mCi) I-131 (A). It disappeared after drinking a glass of water (B).

2.1.2 SPECT/CT

Whole body imaging with SPECT/CT requires long scan time. Therefore, SPECT/CT is usually performed for specific site after whole body scan. The field of view (FOV) of SPECT/CT is usually determined by nuclear medicine physicians based on the planar image findings. So far, many companies have their models of SPECT/CT. This is the one of the usual protocol of SPECT/CT (Infinia Hawkeye 4) of our institution. First, emission SPECT images are acquired with counts from the 10% energy window at 364 KeV, with a matrix size of 128 x 128. A total image of 64 frames is acquired over 360° with an acquisition time of 30 s/frame, angular step of 6°, and zooming factor of 1. After SPECT acquisition, a CT scan is acquired with a low-dose, helical CT scanner. The CT parameters are 140 KeV and 5 mAs, and no intravenous iodinated contrast is administered. The CT data are used for attenuation correction. The Images are reconstructed with a conventional iterative algorithm, ordered subset expectation maximization (OSEM). A workstation providing multiplanar reformatted images are used for image display and analysis.

2.2 Imaging timing of RxWBS

Radioiodine is excreted slowly in hypothyroid patients, especially if they have been on a low iodine diet (Dietlein et al., 2005). Therefore, decreasing background activity is important for visualizing small metastases or remnant thyroid tissue. However, current guidelines for I-131 therapy differ in their recommendations for the optimal time of the RxWBS ranging from 48 – 72 hours (Becker et al., 1996; Luster et al., 2008) to 2 - 10 days (Cooper et al., 2009). Also, there is a lot of discrepancy in the published literature regarding the optimal timing of RxWBS (Cholewinski et al., 2000; Chong et al., 2010; Durante et al., 2006; Hindie et al., 2003; Hung et al., 2009; Khan et al., 1994; Nemec et al., 1979). So far, several studies were done for evaluating efficacy or accuracy of RxWBS which was done at different timing after high-dose I-131 therapy. Khan et al. conducted scans at 2 days and 7 days post-therapy after 3.7–5.6 GBq of I-131 administration (Khan et al., 1994). They reported a higher sensitivity for detection of iodine-avid tissue on RxWBS 7 days post-therapy than earlier RxWBS. Hung et al. analyzed RxWBS at three different time points (first scan performed 3–4 days, second scan 5–6 days, and third scan 10–11 days after I-131 therapy) (Hung et al., 2009). They retrospectively analyzed 239 patients' scans. Twenty-eight percent of lymph node metastases, 17% of lung metastases, and 16% of bone metastases were missed on the late images on 10-11th day. On the other hand, only 5% of the remnants were missed. The ratio of early washout was different between remnants and metastatic lesions. Chong et al. conducted RxWBS on the third and seventh days after I-131 therapy in 60 cases from 52 patients with lung or bone metastases of thyroid cancer (Chong et al., 2010). They showed that 22% of lung metastases and 33% of bone metastases that were not shown on the third day scan were detected on the seventh day scan (Figure 4 and 5). Lee et al. conducted RxWBS on the third and tenth day after I-131 therapy in 81 patients (Lee et al., 2011). They reported that the I-131 avid lesions on the early scan were more easily detected by visual analysis and had higher uptake ratios than those on the delayed scan. The optimal timing for RxWBS is still needed to be clarified.

2.3 Medication and diet after administration of therapeutic dose of I-131

Published guideline for I-131 therapy recommend that low-iodine diet, when possible, <50 μg/day, starting 1-2 weeks prior to radioiodine administration is recommended (Cooper et al., 2009; Luster et al., 2008). However, the duration of this low-iodine diet varies. Usually, regular diet can be started after the treatment. Information about low-iodine diet can be obtained at Thyroid Cancer Survivors Association website, http://www.thyca.org/rai.htm#diet.

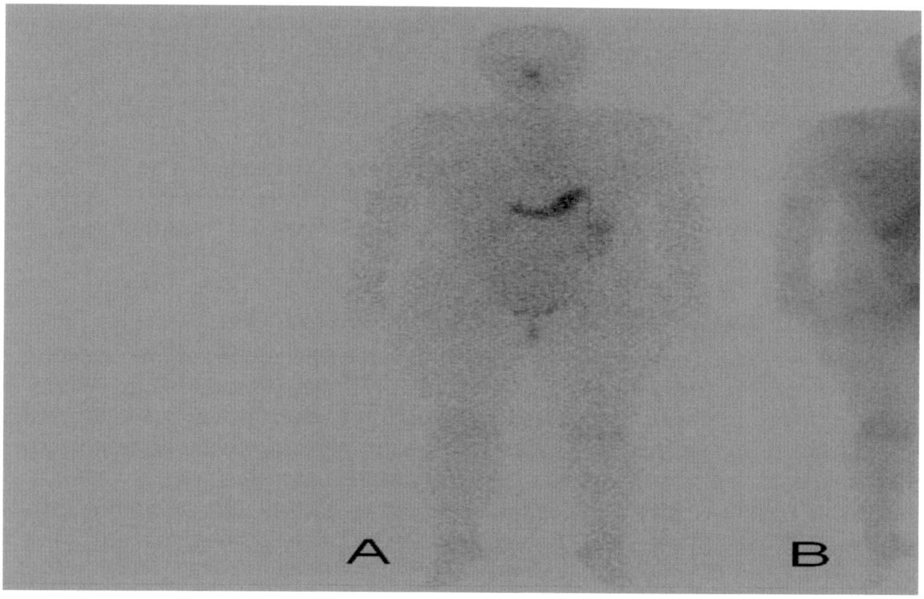

Fig. 4. Diffuse pulmonary metastases. The metastatic uptake is not seen on I-123 DxWBS (A) and early RxWBS (on the third day after therapy) (B). It only appears on the RxWBS which was performed on the seventh day after the administration of 7.4 GBq (200 mCi) I-131 (C).

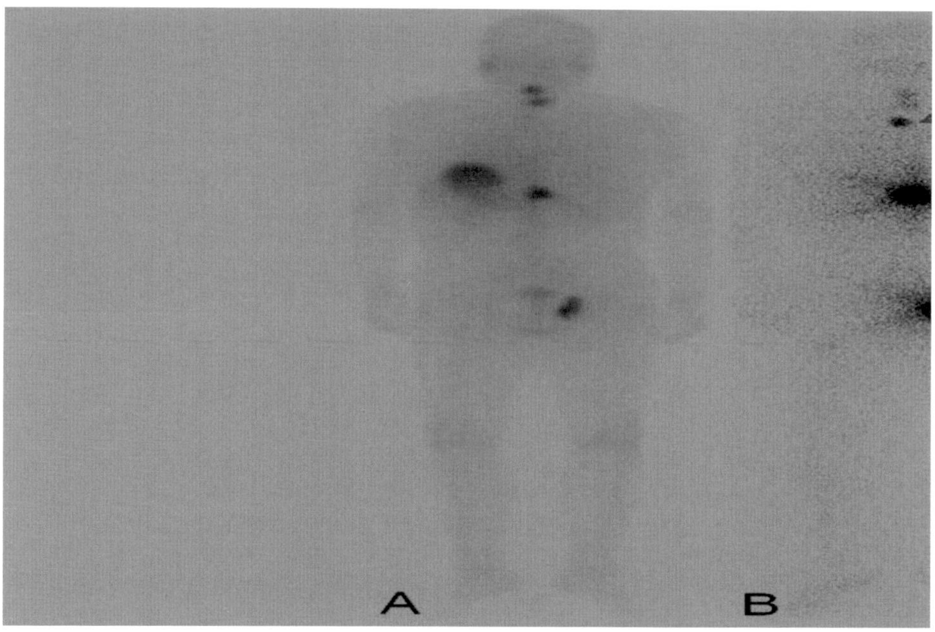

Fig. 5. Multiple osseous metastases. The metastatic lesion in the upper thoracic vertebra (arrow) is only visible on the RxWBS obtained seventh day after administration of 7.4 GBq (200 mCi) I-131 (B). These lesion is not visible on RxWBS obtained third day after therapy (A) or Tc-99m HDP WBS (C).

Thyroid hormone replacement may be resumed on the second or third day after therapy (Cooper et al., 2009; Luster et al., 2008).

3. Findings of RxWBS

The following data are needed to be reported: the name of patient, ID, age, the date of I-131 therapy, I-131 dose, date of RxWBS. When it is available, the serum level of thyroglobulin, thyroid stimulating hormone and anti-thyroglobulin antibody are to be reported. The sites of significant I-131 uptake are needed to be mentioned.

3.1 False positive RxWBS

False positive RxWBS occurs for nonthyroidal I-131 concentration, including external contamination by the saliva, nasal secretions and sweat containing I-131, internal contamination through nasopharyngeal secretion, as well as physiologic uptake in nonthyroidal tissue such as the choroid plexus, salivary glands, gastric mucosa, and urinary tract. Carliscle et al. summarized false positive findings (Carlisle et al., 2003). I-131 uptake can be seen in the nose, salivary glands, mouth, thyroid bed, lactating breast, liver, gall bladder, stomach, esophagus and sweat (Figure 6). Physiologic uptake of I-131 in the salivary glands, nasal mucosa, gastric mucosa, colon, mammary glands and choroid plexus is due to the NIS presence in these tissues (Carlisle et al., 2003; Riedel et al., 2001). Thymic uptake is rare, there is a report that the incidence of thymic uptake was 1-1.2% of cases (Davidson & McDougall, 2000) (Figure 7).

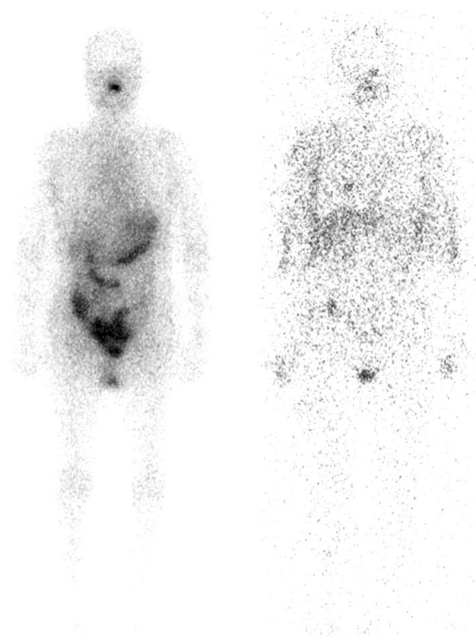

A B

Fig. 6. Diffuse perspiration. (A) On the RxWBS obtained on the third day after I-131 therapy with 3.7 GBq (100 mCi), mild perspiration is noted in both the axillae. (B) On the RxWBS obtained on the seventh day after I-131 therapy, diffuse perspiration is present in both the axillae, chest, upper arms and hands.

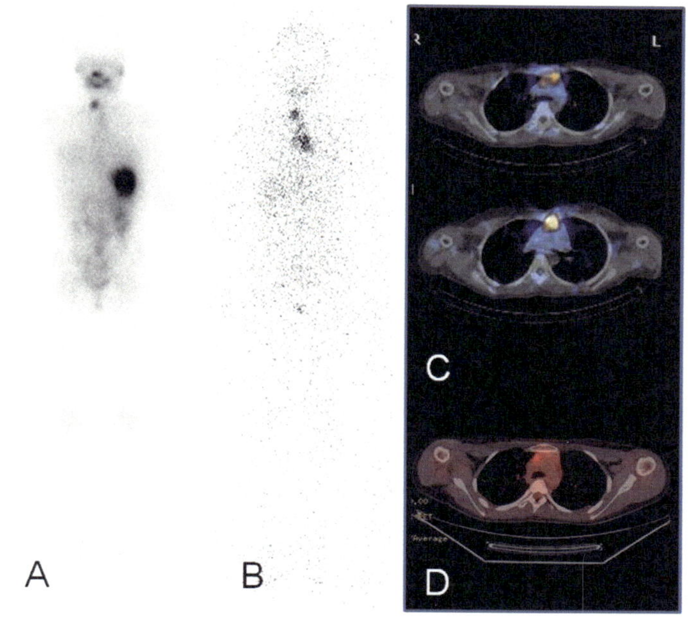

Fig. 7. Thymic uptake. A 12-year-old girl underwent therapy with 3.7 GBq (100 mCi) I-131. RxWBS were obtaind on the third day (A) and seventh day (B) after therapy. Hot uptakes are seen in the right lower neck and upper chest. I-131 SPECT/CT (C) and F-18 FDG PET/CT images (D) confirmed I-131 uptake in the upper chest to be physiologic uptake in the thymus.

Diffuse hepatic uptake of I-131 is rarely found due to occult hepatic metastases but more commonly due to the hepatic de-ionization and conjugation of I-131 which was not incorporated into the thyroid hormone (Carlisle et al., 2003). Chung et al. investigated hepatic uptake on DxWBS or RxWBS. They analyzed scans of 399 patients. They reported that hepatic uptake is more often when higher dose of I-131 was administered. They also reported that the more uptakes appeared in the residual thyroid, the more it appeared in the liver. However, they found that 15 patients showed diffuse hepatic uptake without uptake by the remnant thyroid or metastatic lesion. They followed these patients and metastatic lesions were found in 7 of 15 patients. So, they insisted that diffuse liver uptake indicated functioning thyroid remnant or metastasis (Chung et al., 1997) (Figure 8).

There are some reports I-131 false positive uptake in other pathologic condition unrelated to thyroid cancer: tracheostomy site, bronchiectasis, pulmonary inflammatory disease, pleural effusion, salivary gland tumor, some other carcinoma such as adenocarcinoma, squamous carcinoma, Barrett's esophagus, Meckel's diverticulum (Ain & Shih, 1994; Berquist et al., 1975; Caplan et al., 1987; Carlisle et al., 2003; Fernandez-Ulloa et al., 1976; Hoschl et al., 1988; Misaki et al., 1994; Mitchell et al., 2000; Muratet & Giraud, 1996), and so on. (Figure 9)

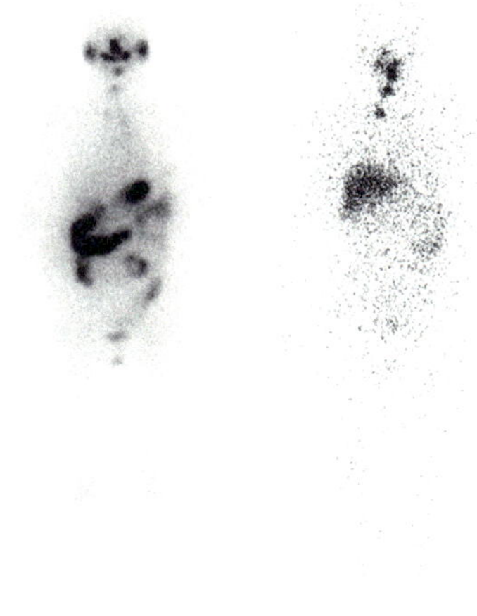

A B

Fig. 8. Diffuse hepatic uptake. A 59-year-old female underwent I-131 therapy with 370 MBq (100 mCi) after total thyroidectomy. On the RxWBS obtained on the third day after therapy, mild focal uptakes in the anterior neck and right lower anterior neck are shown (A). On the RxWBS obtained on the seventh day after therapy, diffuse hepatic uptake appears in addition to the cervical uptakes (B).

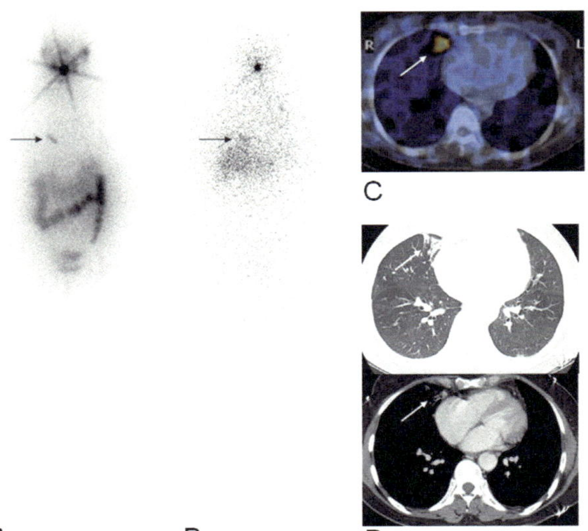

A B D

Fig. 9. I-131 accumulation in the benign pulmonary disease. A 51-year-old female underwent RxWBS on the third day (A) and the seventh day (B) after the administration of 6.66 GBq I-131. Besides the hot uptake in the neck, slightly increased, focal, linear uptake (arrows on A and B) is shown. On SPECT/CT (C), it is on the medial segment of the right middle lobe. Chest CT (D) shows peribronchial cicatrical consolidation and adhesive atelectasis containing mild traction bronchiectatic change in this lesion.

3.2 Diagnostic value of RxWBS

The visualizing functioning metastasis as well as remnant thyroid tissue is related to the dose of I-131. Waxman et al. reported that more lesions were detected when the activity administered was increased from 74 to 370 MBq (2 to 10 mCi) and when even higher yields at 1,110 to 3,700 MBq (30 to 100 mCi) (Waxman et al., 1981). Spies et al. reported that with higher therapeutic dose, RxWBS demonstrated additional findings or more accurate localization compared with a diagnostic dose of 185 MBq (5 mCi) in 46% of cases (Spies et al., 1989).

The diagnostic accuracy of RxWBS is also related with the time interval from the date of administration of I-131 and that of scanning. Khan et al. and Chong et al. reported that earlier scanning might miss the lesions and the effectiveness of the delayed scan on the seventh day from the administration of I-131 (Khan S et al., 1994). Khan et al. performed RxWBS on the second day and seventh day post-therapy (Khan et al., 1994). They reported that the seventh day scan is more sensitive than third day scan. Chong et al. reported that 22% of lung metastasis and 33% of bone metastases that were not shown on the third day scan, though they were detected on the seventh day scan (Chong et al., 2010) (Figure 10).

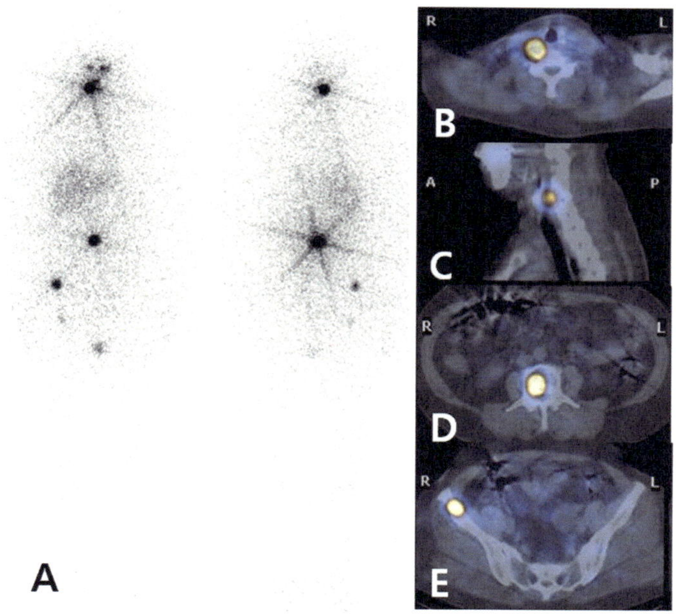

Fig. 10. Vertebral metastasis mimicking remnant thyroid tissue. A 61-year-old female underwent RxWBS after administration of 7.4 GBq (200 mCi) I-131. RxWBS shows multiple uptakes in the abdomen and right pelvic area suggesting distant metastases. Focal uptake in the anterior neck was supposed to be usual remnant thyroid tissue. However, on additional SPECT/CT (B, C), the uptake is detected in the cervical vertebra (C5), not in the thyroidectomy site. SPECT/CT also reveals I-131 uptake on thelumbar vertebra (L3, D) and right iliac bone (E).

Hung et al. conducted different protocol, RxWBS on the third to fourth day, fifth to sixth day and tenth to eleventh day post-therapy (Hung et al., 2009). They reported that there is a trend of decreasing visualization of I-131 uptake in sequential images and that 17% of lung metastasis and 16% of bone metastases were missed on the tenth to eleventh day scans. Lee et al. conducted RxWBS on the third and tenth day post-therapy (Lee et al., 2011). They also reported significant reduction in visual analysis scores and uptake ratios of I-131 avid lesions on the delayed RxWBS.

In addition, diagnostic accuracy of RxWBS is related to the past-history of previous I-131 therapy. Oh et al. reported the sensitivity of RxWBS in detecting distant metastasis after first I-131 therapy is 75% (Oh et al., 2011). In contrast, in patients with history of multiple radioiodine therapy, sensitivity of RxWBS in detecting distant metastasis is only 35%. The sensitivity of RxWBS and SPECT/CT is reported to be similar. However, the specificity of RxWBS is lower than SPECT/CT (Table 1). The sensitivity of FDG PET/CT is lower than RxWBS in detecting distant metastasis and the specificity of FDG PET/CT is much higher than RxWBS or SPECT/CT.

	Sens(%)	Spec(%)	DA(%)	PPV(%)	NPV(%)
All patients (n=140)					
WBS	65	55	59	42	76
SPECT/CT	65	95	85	86	85
PET/CT	61	98	86	93	84
Single therapy (n=101)					
WBS	90	56	63	35	6
SPECT/CT	90	96	95	86	97
PET/CT	48	100	89	100	88
Multiple therapies (n=39)					
WBS	44	50	46	30	33
SPECT/CT	44	86	59	85	46
PET/CT	72	86	77	90	63

Table 1. Diagnostic performance of WBS, SPECT/CT and PET/CT in detecting distant metastasis (patient-based analysis) (adapted and modified from Oh et al., 2011).
Sens, Sensitivity; *Spec*, Specificity; *DA*, diagnostic accuracy; *PPV*, positive predictive value; *NPV*, negative predictive value

Previous radioiodine scanning might be the reason of decreased sensitivity (Rawson et al., 1951). Thyroid stunning has been reported as the temporary impairment of thyroid tissue after a 111 MBq (3 mCi) or greater diagnostic I-131 dose that decreases the final absorbed dose in ablative therapy. However, Rosario et al. reported that diagnostic scanning using a 185 MBq (5 mCi) of I-131 dose does not interfere with uptake of the ablative dose or with treatment efficacy when ablation is performed within 72 hours (Rosario et al., 2005). Dam et al. reported that even though, stunning might occur but there was no significant difference in treatment success rates (Dam et al., 2004).

4. Other imaging modalities

4.1 F-18 Fluorodeoxyglucose PET/CT

Fluorodeoxyglucose (FDG) is a glucose analogue. This is taken into the cell and phosphorylated by the same mechanism as glucose. In thyroid cancer, "Flip-flop phenomenone" is reported (Feine et al., 1996; Khan N. et al., 2003). It means the alternating uptake pattern of I-131 and FDG by the differentiated papillary or follicular thyroid cancer, which thought to be related to the differentiation of tumor (Figure 11 and 12). Bertagna et al. reported that F-18 FDG PET/CT positive results correlated with the serum thyroglobulin level in patients with negative I-131 whole body scan and high serum thyroglobulin level. They also reported that F-18 FDG PET/CT showed highest accuracy when the patient's thyroglobulin level was higher than 21 ng/mL (Bertagna et al., 2009). In addition to that, they also revealed that the levothyroxine therapy regimen does not influence F-18 FDG PET/CT results. Yoshio et al. evaluated 55 cases with differentiated thyroid cancer with F-18 FDG PET/CT and reported that FDG-avid lesions are resistant to radioactive iodine therapy with or without I-131 uptake (Yoshio et al., 2011).

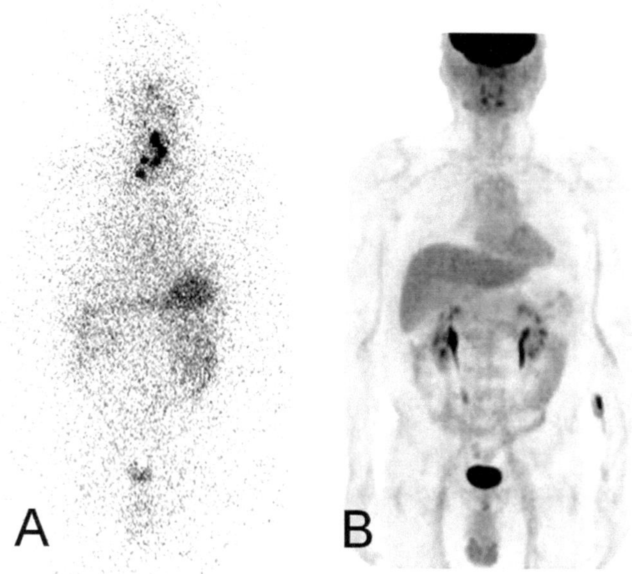

Fig. 11. Flip-flop phenomenone. A 44-year-old male underwent total thyroidectomy due to thyroid papillary carcinoma. I-123 DxWBS (A) shows several hot uptakes in the anterior neck, whereas F-18 FDG PET/CT (B) is negative.

4.2 Tc-99m methoxyisobutylisonitrile (Tc-99m MIBI)

Tc-99m MIBI, a lipophilic cationic molecules, was originally developed as a myocardial perfusion imaging agent. Today Tc-99m MIBI is also used for the study of many neoplastic diseases. The mechanism of Tc-99m MIBI accumulation in tumor has been reported to depend on the size of a tumor, the blood flow and the richness of mitochondria in the tumor

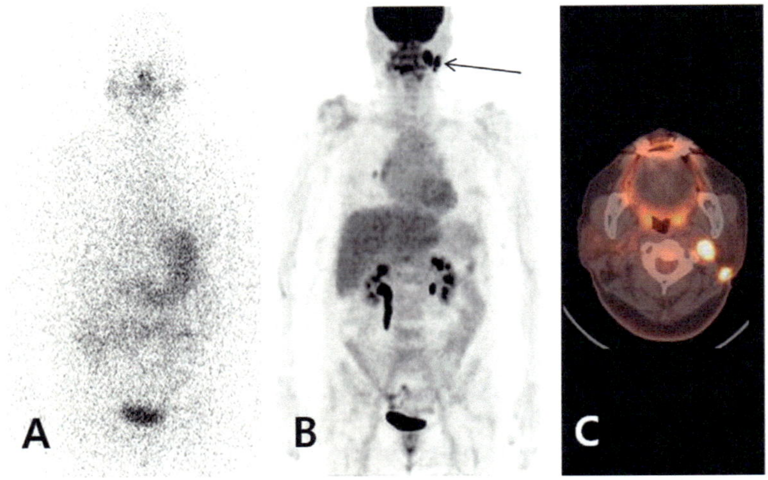

Fig. 12. Iodine negative and F-18 FDG PET positive case. A 65-year-old female underwent I-123 DxWBS (A) and F-18 FDG PET/CT (B,C) for elevated serum thyroglobulin level (3 to 17 ng/ml) after left modified radical lymph node dissection two years ago. I-123 DxWBS (A) does not show abnormal uptake. On F-18 FDG PET/CT (B), focal uptakes were shown in the left lateral neck (arrow). On axial view of fusion image (C), two hypermetabolic lesions were seen in the left cervical level II. Biopsy revealed recurred papillary carcinoma.

cells (Moretti et al., 2005; Piwnica-Worms et al., 1994; Saggiorato et al., 2009). MIBI irreversibly passes into the mitochondria using the electrical gradient generated by a high negative inner transmembrane mitochondrial potential of malignant cells (Chernoff et al., 1993; Moretti et al., 2005; Piwnica-Worms et al., 1994). Also, there is a report that TSH simulates both F-18 FDG PET and Tc-99m MIBI uptake in poorly differentiated papillary thyroid cancer in vitro experiment (Kim et al., 2009). Even though Tc-99m MIBI is inferior to I-131 scintigraphy in detecting I-131 avid lesions (Al Saleh et al., 2007), it can be applied for patients with elevated serum human thyroglobulin levels but negative I-131 whole body scan (Wu et al., 2003). However, there are several reports that F-18 FDG PET is more sensitive than Tc-99m MIBI SPECT in detecting metastatic cervical lymph node in differentiated thyroid cancer patients with elevated serum thyroglobulin level but negative I-131 whole body scan (Iwata et al., 2004; Wu et al., 2003) (Figure 13).

4.3 Tc-99m tetrofosmin

Tetrofosmin is a lipophilic phosphine useful for myocardial perfusion imaging. Significant uptake of Tc-99m tetrofosmin in the thyroid, breast and lung tumors is reported. Tc-99m tetrofosmin is useful in detection of thyroid metastatic disease, particularly when the tumor is not iodine avid. In addition, it does not require withdrawal of thyroid hormone suppression therapy (Sharma et al., 2007). Nishiyama et al. reported that detectability of thyroid cancer metastases using Tc-99m tetrofosmin was 79.4% and that Tc-99m tetrofosmin is more sensitive than I-131 for detection of differentiated thyroid cancer metastasis, particulary for regional lymph node (Nishiyama et al., 2000). Unal et al. reported different results that the sensitivities of Tl-201, Tc-99m tetrofosmin and I-131 in diagnosing distant metastases were comparable (0.85, 0.85, and 0.75, respectively) (Unal et al., 1998).

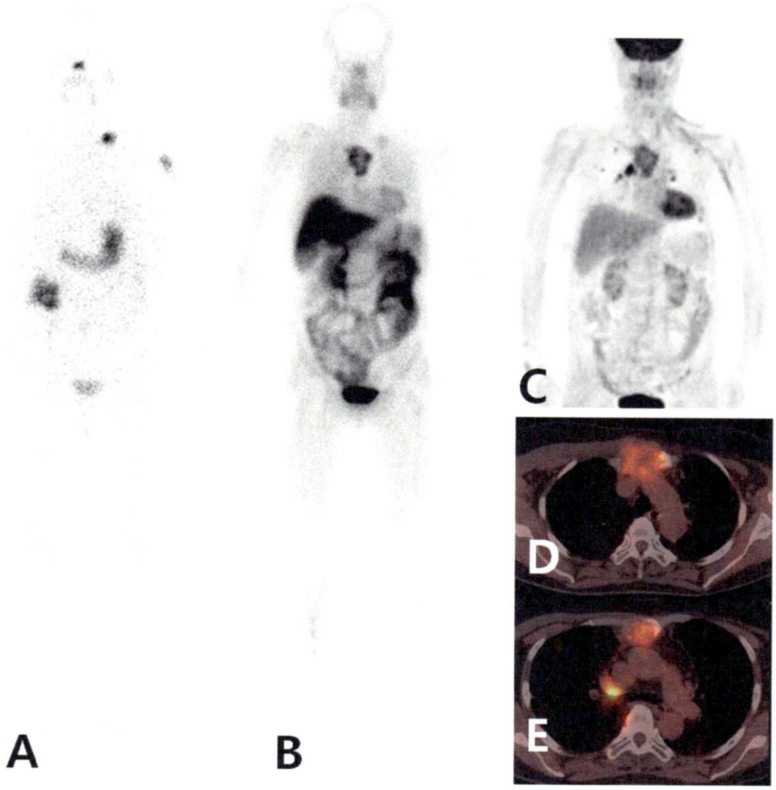

Fig. 13. I-131, Tc-99m MIBI and F-18 FDG images. A 62-year-old woman with metastatic papillary thyroid cancer to the left proximal humerus, clavicle and sternum underwent I-131 therapy with 7.4 GBq (200 mCi). Her serum thyroglobulin level was 260 ng/mL. I-131 RxWBS (A) shows focal hot uptakes in the left clavicle and huemrus. On Tc-99m MIBI WBS, irregular hot uptakes are detected in the sternal area and faint uptake in the left clavicle (B). F-18 FDG PET/CT (C-E) shows multiple hypermetabolic lesions in the sternum, both hilar lymph nodes and lungs.

4.4 Thallium-201

Thallium-201 (Tl-201) is a monovalemt cationic radioisotope listed in same group with gallium in the periodic table. The membrane permeability for Tl-201 is almost equal to that for potassium (Elgazzar et al., 1993). It is suggested that intracellular accumulation of thallous ions is due to the transmembrane electropotential gradient (Mullins & Moore, 1960). The primary role of Tl-201 in nuclear medicine is for imaging of myocardial perfusion and viability (Pauwels et al., 1998). Also, Tl-201 chloride has affinity for various malignant tumors, although it is not specific for malignant tumor (Senga et al., 1982). Uptake of Tl-201 in tumor seems to be determined by blood flow, grade of malignancy, viability of tumor cells and tumor necrosis (Pauwels et al., 1998). There are several reports regarding Tl-201 and thyroid cancer. Shiga et al. compared FDG PET with I-131 and Tl-201 scintigraphy and reported that FDG uptake was concordant with I-131 in 38% and with Tl-201 uptake in 94% (Shiga et al., 2001). Senga et al. reported that when tumor showed a positive scan with Tl-

201 chloride but negative results using Ga-67 citrate, it was differentiated thyroid carcinoma or poorly differentiated adenoma (Senga et al., 1982). Carril et al. analyzed Tl-201 and I-131 in ablated thyroid cancer patients. They reported that the sensitivity and specificity were 94% and 96% for Tl-201 and 29% and 100% for I-131 (Carril et al., 1997). Nakada et al. reported that Tl-201 uptake correlated well with the proliferating cell nuclear antigen index, which represents proliferative activity (Nakada et al., 1999).

4.5 I-124 PET/CT

I-124 is a positron emitter with a half-life of 4.18 days, produced by a cyclotron. It can be used to directly image thyroid cancer using PET scanner. Van Nostrand et al. compared I-124 PET with I-131 DxWBS in detecting residual thyroid tissue and/or metastatic lesion. They reported that I-124 PET identified as many as 50% more foci of radioiodine uptake suggestive of additional residual thyroid tissue and/or metastasis (Van Nostrand et al., 2010). They suggest that I-124 PET produced superior results because the PET scanner provides images with reduced background noise and enhanced spatial and contrast resolution compared with I-131 DxWBS. The longer half-life of I-124 is useful for dose monitoring over an extended time period (Surti et al., 2009). It can be also used for lesion-specific dosimetry. I-131 mean absorbed dose distributions can be calculated from serial I-124 PET image (Erdi et al., 1999; Larson & Robbins, 2002).

5. Conclusion

The I-123 DxWBS or I-131 DxWBS is sensitive and specific for treatable remnant or metastatic lesion. About 25% of RxWBS detect lesions missed by DxWBS. For this reason, following administration of a therapeutic I-131 dose, RxWBS should always be performed in patients with well differentiated thyroid cancer. The timing of RxWBS is currently still controversial. Based on several studies, the timing of post-therapeutic I-131 WBS is within 5th to 10th day, especially more opportune around 7th day after therapy. I-131 WBS with SPECT/CT may be the highly tailored approach for assessing distant metastatic lesions in patients who received a radioiodine therapy if SPECT/CT is available. RxWBS is especially likely to provide the useful information when DxWBSs are negative and the serum thyroglobulin levels are elevated. Other imaging modalities including F-18 FDG PET/CT is useful in detecting remnant thyroid tissues or metastatic thyroid cancer in patient with the elevated serum thyroglobulin level and negative iodine images. I-124 can be also useful in detection of the lesion and evaluation of lesional and whole-body dosimetry in patients with well-differentiated thyroid cancer.

6. References

Ain, K.B. & Shih, W.J. (1994). False-positive I-131 uptake at a tracheostomy site. Discernment with Tl-201 imaging. *Clinical Nuclear Medicine*, Vol. 19, No. 7, (July 1994), pp. 619-621, ISSN 0363-9762

Al Saleh, K.; Safwat, R.; Al-Shammeri, I.; Abdul Naseer, M.; Hooda, H. & Al-Mohannadi, S. (2007). Comparison of whole body scintigraphy with Tc-99m-methoxyisobutylisonitrile and iodine-131 NA in patients with differentiated thyroid cancer. *The Gulf Journal of Oncology*, Vol. 1, No. 1, (January 2007), pp. 29-33, ISSN 2078-2101

Alzahrani, A.S.; Bakheet, S.; Al Mandil, M.; Al-Hajjaj, A.; Almahfouz, A. & Al Haj, A. (2001). ^{123}I isotope as a diagnostic agent in the follow-up of patients with differentiated thyroid cancer: comparison with post 131I therapy whole body scanning. *The Journal of Clinical Endocrinology & Metabolism*, Vol. 86, No. 11, (November 2001), pp. 5294-5300, ISSN 1945-7197

Becker, D.; Charkes, N.D.; Dworkin, H.; Hurley, J.; McDougall, I.R.; Price, D.; Royal, H. & Sarkar, S. (1996). Procedure guideline for extended scintigraphy for differentiated thyroid cancer: 1.0. Society of Nuclear Medicine. *Journal of Nuclear Medicine*, Vol. 37, No. 7, (July 1996), pp. 1269-1271, ISSN 0161-5505

Berquist, T.H.; Nolan, N.G.; Stephens, D.H. & Carlson, H.C. (1975). Radioisotope scintigraphy in diagnosis of Barrett's esophagus. *The American journal of roentgenology, radium therapy, and nuclear medicine*, Vol. 123, No. 2, (February 1975), pp. 401-411, ISSN 0002-9580

Bertagna, F.; Bosio, G.; Biasiotto, G.; Rodella, C.; Puta, E.; Gabanelli, S.; Lucchini, S.; Merli, G.; Savelli, G.; Giubbini, R.; Rosenbaum, J. & Alavi, A. (2009). F-18 FDG-PET/CT evaluation of patients with differentiated thyroid cancer with negative I-131 total body scan and high thyroglobulin level. *Clinical Nuclear Medicine*, Vol. 34, No. 11, (October 2009), pp. 756-761, ISSN 0363-9762

Caplan, R.H.; Gundersen, G.A.; Abellera, R.M. & Kisken, W.A. (1987). Uptake of iodine-131 by a Meckel's diverticulum mimicking metastatic thyroid cancer. *Clinical Nuclear Medicine*, Vol. 12, No. 9, (September 1987), pp. 760-762, ISSN 0363-9762

Carlisle, M.R.; Lu, C. & McDougall, I.R. (2003). The interpretation of ^{131}I scans in the evaluation of thyroid cancer, with an emphasis on false positive findings. *Nuclear Medicine Communications*, Vol. 24, No. 6, (June 2003), pp. 715-735, ISSN 0143-3636

Carril, J.M.; Quirce, R.; Serrano, J.; Banzo, I.; Jimenez-Bonilla, J.F.; Tabuenca, O. & Barquin, R.G. (1997). Total-body scintigraphy with thallium-201 and iodine-131 in the follow-up of differentiated thyroid cancer. *Journal of Nuclear Medicine*, Vol. 38, No. 5, (May 1997), pp. 686-692, ISSN 0161-5505

Casara, D.; Rubello, D.; Saladini, G.; Gallo, V.; Masarotto, G. & Busnardo, B. (1991). Distant metastases in differentiated thyroid cancer: long-term results of radioiodine treatment and statistical analysis of prognostic factors in 214 patients. *Tumori*, Vol. 77, No. 5, (October 1991), pp. 432-436, ISSN 0300-8916

Chernoff, D.M.; Strichartz, G.R. & Piwnica-Worms, D. (1993). Membrane potential determination in large unilamellar vesicles with hexakis(2-methoxyisobutylisonitrile)technetium(I). *Biochimica et Biophysica Acta*, Vol. 1147, No. 2, (April 1993), pp. 262-266, ISSN 0006-3002

Cholewinski, S.P.; Yoo, K.S.; Klieger, P.S. & O'Mara, R.E. (2000). Absence of thyroid stunning after diagnostic whole-body scanning with 185 MBq 131I. *Journal of Nuclear Medicine*, Vol. 41, No. 7, (July 2000), pp. 1198-1202, ISSN 0161-5505

Chong, A.; Song, H.C.; Min, J.J.; Jeong, S.Y.; Ha, J.M.; Kim, J.; Yoo, S.U.; Oh, J.R. & Bom, H.S. (2010). Improved Detection of Lung or Bone Metastases with an I-131 Whole Body Scan on the 7th Day After High-Dose I-131 Therapy in Patients with Thyroid Cancer. *Nuclear Medicine and Molecular Imaging*, Vol. No. (October 2010), pp. 1-9, ISSN 1869-3474

Chung, J.K.; Lee, Y.J.; Jeong, J.M.; Lee, D.S.; Lee, M.C.; Cho, B.Y. & Koh, C.S. (1997). Clinical significance of hepatic visualization on iodine-131 whole-body scan in patients with thyroid carcinoma. *Journal of Nuclear Medicine*, Vol. 38, No. 8, (August 1997), pp. 1191-1195, ISSN 0161-5505

Cooper, D.S.; Doherty, G.M.; Haugen, B.R.; Kloos, R.T.; Lee, S.L.; Mandel, S.J.; Mazzaferri, E.L.; McIver, B.; Pacini, F.; Schlumberger, M.; Sherman, S.I.; Steward, D.L. & Tuttle, R.M. (2009). Revised American Thyroid Association management guidelines for patients with thyroid nodules and differentiated thyroid cancer. *Thyroid*, Vol. 19, No. 11, (November 2009), pp. 1167-1214, ISSN 1557-9077

Dam, H.Q.; Kim, S.M.; Lin, H.C. & Intenzo, C.M. (2004). 131I therapeutic efficacy is not influenced by stunning after diagnostic whole-body scanning. *Radiology*, Vol. 232, No. 2, (August 2004), pp. 527-533, ISSN 0033-8419

Davidson, J. & McDougall, I.R. (2000). How frequently is the thymus seen on whole-body iodine-131 diagnostic and post-treatment scans? *European Journal of Nuclear Medicine*, Vol. 27, No. 4, (May 2000), pp. 425-430, ISSN 0340-6997

Dietlein, M.; Moka, D. & Schicha, H. (2005). Radioiodine therapy for thyroid cancer, In: *Thyroid cancer*, H. J. Biersack & F. Grunwald, pp. 93, Springer, ISBN 3540413901, New York

Donahue, K.P.; Shah, N.P.; Lee, S.L. & Oates, M.E. (2008). Initial staging of differentiated thyroid carcinoma: continued utility of posttherapy 131I whole-body scintigraphy. *Radiology*, Vol. 246, No. 3, (March 2008), pp. 887-894, ISSN 0033-8419

Durante, C.; Haddy, N.; Baudin, E.; Leboulleux, S.; Hartl, D.; Travagli, J.P.; Caillou, B.; Ricard, M.; Lumbroso, J.D.; De Vathaire, F. & Schlumberger, M. (2006). Long-term outcome of 444 patients with distant metastases from papillary and follicular thyroid carcinoma: benefits and limits of radioiodine therapy. *The Journal of Clinical Endocrinology & Metabolism*, Vol. 91, No. 8, (August 2006), pp. 2892-2899, ISSN 0021-972X

Elgazzar, A.H.; Fernandez-Ulloa, M. & Silberstein, E.B. (1993). 201Tl as a tumour-localizing agent: current status and future considerations. *Nucl Med Commun*, Vol. 14, No. 2, (February 1993), pp. 96-103, ISSN 0143-3636 (Print) 0143-3636 (Linking)

Erdi, Y.E.; Macapinlac, H.; Larson, S.M.; Erdi, A.K.; Yeung, H.; Furhang, E.E. & Humm, J.L. (1999). Radiation Dose Assessment for I-131 Therapy of Thyroid Cancer Using I-124 PET Imaging. *Clin Positron Imaging*, Vol. 2, No. 1, (October 2003), pp. 41-46, ISSN 1095-0397

Fatourechi, V.; Hay, I.D.; Mullan, B.P.; Wiseman, G.A.; Eghbali-Fatourechi, G.Z.; Thorson, L.M. & Gorman, C.A. (2000). Are posttherapy radioiodine scans informative and do they influence subsequent therapy of patients with differentiated thyroid cancer? *Thyroid*, Vol. 10, No. 7, (August 2000), pp. 573-577, ISSN 1050-7256

Feine, U.; Lietzenmayer, R.; Hanke, J.P.; Held, J.; Wohrle, H. & Muller-Schauenburg, W. (1996). Fluorine-18-FDG and iodine-131-iodide uptake in thyroid cancer. *Journal of Nuclear Medicine*, Vol. 37, No. 9, (September 1996), pp. 1468-1472, ISSN 0161-5505

Fernandez-Ulloa, M.; Maxon, H.R.; Mehta, S. & Sholiton, L.J. (1976). Iodine-131 uptake by primary lung adenocarcinoma. Misinterpretation of 131I scan. *JAMA*, Vol. 236, No. 7, (August 1976), pp. 857-858, ISSN 0098-7484

Hindie, E.; Melliere, D.; Lange, F.; Hallaj, I.; de Labriolle-Vaylet, C.; Jeanguillaume, C.; Lange, J.; Perlemuter, L. & Askienazy, S. (2003). Functioning pulmonary metastases of thyroid cancer: does radioiodine influence the prognosis? *European*

Journal of Nuclear Medicine and Molecular Imaging, Vol. 30, No. 7, (March 2003), pp. 974-981, ISSN 1619-7070

Hoschl, R.; Choy, D.H. & Gandevia, B. (1988). Iodine-131 uptake in inflammatory lung disease: a potential pitfall in treatment of thyroid carcinoma. *Journal of Nuclear Medicine*, Vol. 29, No. 5, (May 1988), pp. 701-706, ISSN 0161-5505

Hung, B.T.; Huang, S.H.; Huang, Y.E. & Wang, P.W. (2009). Appropriate time for post-therapeutic I-131 whole body scan. *Clinical Nuclear Medicine*, Vol. 34, No. 6, (June 2009), pp. 339-342, ISSN 1536-0229

Iwano, S.; Kato, K.; Nihashi, T.; Ito, S.; Tachi, Y. & Naganawa, S. (2009). Comparisons of I-123 diagnostic and I-131 post-treatment scans for detecting residual thyroid tissue and metastases of differentiated thyroid cancer. *Annals of Nuclear Medicine*, Vol. 23, No. 9, (September 2009), pp. 777-782, ISSN 1864-6433 (Electronic)

Iwata, M.; Kasagi, K.; Misaki, T.; Matsumoto, K.; Iida, Y.; Ishimori, T.; Nakamoto, Y.; Higashi, T.; Saga, T. & Konishi, J. (2004). Comparison of whole-body 18F-FDG PET, 99mTc-MIBI SPET, and post-therapeutic 131I-Na scintigraphy in the detection of metastatic thyroid cancer. *European Journal of Nuclear Medicine and Molecular Imaging*, Vol. 31, No. 4, (April 2004), pp. 491-498, ISSN 1619-7070

Khan, N.; Oriuchi, N.; Higuchi, T.; Zhang, H. & Endo, K. (2003). PET in the follow-up of differentiated thyroid cancer. *British Journal of Radiology*, Vol. 76, No. 910, (October 2003), pp. 690-695, ISSN 0007-1285

Khan, S.; Waxman, A.; Nagaraj, N. & G, B. Optimization of post ablative I-131 scintigraphy: comparison of 2 day vs. 7 day post therapy study in patients with differentiated thyroid cancer (DTC), *Proceedings of 41st Annual Meeting of the Society of Nuclear Medicine.*, Cedars-sinai Medical center, Los Angeles, CA, 1994

Kim, C.H.; Yoo Ie, R.; Chung, Y.A.; Park, Y.H.; Kim, S.H.; Sohn, H.S. & Chung, S.K. (2009). Influence of thyroid-stimulating hormone on 18F-fluorodeoxyglucose and 99mTc-methoxyisobutylisonitrile uptake in human poorly differentiated thyroid cancer cells in vitro. *Annals of Nuclear Medicine*, Vol. 23, No. 2, (February 2009), pp. 131-136, ISSN 0914-7187

Larson, S.M. & Robbins, R. (2002). Positron emission tomography in thyroid cancer management. *Seminars in Roentgenology*, Vol. 37, No. 2, (July 2002), pp. 169-174, ISSN 0037-198X

Lee, J.W.; Lee, S.M.; Koh, G.P. & Lee, D.H. (2011). The comparison of (131)I whole-body scans on the third and tenth day after (131)I therapy in patients with well-differentiated thyroid cancer: preliminary report. *Annals of Nuclear Medicine*, Vol. No. (April 2011), pp. ISSN 1864-6433

Luster, M.; Clarke, S.E.; Dietlein, M.; Lassmann, M.; Lind, P.; Oyen, W.J.; Tennvall, J. & Bombardieri, E. (2008). Guidelines for radioiodine therapy of differentiated thyroid cancer. *European Journal of Nuclear Medicine and Molecular Imaging*, Vol. 35, No. 10, (August 2008), pp. 1941-1959, ISSN 1619-7070

Mazzaferri, E. L. (1986). In: *Treatment of carcinoma of follicular epithelium*, pp. 1342-1343, Lippincott, ISBN 0397508026 Philadelphia

Mazzaferri, E.L. & Jhiang, S.M. (1994). Long-term impact of initial surgical and medical therapy on papillary and follicular thyroid cancer. *American Journal of Medicine*, Vol. 97, No. 5, (November 1994), pp. 418-428, ISSN 0002-9343

Misaki, T.; Takeuchi, R.; Miyamoto, S.; Kasagi, K.; Matsui, Y. & Konishi, J. (1994). Radioiodine uptake by squamous-cell carcinoma of the lung. *Journal of Nuclear Medicine*, Vol. 35, No. 3, (March 1994), pp. 474-475, ISSN 0161-5505

Mitchell, G.; Pratt, B.E.; Vini, L.; McCready, V.R. & Harmer, C.L. (2000). False positive ^{131}I whole body scans in thyroid cancer. *The British Journal or Radiology*, Vol. 73, No. 870, (July 2000), pp. 627-635, ISSN 0007-1285

Moretti, J.L.; Hauet, N.; Caglar, M.; Rebillard, O. & Burak, Z. (2005). To use MIBI or not to use MIBI? That is the question when assessing tumour cells. *European Journal of Nuclear Medicine and Molecular Imaging*, Vol. 32, No. 7, (July 2005), pp. 836-842, ISSN 1619-7070

Mullins, L.J. & Moore, R.D. (1960). The movement of thallium ions in muscle. *J Gen Physiol*, Vol. 43, No. 4, (March 1960), pp. 759-773, ISSN 0022-1295 (Print) 0022-1295 (Linking)

Muratet, J.P. & Giraud, P. (1996). Thymus accumulation of I-131 after therapeutic dose for thyroid carcinoma. *Clinical Nuclear Medicine*, Vol. 21, No. 9, (September 1996), pp. 736-737, ISSN 0363-9762

Nakada, K.; Katoh, C.; Morita, K.; Kanegae, K.; Tsukamoto, E.; Shiga, T.; Mochizuki, T. & Tamaki, N. (1999). Relationship among 201T1 uptake, nuclear DNA content and clinical behavior in metastatic thyroid carcinoma. *Journal of Nuclear Medicine*, Vol. 40, No. 6, (August 1999), pp. 963-967, ISSN 0161-5505

Nemec, J.; Rohling, S.; Zamrazil, V. & Pohunkova, D. (1979). Comparison of the distribution of diagnostic and thyroablative I-131 in the evaluation of differentiated thyroid cancers. *Journal of Nuclear Medicine*, Vol. 20, No. 2, (February 1979), pp. 92-97, ISSN 0161-5505

Nishiyama, Y.; Yamamoto, Y.; Ono, Y.; Takahashi, K.; Nakano, S.; Satoh, K.; Ohkawa, M. & Tanabe, M. (2000). Comparison of ^{99m}Tc-tetrofosmin with ^{201}Tl and ^{131}I in the detection of differentiated thyroid cancer metastases. *Nuclear Medince Communications*, Vol. 21, No. 10, (October 2000), pp. 917-923, ISSN 0143-3636

Oh, J.R.; Byun, B.H.; Hong, S.P.; Chong, A.; Kim, J.; Yoo, S.W.; Kang, S.R.; Kim, D.Y.; Song, H.C.; Bom, H.S. & Min, J.J. (2011). Comparison of (131)I whole-body imaging, (131)I SPECT/CT, and (18)F-FDG PET/CT in the detection of metastatic thyroid cancer. *European Journal of Nuclear Medicine and Molecular Imaging*, Vol. 38, No. 8, (August 2011), pp. 1459-1468, ISSN 1619-7089

Pauwels, E.K.; McCready, V.R.; Stoot, J.H. & van Deurzen, D.F. (1998). The mechanism of accumulation of tumour-localising radiopharmaceuticals. *European Journal of Nuclear Medicine*, Vol. 25, No. 3, (March 1998), pp. 277-305, ISSN 0340-6997

Piwnica-Worms, D.P.; Kronauge, J.F.; LeFurgey, A.; Backus, M.; Hockett, D.; Ingram, P.; Lieberman, M.; Holman, B.L.; Jones, A.G. & Davison, A. (1994). Mitochondrial localization and characterization of ^{99m}Tc-SESTAMIBI in heart cells by electron probe X-ray microanalysis and 99Tc-NMR spectroscopy. *Magnetic Resonance Imaging*, Vol. 12, No. 4, (January 1994), pp. 641-652, ISSN 0730-725X

Rawson, R.W.; Rall, J.E. & Peacock, W. (1951). Limitations and indications in the treatment of cancer of the thyroid with radioactive iodine. *The Journal of Clinical Endocrinology & Metabolism*, Vol. 11, No. 10, (October 1951), pp. 1128-1142, ISSN 0021-972X

Riedel, C.; Dohan, O.; De la Vieja, A.; Ginter, C.S. & Carrasco, N. (2001). Journey of the iodide transporter NIS: from its molecular identification to its clinical role in cancer.

Trends in Biochemical Sciences, Vol. 26, No. 8, (August 2001), pp. 490-496, ISSN 0968-0004

Rosario, P.W.; Barroso, A.L.; Rezende, L.L.; Padrao, E.L.; Maia, F.F.; Fagundes, T.A. & Purisch, S. (2005). 5 mCi pretreatment scanning does not cause stunning when the ablative dose is administered within 72 hours. *Arquivos Brasileiros de Endocrinologia & Metabologia*, Vol. 49, No. 3, (March 2006), pp. 420-424, ISSN 0004-2730

Saggiorato, E.; Angusti, T.; Rosas, R.; Martinese, M.; Finessi, M.; Arecco, F.; Trevisiol, E.; Bergero, N.; Puligheddu, B.; Volante, M.; Podio, V.; Papotti, M. & Orlandi, F. (2009). ^{99m}Tc-MIBI Imaging in the presurgical characterization of thyroid follicular neoplasms: relationship to multidrug resistance protein expression. *Journal of Nuclear Medicine*, Vol. 50, No. 11, (November 2009), pp. 1785-1793, ISSN 1535-5667

Samaan, N.A.; Schultz, P.N.; Haynie, T.P. & Ordonez, N.G. (1985). Pulmonary metastasis of differentiated thyroid carcinoma: treatment results in 101 patients. *The Journal of Clinical Endocrinology & Metabolism*, Vol. 60, No. 2, (February 1985), pp. 376-380, ISSN 0021-972X

Samaan, N.A.; Schultz, P.N.; Hickey, R.C.; Goepfert, H.; Haynie, T.P.; Johnston, D.A. & Ordonez, N.G. (1992). The results of various modalities of treatment of well differentiated thyroid carcinomas: a retrospective review of 1599 patients. *The Journal of Clinical Endocrinology & Metabolism*, Vol. 75, No. 3, (September 1992), pp. 714-720, ISSN 0021-972X

Schlumberger, M.; Tubiana, M.; De Vathaire, F.; Hill, C.; Gardet, P.; Travagli, J.P.; Fragu, P.; Lumbroso, J.; Caillou, B. & Parmentier, C. (1986). Long-term results of treatment of 283 patients with lung and bone metastases from differentiated thyroid carcinoma. *The Journal of Clinical Endocrinology & Metabolism*, Vol. 63, No. 4, (October 1986), pp. 960-967, ISSN 0021-972X

Senga, O.; Miyakawa, M.; Shirota, H.; Makiuchi, M.; Yano, K.; Miyazawa, M. & Takizawa, M. (1982). Comparison of Tl-201 chloride and Ga-67 citrate scintigraphy in the diagnosis of thyroid tumor: concise communication. *Journal of Nuclear Medicine*, Vol. 23, No. 3, (March 1982), pp. 225-228, ISSN 0161-5505

Sharma, R.; Chakravarty, K.L.; Tripathi, M.; Kaushik, A.; Bharti, P.; Sahoo, M.; Chopra, M.K.; Rawat, H.; Misra, A.; Mondal, A. & Kashyap, R. (2007). Role of 99mTc-Tetrofosmin delayed scintigraphy and color Doppler sonography in characterization of solitary thyroid nodules. *Nuclear Medicine Communcations*, Vol. 28, No. 11, (September 2007), pp. 847-851, ISSN 0143-3636

Shiga, T.; Tsukamoto, E.; Nakada, K.; Morita, K.; Kato, T.; Mabuchi, M.; Yoshinaga, K.; Katoh, C.; Kuge, Y. & Tamaki, N. (2001). Comparison of (18)F-FDG, (131)I-Na, and (201)Tl in diagnosis of recurrent or metastatic thyroid carcinoma. *Journal of Nuclear Medicine*, Vol. 42, No. 3, (March 2001), pp. 414-419, ISSN 0161-5505

Souza Rosario, P.W.; Barroso, A.L.; Rezende, L.L.; Padrao, E.L.; Fagundes, T.A.; Penna, G.C. & Purisch, S. (2004). Post I-131 therapy scanning in patients with thyroid carcinoma metastases: an unnecessary cost or a relevant contribution? *Clinical Nuclear Medicine*, Vol. 29, No. 12, (Novemeber 2004), pp. 795-798, ISSN 0363-9762

Spies, W.G.; Wojtowicz, C.H.; Spies, S.M.; Shah, A.Y. & Zimmer, A.M. (1989). Value of post-therapy whole-body I-131 imaging in the evaluation of patients with thyroid carcinoma having undergone high-dose I-131 therapy. *Clinical Nuclear Medicine*, Vol. 14, No. 11, (November 1989), pp. 793-800, ISSN 0363-9762

Surti, S.; Scheuermann, R. & Karp, J.S. (2009). Correction technique for cascade gammas in I-124 imaging on a fully-3D, Time-of-Flight PET Scanner. *IEEE Trans Nucl Sci*, Vol. 56, No. 3, (August 2009), pp. 653-660, ISSN 0018-9499

Thyroid cancer survivors' Association, Inc. (05.23.2011). Radioactive iodine (RAI), In: *Thyroid Cancer Survivors Association website*, 06.22.2011, Available from: <http://www.thyca.org/rai.htm#diet>

Unal, S.; Menda, Y.; Adalet, I.; Boztepe, H.; Ozbey, N.; Alagol, F. & Cantez, S. (1998). Thallium-201, technetium-99m-tetrofosmin and iodine-131 in detecting differentiated thyroid carcinoma metastases. *Journal of Nuclear Medicine*, Vol. 39, No. 11, (November 1998), pp. 1897-1902, ISSN 0161-5505

Van Nostrand, D.; Moreau, S.; Bandaru, V.V.; Atkins, F.; Chennupati, S.; Mete, M.; Burman, K. & Wartofsky, L. (2010). (124)I positron emission tomography versus (131)I planar imaging in the identification of residual thyroid tissue and/or metastasis in patients who have well-differentiated thyroid cancer. *Thyroid*, Vol. 20, No. 8, (August 2010), pp. 879-883, ISSN 1050-7256

Waxman, A.; Ramanna, L.; Chapman, N.; Chapman, D.; Brachman, M.; Tanasescu, D.; Berman, D.; Catz, B. & Braunstein, G. (1981). The significance of 1-131 scan dose in patients with thyroid cancer: determination of ablation: concise communication. *Journal of Nuclear Medicine*, Vol. 22, No. 10, (October 1981), pp. 861-865, ISSN 0161-5505

Wu, H.S.; Huang, W.S.; Liu, Y.C.; Yen, R.F.; Shen, Y.Y. & Kao, C.H. (2003). Comparison of FDG-PET and technetium-99m MIBI SPECT to detect metastatic cervical lymph nodes in well-differentiated thyroid carcinoma with elevated serum HTG but negative I-131 whole body scan. *Anticancer Research*, Vol. 23, No. 5b, (December 2003), pp. 4235-4238, ISSN 0250-7005

Yoshio, K.; Sato, S.; Okumura, Y.; Katsui, K.; Takemoto, M.; Suzuki, E.; Katayama, N.; Kaji, M. & Kanazawa, S. (2011). The local efficacy of I-131 for F-18 FDG PET positive lesions in patients with recurrent or metastatic thyroid carcinomas. *Clincal Nuclear Medicine*, Vol. 36, No. 2, (February 2011), pp. 113-117, ISSN 0363-9762

10

Apoptosis Imaging in Diseased Myocardium

Junichi Taki, Hiroshi Wakabayashi, Anri Inaki,
Ichiro Matsunari and Seigo Kinuya
Kanazawa University & Medical and Pharmacological Research Center Foundation,
Japan

1. Introduction

In various myocardial disorders including myocardial ischemia, infarction and subsequent cardiac remodelling and heart failure, myocarditis, cardiomyopathy, cardiac allograft rejection, chemotherapy induced cardiotoxicity, both necrosis and apoptosis are considered to play an important role in the underling pathophysioloy. Molecular and cellular dysfunction has been widely investigated in cardiovascular fields using various modalities. Of particular, radionuclide imaging technique has advantage for quantitative assessment of molecular function in vivo in patients. Especially in patients with coronary artery disease, perfusion imaging agents such as ^{201}Tl, ^{99m}Tc-MIBI and tetrofosmin with combination of stress testing and ECG-gated data acquisition have been used for the simultaneous assessment of the ventricular function and severity of myocardial perfusion abnormality including its location and size in stress and resting condition. From these data, status of myocardial ischemia or jeopardized myocardium, myocardial viability and reversibility of wall motion abnormality can be diagnosed to some extent but still insufficiently. Molecular imaging may play an important role for assessing the pathophysiology and its severity in these various cardiovascular diseases beyond perfusion imaging. This chapter focuses on the apoptosis imaging that is one of the most possible nuclear molecular imaging in-vivo at this stage, and its clinical application might permit more precise assessment of the pathophysiology in various myocardial abnormalities beyond perfusion imaging.

Four decades ago, the term apoptosis has been introduced by Kerr et. al. as a special form of cell death different from necrosis (Kerr, et al., 1972). Necrosis is passive and unregulated form of cell death, characterized by irreversible loss of plasma membrane integrity with cell swelling and rupture after sudden severe insults which preclude adequate homeostatic energy-dependent cell functions, leading to release of intracellular contents and a subsequent inflammatory response. Apoptosis on the other hand is characterized morphologically by the condensation of nuclear chromatin, cytoplasmic condensation, cell shrinkage, followed by the nuclear and cellular fragmentation and phagocytosis of apoptotic bodies by neighboring cells in the absence of inflammation. Apoptosis is considered to be an active and highly regulated ATP dependent programmed cell daeth process and plays an important roles in embryonic developement and maintenace of postnatal tissues and contributes to both normal physiology and pathology. Dysregulation of apoptosis results in either too littel or too much cell death and implicated in various diseases. For instance, insufficient apoptosis may contribute carcinogenesis, on the otherhand, eccessive apoptosis may account for substantial portion of pathogenesis of myocardial infarction and heart failure.

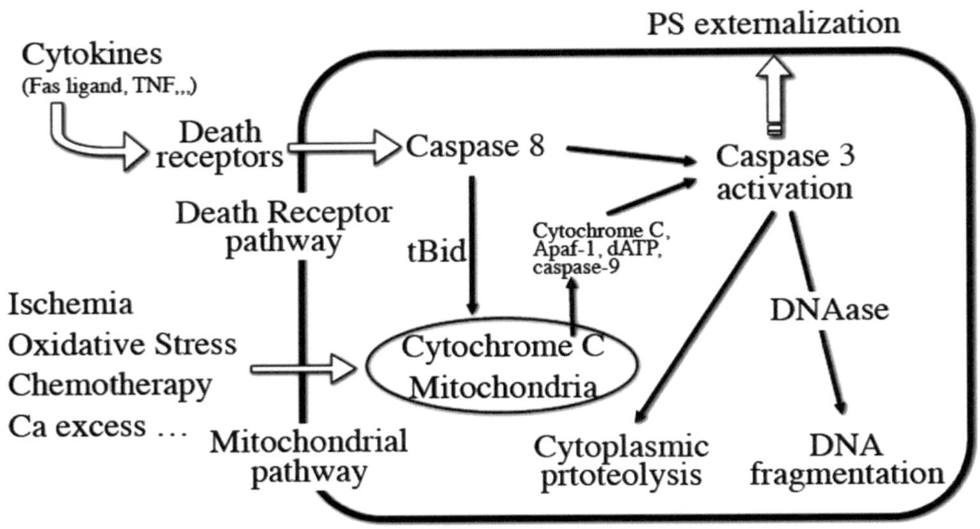

Fig. 1. Schema of two major pathway for apoptosis.
Apoptosis can be mediated through the death receptor pathway, or by mitochondrial pathway that is initiated by the release of cytochrome c into the cytosol. Both pathways result in activation of caspase-3, the final effector enzyme of apoptosis, leading to the cleavage of numerous structural and regulatory cellular proteins, thereby producing the apoptotic phenotype characterized by cell shrinkage, chromatin condensation, nucleus fragmentation, and externalization of phosphatidylserin (PS) on the outside of the cell membrane.

Apoptosis is mediated by 2 central pathway: the extrinsic (or death receptor) pathway that utilizes cell surface receptors (e.g. Fas) and the intrinsic (or mitochondrial) pathway that involves the mitochondria and cytoplasmic reticulum (Fig. 1.). The extrinsic or death receptor pathway relies on the binding of specific cytokines expressed by other cells, including Fas ligand, tumor necrosis factor alfa, or other factors that binds to specific cellular receptors. Ligand binding initiates the activation of caspase-8, which in turn activates downstream effector caspases including caspase-3, the final effector enzyme of apoptosis. In contrast to extrinsic pathway that transduces a specialized set of death stimuli, the intrinsic or mitochondrial pathway integrates a broad spectrum of extracellular and intracellular stresses such as ischemia, reperfusion injury, chemotherapy, oxidative stress etc. These stimuli converges on the mithochondria leading to the release of several factors into cytosol including cytochrome c, which activates the initiator caspase-9 via the apoptosome followed by the activation of effector caspases. The activation of down stream caspases leads to the cleavage of numerous structural and regulatory cellular proteins, thereby producing the apoptotic phenotype characterized by cell shrinkage, chromatin condensation, nucleus fragmentation, and externalization of phosphatidylserin (PS) on the outside of the cell membrane which serves as an "eat me" signal for phagocyte. Intracellular components are packaged by blebbing and the cell is fragmentated into apoptotic bodies and designated to be engulfed and phagocytosed by macrophages and neighbouring cells without causing inflammation.

2. Radipharmaceuticals for molecular imaging of apoptosis

After the initial description of apoptosis based on the morphological features, several useful biochemical and immunohistochemical detection methods were subsequently introduced based on the understanding of the basic mechanisms of apoptosis. As a histochemical technique for the detection of apoptosis, terminal deoxynucleotidyltransferase-dUTP-nick end-labeling (TUNEL) assays has become a standard technique for in situ labeling and localization of DNA breaks in individual nuclei on tissue section (Gavrieli, et al.,1992). TUNEL is based on the specific binding of terminal deoxynucleotidyltransferase (TdT) to 3′-OH ends of fragmented DNA. As DNA ladder formation is quite a late feature of apoptosis, TUNEL assay appears to be uniquely associated with apoptotic cell death. For the in-vivo imaging initiator caspases and effector caspases can be distinguished and serve as potential targets inside the apoptotic cells. However, for molecular target for in-vivo imaging, it is favorable that the target exists on cell surface rather than in cytoplasm or nucleus. Accordingly, to date, most noninvasive imagings of apoptosis target PS on the cell membrane, which is a membrane aminophospholipid that is normally located on the inner leaflet of cell membrane but is rapidly trnaslocated to the outer leaflet of cell membrane once the cell become apoptotic. Annexin V, a 36-kD physiologic protein, binds with nanomolar affinity to PS in a calcium dependent manner, therefore, ^{99m}Tc labeled annexin V permits imaging of apoptosis in vivo in its early stage (Blankenberg, et al., 1998; Hofstra, et al., 2000; Kemerink, et al., 2003).

2.1 Radiolabeled annexin V

Annexin V (also known as annexin A5) is consisted of 319 amino acids and a 36-kD endogeneous human protein that is mainly distributed intracellularly with very high concentrations in placenta, and lower concentrations in endothelial cells, myocardium, skeletal muscle, kidneys, skin, red blood cells, platelets, and monocytes. Very low concentrations of annexin V (1-6 ng/ml) circulate in blood of healthy humans (Andree et al., 1992). Several advantages for the use of annexin V for apoptotic imaging have been described including very high affinity for PS with low nanomolar to subnanomolar dissociation constant values, ready production by recombinant DNA technology, and lack of toxicity of the protein.

In healthy cells, anionic phospholipid PS and phosphatidylethanolamine (PE) confined to the inner leaflet of the lipid bilayer plasma membrane by an ATP dependent enzyme called translocase. On the other hand, ATP dependent enzyme, floppase, pumps cationic phospholipids such as phosphatidylcholine (PC) and sphingomyelin to the cell surface. Therefore, an asymmetric distribution of different phospholipids between the inner and outer leaflet of the plasma membrane is maintained in normal cells. However, at the beginning of the execution phase of apoptosis, rapid redistribution of PS and PC across the cell membrane is facilitated by a calcium ion-dependent deactivation of translocase and floppase and activation of scramblase. Then, PS exposes on the cell surface and annexin V become accessible to PS. This PS exposure is attractive target for imaging apoptosis, since it is a near universal event in apoptosis, it occurs early after the apoptotic stimulus, and it presents millions of binding sites per cell on the cell surface.

Annexin V and its derivatives have been labeled with ^{123}I, ^{124}I, ^{125}I, ^{99m}Tc, ^{18}F, thereby providing a broad range of imaging applications in apoptosis research from autoradiography and single photon imaging including SPECT, and to PET. However, most of the radiolabeled annexin V used in clinical trials are ^{99m}Tc labeled annexin V, because ^{99m}Tc is characterized by the most suitable radionuclide properties for SPECT imaging in human and is inexpensive and easily available.

^{99m}Tc-BTAP-annexin V using a diamide dimercaptide N_2S_2 chelate for labeling (^{99m}Tc- N_2S_2-annexin V) was introduced in early 1990s and examined to detect left atrial thrombi in vivo in swine (Stratton et al., 1995). Biodistribution and dosimetry study of ^{99m}Tc-BTAP-annexin V in patients revealed that the radioactivity predominates in kidney, liver and urine bladder and fast and extensive bowel excretion of the tracer precludes the assessment of abdominal region (Kemerink, et al., 2001a). N_2S_2 labeling method is cumbersome but radiochemical yield is low and had a high degree of non specific tracer excretion into bowel via excretion to bile.

Accordingly, an improved labeling method using the bifunctional agent hydrazinonicotinamide (HYNIC) was introduced (Blankenberg, et al., 1998). ^{99m}Tc-labeling of reconstituted HYNIC-annexin V can be performed by simply reacting the conjugate with ^{99m}Tc-pertechnetate in the presence of stannous tricine for 5-10min in room temperature and it provides ^{99m}Tc-HYNIC-annexin V in high radiochemical yield (usually 92-95%) without requiring any additional purification step. Phase I clinical trial with ^{99m}Tc-HYNIC-annexin V also demonstrated strongest uptake in kidney, liver and urine bladder. However, in contrast to ^{99m}Tc-BTAP-annexin V no bowel excretion was observed in ^{99m}Tc-HYNIC-annexin V, having a favorable biodistribution for imaging of the abdominal as well as thoracic area.

As an alternative methods for radiolabeling annexin V, self chelating annexin V mutants had been introduced (Tait, et al., 2000, 2005). Annexin V mutants with endogeneous site for ^{99m}Tc chelation such as V-117 and V-128 have major advantages over the HYNIC chelatior in terms with lower renal retention. Many other kind of ^{99m}Tc-labeled annexin V have been introduced, however, only ^{99m}Tc-i-annexin V (Kemerink, et al., 2001b) was tested in clinical trial in addition to ^{99m}Tc-BTAP-annexin V and ^{99m}Tc-HYNIC-annexin V.

As a PET tracer, several approaches to label annexin V with ^{18}F have been developed (Grierson, et al. 2004; Murakami et al., 2004).^{18}F-annexin V has lower uptake in the liver, spleen, and kidneys than ^{99m}Tc-HYNIC-annexin V.

2.2 Radiolabeled C2A

C2A domain of synaptotagmin I also binds PS with nanomolar affinity in a calcium-dependent manner. The C2A is labeled in the form of C2A-GST (GST: glutathione S-transferase) fusion protein. The fusion protein can be stably labeled with ^{99m}Tc at a reasonably high radiochemical yield and purity through thiolation using 2-iminothiolane (Zhao, et al., 2006). ^{99m}Tc-C2A-GST accumulates well in the area at risk in a rat model of acute myocardial infarction in both in-vivo imaging and autoradiography. Recently, ^{18}F-C2A-GST was synthesized and significant uptake in the VX2 rabbit lung cancer with paclitaxel induced apoptosis was observed in small animal PET/CT (Wang, et al., 2011). Radiochemical purity of ^{18}F-C2A-GST was more than 95% and stable for 4 h after formulation. Biodistribution in mice was favorable with major excretion from the kidneys and rapid clearance from blood and nonspecific organs.

2.3 Radiolabeled caspase targeted tracer

Caspase activation is the central role in the execution of cell death, therefore, caspases are the attractive targets for apoptosis imaging. Non-peptide based isatin sulfonamide analogs were synthesized with nanomolar potency for inhibiting caspase-3 and caspase-7 and one of the analogs, WC-II-89 was labeled with ^{18}F (Zhou et al., 2006). ^{18}F- WC-II-89 showed a high uptake in the liver of chemically induced apoptosis. Although molecules that target caspase-3 is attractive, there are limited animal data and it is not yet known how sensitive this kind of agents will be for actual imaging in humans.

2.4 Uncategorized tracer

Recently a novel family of low molecular mass amphipatic apoptosis markers (ApoSense) was developed targeting the cell membrane of apoptotic cells. ^{18}F-labeled 5-fluoropentyl-2-methyl-malonic acid (^{18}F-ML-10) belongs to this family of low-molecular-weight compounds used for the imaging of cell death in vivo. This compound responds to alterations in plasma membrane potential and phospholipid scrambling, which are hallmarks of apoptotic cells. To which cell membrane targets this probe binds is unknown. After systemic administration, the compound can detect apoptotic cells from the early stages of the death process, cross the intact plasma membrane, and accumulate in the cytoplasm. In animal model of cerebral infarction, selective uptake was observed in the region of ischemia at 24 hr after the middle cerebral artery occlusion (Reshef et al., 2008).

3. Apoptosis imaging in acute myocardial ischemia

It has been believed that myocardium directly start to die via necrosis shortly after the onset of myocardial infarction that march of necrosis spread as a wavefront from endocardium to epicardium. However, recent animal experiments with permanent coronary artery occlusion revealed that cell death process starts as apoptosis and severe ATP depletion due to ischemia may preclude the execution of apoptosis and lead to plasma membrane permeability barrier breakdown and secondary necrosis. Therefore, apoptosis imaging might play important role in the assessment of myocardial cell death process in acute myoacrdial infarction, especially in its early stage.

3.1 Animal experiment in permanent occlusion of coronary artery

In a rat model of permanent coronary artery ligation, Kajstura et al. investigated the contribution of the apoptosis and necrosis to cardiomyocyte death using TUNEL method and DNA laddering for apoptosis and antimyosin monoclonal antibody labeling (Kajstura, et a., 1996). After 2 h of the left main coronary artery ligation, TUNEL positive myocytes appeared in the central portion of the left ventricular free wall and peaked at 4.5 h. Myosin labeled cells also appeared at 2 h after ligation and significantly increased after 6 h to 2 days. However, at 2 h after coronary ligation, number of apoptotic cells was 2.8×10^6 and number of necrotic cells was 9×10^4. Therefore, early after myocardial infarction, apoptosis is the predominant form of cell death, and 1 to 2 days after infarction, necrosis is the dominant form of cell death followed by low levels of both apoptosis and necrosis at 7 days after infarction. If cells undergoing apoptosis are not cleared before they deplete their intracellular ATP stores that are necessary to maintain plasma membrane integrity, plasma membrane permeability barrier breakdown occurs and cells are converted from apoptosis to necrosis as known as secondary necrosis, results in inflammation.

3.2 Animal experiment in acute ischemia and reperfusion

In a mouse model of 15 and 30 min of ischemia and 90 min of reperfusion, percentage of cardiomyocytes staining positivity for biotinylated annexin V was far greater than the

percentage staining positivity for IgG, which indicates plasma cell membrane leakage (Dumont et al., 2000). Accordingly, at least 90 min of reperfusion, most of the annexin V uptake might represent PS externalization.
We investigated the temporal and spatial change of ^{99m}Tc-annexin V accumulation in a rat model of 20 min coronary artery occlusion and reperfusion. ^{99m}Tc-annexin V uptake was imaged at 30 min, 90 min, 6 h, 24 h, 3 day, 2 weeks after reperfusion. The strongest ^{99m}Tc-annexin V uptake was observed in the mid myocardium of the area at risk at 30 m and 90 m of reperfusion and the uptake expanded to subendocardial and subepicardial layer at 6 h after reperfusion, followed by gradual reduction of the uptake over 3 days (Fig. 2) (Taki, et al., 2004). On the other hand, TUNEL positivity peaked at 6 h to 1 day after reperfusion. These findings are in keeping with the known temporal sequence of apoptosis, in which one of the earliest events is externalization of phosphatidylserine, followed by DNA fragmentation. Using fluorescent labeled annexin V, real time monitoring of annexin V binding to cardiomyocytes after 30 m ischemia and reperfusion demonstrated that cardiomyocytes started to bind annexin V within minute and the amount of binding reached a maximum within 20-25 m (Dumont, et al., 2001). These finding indicate that apoptosis commences just after ischemia and reperfusion and PS externalization reaches plateau around 30 m after reperfusion.

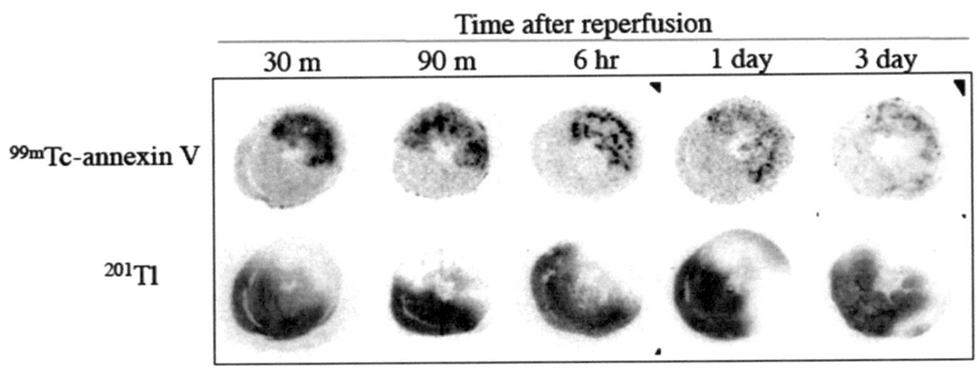

Fig. 2. Autoradiography of ^{99m}Tc-annexin V and ^{201}Tl at various reperfusion time after 20 min of coronary artery occlusion.
At a examination time after 20 min ischemia and reperfusion, ^{99m}Tc-annexin V (80-150 MBq) was injected and 1 h later ^{201}Tl (0.74 MBq) was injected just after the coronary artery reocclusion to verify the area at risk. Upper low demonstrated ^{99m}Tc-annexin V images and lower low shows ^{201}Tl image that represents area at risk.

The amount of annexin V binding to apoptotic cardiomyocytes after reperfusion depends on the severity of ischemia and reperfusion time (Taki, et al., 2007a). In a rat model of 5 min, 10 min, 15 min ischemia and reperfusion model, degree of ^{99m}Tc-annexin V accumulation depend on the length of the coronary artery occlusion time and time period after reperfusion: significant uptake of ^{99m}Tc-annexin V accumulation was observed in 15 min and 10 min ischemia (uptake ratio was 4.46±3.16 and 2.02±0.47, respectively), whereas, no significant uptake was observed in 5 min ischemia at 30 min after reperfusion. ^{99m}Tc-annexin V uptake in 15 min and 10 min ischemia reduced at 90 min (uptake ratio was 3.49±1.78 and

1.47±0.11, respectively) and only mild uptake was observed at 6 h and 24 h after reperfusion. Interestingly, no morphological sign of necrosis and apoptosis was observed until 24 h after reperfusion in 10 min ischemia and only micro foci of cell degeneration and cell infiltration were observed until 24 h after reperfusion in 15 min ischemia, with mild TUNEL positivity which peaked at 6 hr (1.03±0.40% in 10 min ischemia and 2.84±0.94% in 15 min ischemia). These data indicate that ^{99m}Tc-annexin V uptake can be observed after mild ischemic insults those do not result in myocardial infarction.

Several cardioprotective interventions such as ischemic preconditioning, postconditioning, and caspase inhibitor preparation attenuate ^{99m}Tc-annexin V uptake (Taki, et al., 2007). Ischemic preconditioning suppressed ^{99m}Tc-annexin V binding by 90 % of control and postoconditioning and caspase inhibitor attenuate the binding by around 70 %.

Reversibility of PS externalization in brief ischemia was demonstrated (Kenis, et al., 2010). In murine myocardium with 5 min ischemia and 90 min and 6 h of reperfusion, fluorescent labeled annexin V injected before 10 min of sacrifice binds cell surface, but not at 24 h after reperfusion. On the other hand fluorescent-annexin V injected at the onset of reperfusion exclusively localized intracellularly at 90 min, 6 h, and 24h after reperfusion. No TUNEL positivity was observed in this 5 min ischemia and reperfusion model. These data indicate that in brief ischemia, PS externalizes transiently, which is amenable to targeting by annexin V for at least 6 h after reperfusion, and internalize after annexin V binding (reversibility of the apoptotic process).

3.3 Clinical findings and potential future application

In human pathological study by TUNEL staining and DNA electrophoresis, widespread apoptosis in infarcts was observed only a few hours in age before the appearance of coagulative necrosis (Veinot, et al. 1997). In addition, TUNEL positibity was observed primarily in myocytes containing contraction bands, which occur predominantly in regions of reperfused myocardium. These findings are consistent with animal experiment, and in infarcted human myocardium, apoptosis is the early and predominant form of cell death and its appearance is accelerated in reperfused myocardium.

First clinical imaging with ^{99m}Tc-annexin V in 7 patients with acute myocardial infarction demonstrated significant uptake of ^{99m}Tc-annexin V (injected 2 h after reperfusion) in the area corresponding to the perfusion defect in 6 patients (Hofstra, et al., 2000). Subsequent study in 9 patients with acute myocardial infarction, ^{99m}Tc-annexin V uptake (injected within 1.5 - 7 h after reperfusion) was again clearly visualized on SPECT performed at 15 h later in infracted areas with a matching perfusion defect confirmed by ^{99m}Tc-sestamibi SPECT before reperfusion. Repeat ^{99m}Tc-sestamibi SPECT at 1 – 3 week after the onset of infarction demonstrated that the perfusion defects were significantly smaller than the defects in acute phase, suggesting that the significant amount of myocardium in perfusion defect with ^{99m}Tc-annexin V uptake in acute phase might be in reversible damage rather than irreversible necrosis. Imaging of the extent of apoptosis resulting from acute coronary syndromes could be a valuable tool to help guide revascularization strategies and therapy with anti-apoptotic drugs if available in near future. Other potential application of ^{99m}Tc-annexin V imaging would be in the detection of myocardial ischemic insults in patients with acute coronary syndrome without ST elevation and troponin leakage, in assessment of the effect of revascularization in acute coronary syndrome, in evaluation of the effect of postconditioning at reperfusion therapy, in detection of transient PS exetrnalization due to brief spontaneous or stress induced ischemia. However, several questions yet to be answered concerning the clinical application of ^{99m}Tc-annexin V imaging. In vivo imaging 1 hr after tracer injection is feasible in rats because blood clearance of ^{99m}Tc-annexin V was rather fast, although, the earliest optimal time for imaging after tracer injection should be investigate in human. In heart transplantation patients, it was revealed that ^{99m}Tc-annexin V SPECT imgaing was possible 1 h after tracer injection (Narula, et al., 2001). Speedy imaging after tracer injection is crucial especially in emergency situation. Are therapeutic interventions beneficial for all annexin-positive myocardium, or in only specific pathological status, or in only limited time window? How much of the shift from necrosis to apoptosis by therapeutic intervention is cardioprotective (Narula, et al., 2003)? Necrosis is more harmful than apoptosis, because cells are removed without inflammation in apoptosis but cells are removed with inflammation and fibrosis follows in necrosis. Is annexin V positive scan in stress induced ischemia related to subsequent prognosis, or indication of PCI? These potential imaging concepts of the assessment of myocardial injury, stress, cell death in acute ischemia should be validated in clinical studies.

It has been increasingly clear that apoptosis is a major contributor to early cardiomyocyte cell death after acute myocardial infarction, and is involved in post myocardial infarction ventricular dysfunction and adverse remodeling that develop heart failure. These findings emphasize the need for the reliable in-vivo imaging of apoptosis that assess the ongoing pathology so that rational preventive therapies can be applied and to assess the consequence of therapies. ^{99m}Tc-annexin V imaging might be applied to assess myocardium at risk or cell death in acute coronary syndrome and prediction of the ventricular remodeling after myocardial infarction and heart failure by allowing visualization of ongoing PS externalization that might precede or underlie change in pathophysiology, morphology, and LV dysfunction.

4. Apoptosis imaging in heart failure and cardiomyopathy

In spite of dramatic improvement of therapies in acute coronary syndrome, post acute myocardial infarction mortality has reached a plateau and post infarction heart failure due to ventricular remodeling is on the increase. About 15 to 25 % of acute myocardial infarction patients develop heart failure that remains a progressive despite of continuous pharmacological therapy. It has been reported that myocardial apoptosis shortly after acute myocardial infarction might be a strong predictor of unfavorable LV remodeling and early post infarction symptomatic heart failure in 16 patients dying ≥10 days after myocardial infarction (Abbate, et al., 2003).

In rats with anterior myocardial infarction, 28-day infusion of caspase inhibitor after infarction ameliorated apoptosis, preserved myocardial contractile proteins, decreased myocardial interstitial collagen deposite, reduced systolic dysfunction, and attenuated LV remodeling (Chandrashekhar, et al., 2004). If so, apoptosis imaging could be a promising noninvasive method to identify patients at risk of heart failure development due to LV remodeling and to monitor the treatment effect if some specific anti-apoptotic agents will reach the stage of clinical study.

In patients with advanced heart failure, low but abnormal rate of cardiac myocyte apoptosis persist for months (0.08% to 0.25% in heart failure vs 0.001% to 0.002% in normal subjects), thereby ultimately might result in a large loss of functional cardimyocytes (Olivetti, et al.,

1997; Saraste, et al., 1999; Guerra, et al., 1999). In study with transgenic mice that express a conditionally active caspase exclusively in the myocardium, low rate of cardiomyocyte apoptosis as 0.023% is sufficient to cause a lethal dilated cardiomyopathy. Conversely, inhibition of cardiac myocyte apoptosis by caspase inhibitor in this murine model largely prevents the development of cardiac dilation and contractile dysfunction, indicating that myocyte apoptosis may be a causal mechanism of heart failure, and inhibition of this cell death process may constitute the basis for novel therapies (Wencker, et al., 2003). The low level of cell death due to apoptosis in heart failure makes detection of apoptosis with the current techniques very challenging.

In recent study in 9 consecutive patients with advanced nonischemic cardiomyopathy (8 dilated and 1 hypertrophic cardiomyopathy) and 2 relatives, 5 patients showed focal or global ^{99m}Tc-annexin V uptake in the left ventricular myocardium. Interestingly, these 5 patients with ^{99m}Tc-annexin V uptake had experienced a significant worsening or a recent onset of heart failure, on the contrary, 4 patients without ^{99m}Tc-annexin V uptake had no recent evidence of worsening of heart failure. In addition, during a follow up of 1 year, 4 patients with ^{99m}Tc-annexin V uptake showed a decline of LVEF, on the other hand, in patients without ^{99m}Tc-annexin V uptake, clinical status and LVEF remained stable (Kietselaer, et al., 2007). These data indicate that the ^{99m}Tc-annexin V imaging in advanced non-ischemic cardiomyopathy, may identify the patients with high risk who might benefite from cell death blocking therapies.

5. Apoptosis imaging in myocarditis

In a rat model of autoimmune myocarditis, ^{99m}Tc-annexin V (HYNIC annexin V) and ^{14}C-deoxyglucose (DG) uptakes were examined (Tokita, et al.,2003). Myocarditis was triggered by an immunization of rats by infusing porcine cardiac myosine and the rats formed antibodies against the myosin and developed myocarditis. In acute phase of myocarditis, both ^{99m}Tc-annexin V (2.8 time more than normal rats) and ^{14}C-DG (2.7 time more than normal rats) uptake increased significantly, however, only ^{99m}Tc-annexin V distribution correlated with the TUNEL positive area, and the distribution of ^{14}C-DG correlated with inflammatory cell infiltration. In subacute phase, ^{99m}Tc-annexin V uptake returned normal level, on the other hand, ^{14}C-DG uptake decreased but still higher uptake reflecting prolonged mild inflammatory cell infiltration. In this model of immune myocarditis, there was a marked difference in distribution of apoptotic cell death and inflammation. The data indicates that ^{99m}Tc-annexin V uptake is specific in myocardial apoptotic process induced by inflammation and is independent of inflammatory cell infiltration.

Another animal experiment in a rat model that develops spontaneous myocarditis mimicking catecholamine induced subacute myocarditis demonstrated significantly increased ^{99m}Tc-annexin V uptake in planar scinitgraphy. Autoradiogrpahy confirmed increased ^{99m}Tc-annexin V uptake. Histopatology demonstrated patchy areas of interstitial edema with inflammatory cells in the perivascular areas and at cardiocyte layers, and myocyte necrosis with nuclear extrusion, scattered throughout the myocardium and apostatin-positive cells were diffusely but inhomogeneously distributed throughout the myocardium (Peker, et al., 2004).

In myocarditis, apoptosis imaging might play an important role, in confirming the diagnosis in terms of the extent of the involvement and disease activity, selecting patients with antiapoptotic therapy and monitoring the effect of therapy.

6. Apoptosis imaging in cardiotoxicity induced by chemotherapy

The development of chemotherapy has played a significant role in the management of cancer patients. Of the classic cytotoxic agents, antracyclines are the still one of the most important agents for cancer therapy and are well known for their dose dependent acute and chronic cardiotoxicity, resulting in irreversible and progressive cardiac dysfunction and heart failure. Although new anticancer molecular targeting agents improved the prognosis of cancer patients, some agents may have serious cardiovascular side effect. Standard clinical approaches utilize the serial monitoring of the left ventricular ejection fraction to identify chemotherapy induced cardiotoxicity. For this purpose, radionuclide ECG gated blood-pool scintigraphy has been used as a gold standard technique. However, ejection fraction impairment is relatively late manifestation of myocardial damage. Therefore, the development of more sensitive methods is required to identify the cardiotoxicity before the onset of ventricular dysfunction.

In a rat model of doxorubicin cardiotoxicity (cumulative dose: 7.5mg/Kg, 10mg/Kg, 12.5mg/Kg), planar scintigraphy detected the increase of ^{99m}Tc-annexin V uptake dose dependently and correlated with expression of left ventricular atrial natriuretic factor messenger RNA (Bennink, et al., 2004). Another study with doxorubicin treated rats (cumulative dose: 7.5mg/Kg and 15mg/Kg) demonstrated that dose dependent increase in ^{99m}Tc-annexin V uptake by SPECT/CT and TUNEL positivity. In contrast in this syudy, echocardiography detected ventricular dysfunction only at the highest doxorubicin dose (Gabrielson, et al., 2008). These data suggest that apoptosis imaging could serve as a more sensitive early marker of doxorubicin cardiotoxixity than left ventricular dysfunction, might providing the opportunity to modify or stop the chemotherapy before clinically overt heart failure.

7. Apoptosis imaging heart transplantation

Acute rejection remains a limiting factor of cardiac transplantation. The histopathologic manifestation of transplant rejection comprises perivascular and interstitial mononuclear inflammatory cell infiltration associated with myocyte apoptosis and necrosis. To monitor the acute rejection, endomyocardial biopsies are required frequently. Current guidelines recommend 15-20 endomyocardial biopsies in the first year after transplantation to monitor potential allograft rejection. However, invasive endomyocardial biopsy may be associated with a small risk of complications. If non-invasive imaging for the detection of transplant rejection is feasible, endomyocardial biopsies might be reduced.

Study with rat model of allograft rejection demonstrated that significant ^{99m}Tc-annexin V uptake correlated well with the histologic grade of rejection and scattered positive TUNEL stainings were observed in graft-infiltrating inflammatory cells, endothelial cells, and myocytes. In addition, after the treatment of rejection with cyclosporine, no TUNEL positivity was observed and ^{99m}Tc-annexin V uptake decreased to baseline (Vriens, et al., 1998). In 18 patients with cardiac allograft recipients, 5 had positive myocardial uptake of ^{99m}Tc-annexin V at 1 h after the tracer injection and all these 5 patients showed at least moderate transplant rejection and caspase-3 staining in their biopsy specimens. On the other hand, 11 of 13 patients with no cardiac uptake of ^{99m}Tc-annexin V demonstrated no finding of rejection and other 2 patients showed only focal lymphomononuclear cell infiltration (Narula, et al., 2001). In another clinical study with 10 patients with cardiac transplant, 2 patients with moderate acute rejection by endomyocardial biopsy showed significant ^{99m}Tc-annexin V uptake, however, specificity was suboptimal with 4 of 8 patients without rejection demonstrating significant ^{99m}Tc-annexin V uptake.

All these animal and clinical studies revealed that the apoptosis imaging has potential to noninvasively identify patients with transplant rejection and monitor the response to immune modulation therapy.

8. Conclusions

For the imaging apoptosis, for the time being, it appears that agents that bind to markers expressing cell surface of apoptotic cells, such as annexin V and its derivatives, have advantage in terms of the sensitivity and specificity over other tracers. Based on the research achievement to date including experiences with ^{99m}Tc-annexin V imaging in patients, ^{99m}Tc-annexin V and its related tracers are considered as one of the most suitable tracers for clinical application at this stage, and also the positron labeled tracers such as ^{18}F-annexin V are desired to apply clinical imaging. In cardiac diseases that involve cardiomyocytes, myocytes loss implies loss of cardiac function because cardiomyctes cannot be regenerated through cell division. In acute coronary syndrome, measurement of cardiac biomarkers are standard diagnostic tool, but they reflect the results of cardiomyocytes death. Whereas, apoptosis imaging such as ^{99m}Tc-annexin V can identify the cells starting or undergoing apoptosis, however, part of PS exposure of these cells might be reversible and some cells are capable of surviving. Therefore, apoptosis imaging might be beneficial for future strategy of the patient's management. Other than acute coronary syndrome, including heart failure, myocarditis, cardiomyopathies, and transplanted rejection, apoptotic cell death has turned out one of the crucial players in underlying pathophysiologies. Hence, apoptosis imaging in patients with various cardiac diseases will enhance the understanding of the ongoing pathophysiology, identification of high risk patients, and lead to effective therapies to salvage the myocardium in risk and be helpful in monitoring the effect of therapy.

9. References

Abbate A, Biondi-Zoccai GG, Bussani R, Dobrina A, Camilot D, Feroce F, Rossiello R, Baldi F, Silvestri F, Biasucci LM & Baldi, A. (2003). Increased myocardial apoptosis in patients with unfavorable left ventricular remodeling and early symptomatic post-infarction heart failure. *J Am Coll Cardiol* Vol.41(No. 5):753-760.

Andree HA, Stuart MC, Hermens WT, Reutelingsperger CP, Hemker HC, Frederik PM, Willems G.M. (1992). Clustering of lipid-bound annexin V may explain its anticoagulant effect. *J Biol Chem* Vol.267(No. 25),:17907-17912.

Bennink RJ, van den Hoff MJ, van Hemert FJ, de Bruin KM, Spijkerboer AL, Vanderheyden JL, Steinmetz N & van Eck-Smit BL. (2004) Annexin V imaging of acute doxorubicin cardiotoxicity (apoptosis) in rats. *J Nucl Med* Vol.45(No. 5):842-848.

Blankenberg FG, Katsikis PD, Tait JF, *et al.* (1998). In vivo detection and imaging of phosphatidylserine expression during programmed cell death. *Proc. Natl. Acad. Sci. U S A.* Vol.95(No. 111): 6349-6354

Chandrashekhar Y, Sen S, Anway R, Shuros A & Anand I. (2004). Long-term caspase inhibition ameliorates apoptosis, reduces myocardial troponin-I cleavage, protects left ventricular function, and attenuates remodeling in rats with myocardial infarction. *J Am Coll Cardiol* Vol. 43(No.2): 295-301.

Dumont EA, Hofstra L, van Heerde WL, van den Eijnde S, Doevendans PA, DeMuinck E, Daemen MA, Smits JF, Frederik P, Wellens HJ, Daemen MJ & Reutelingsperger CP. (2000). Cardiomyocyte death induced by myocardial ischemia and reperfusion: measurement with recombinant human annexin-V in a mouse model. *Circulation* Vol.102(No. 13):1564-1568.

Dumont EA, Reutelingsperger CP, Smits JF, Daemen MJ, Doevendans PA, Wellens HJ & Hofstra L. (2001). Real-time imaging of apoptotic cell-membrane changes at the single-cell level in the beating murine heart. *Nat Med* Vol.7(No.12):1352-1355.

Gabrielson KL, Mok GS, Nimmagadda S, Bedja D, Pin S, Tsao A, Wang Y, Sooryakumar D, Yu SJ, Pomper MG & Tsui BM. (2008). Detection of dose response in chronic doxorubicin-mediated cell death with cardiac technetium 99m annexin V single-photon emission computed tomography. *Mol Imaging* Vol.7(No. 3):132-138.

Gavrieli Y, Sherman Y & Ben-Sasson S. (1992). Identification of programmed cell death in situ via specific labeling of nuclear DNA fragmentation. *J Cell Biol* Vol.119(No. 3):493-501

Grierson JR, Yagle KJ, Eary JF, Tait JF, Gibson DF, Lewellen B, Link JM, & Krohn KA. (2004). Production of [F-18]fluoroannexin for imaging apoptosis with PET. *Bioconjug Chem.* Vol.15(No.2):373-379.

Guerra S, Leri A, Wang X, Finato N, Di Loreto C, Beltrami CA, Kajstura J & Anversa P. (1999) Myocyte death in the failing human heart is gender dependent. *Circ Res* Vol.85(No.9):856-866.

Hofstra L, Liem IH, Dumont EA, Boersma HH, van Heerde WL, Doevendans PA, De Muinck E, Wellens HJ, Kemerink GJ, Reutelingsperger CP & Heidendal GA. (2000). Visualisation of cell death in vivo in patients with acute myocardial infarction. *Lance.* Vol.356(No. 9225):209-212.

Kajstura J, Cheng W, Reiss K, Clark WA, Sonnenblick EH, Krajewski S, Reed JC, Olivetti G & Anversa, P. (1996). Apoptotic and necrotic myocyte cell deaths are independent contributing variables of infarct size in rats. *Lab Invest* Vol.74(No. 1):86-107.

Kemerink GJ, Boersma HH, Thimister PW, Hofstra L, Liem IH, Pakbiers MT, Janssen D, Reutelingsperger CP & Heidendal, GA. (2001a). Biodistribution and dosimetry of 99mTc-BTAP-annexin-V in humans. *Eur J Nucl Med* Vol.28(No. 9): 1373-1378.

Kemerink GJ, Liem IH, Hofstra L, Boersma HH, Buijs WC, Reutelingsperger CP & Heidendal, G. A. (2001b). Patient dosimetry of intravenously administered 99mTc-annexin V. *J Nucl Med* Vol.42(No. 2):382-387.

Kemerink GJ, Liu X, Kieffer D, Ceyssens S, Mortelmans L, Verbruggen AM, Steinmetz, ND, Vanderheyden, JL, Green, AM & Verbeke, K. (2003). Safety, biodistribution, and dosimetry of ^{99m}Tc-HYNIC-annexin V, a novel human recombinant annexin V for human application. *J Nucl Med* Vol.44(No. 6): 947-952.

Kenis H, Zandbergen HR, Hofstra L, Petrov AD, Dumont EA, Blankenberg FD, Haider, N, Bitsch, N, Gijbels, M, Verjans, JW, Narula, N, Narula, J & Reutelingsperger, CP. (2010) Annexin A5 uptake in ischemic myocardium: demonstration of reversible phosphatidylserine externalization and feasibility of radionuclide imaging. *J Nucl Med* Vol.51(No. 2):259-267.

Kerr JF., Wyllie AH. & Currie AR. (1972). Apoptosis: a basic biological phenomenon with wide ranging implications in tissue kinetics. *Br J Cancer* Vol.26(No. 4):239 -257

Kietselaer BL, Reutelingsperger CP, Boersma HH, Heidendal GA, Liem IH, Crijns HJ, Narula J & Hofstra L. (2007) Noninvasive detection of programmed cell loss with 99mTc-labeled annexin A5 in heart failure. *J Nucl Med* Vol.48(No. 4):562-567.

Kown MH, Strauss HW, Blankenberg FG, Berry GJ, Stafford-Cecil S, Tait JF, Goris ML & Robbins RC. (2001). In vivo imaging of acute cardiac rejection in human patients using (99m)technetium labeled annexin V. *Am J Transplant* Vol.1(No. 3):270-277.

Murakami Y, Takamatsu H, Taki J, Tatsumi M, Noda A, Ichise R, Tait JF, Nishimura S. (2004). 18F-labelled annexin V: a PET tracer for apoptosis imaging. *Eur J Nucl Med Mol Imaging* Vol.31(No. 4):469-474.

Narula J, Acio ER, Narula N, Samuels LE, Fyfe B, Wood D, Fitzpatrick JM, Raghunath PN, Tomaszewski JE, Kelly C, Steinmetz N, Green A, Tait JF, Leppo J, Blankenberg FG, Jain D & Strauss HW. (2001). Annexin-V imaging for noninvasive detection of cardiac allograft rejection. *Nat Med* Vol.7(No. 12):1347-1352.

Narula J & Strauss HW. (2003). Invited commentary: P.S.* I love you: implications of phosphatidyl serine (PS) reversal in acute ischemic syndromes. *J Nucl Med* Vol.44(No. 3):397-399.

Olivetti G, Abbi R, Quaini F, Kajstura J, Cheng W, Nitahara JA, Quaini E, Di Loreto C, Beltrami CA, Krajewski S, Reed JC & Anversa P. (1997). Apoptosis in the failing human heart. N *Engl J Med* Vol.336(No. 16):1131-1141.

Peker C, Sarda-Mantel L, Loiseau P, Rouzet F, Nazneen L, Martet G, Vrigneaud JM, Meulemans A, Saumon G, Michel JB & Le Guludec D. (2004). Imaging apoptosis with (99m)Tc-annexin-V in experimental subacute myocarditis. *J Nucl Med* Vol.45(No. 6):1081-1086.

Reshef A, Shirvan A, Waterhouse RN, Grimberg H, Levin G, Cohen A, Ulysse LG, Friedman G, Antoni G & Ziv I. (2008). Molecular imaging of neurovascular cell death in experimental cerebral stroke by PET. *J Nucl Med* Vol.49(No. 9):1520-1528.

Saraste A, Pulkki K, Kallajoki M, Heikkila P, Laine P, Mattila S, Nieminen MS, Parvinen M & Voipio-Pulkki LM. (1999). Cardiomyocyte apoptosis and progression of heart failure to transplantation. *Eur J Clin Invest* Vol.29(No. 5):380-386.

Stratton JR, Dewhurst TA, Kasina S, Reno JM, Cerqueira MD, Baskin DG, et al. (1995). Selective uptake of radiolabeled annexin V on acute porcine left atrial thrombi. *Circulation.* Vol.92(No.10):3113-3121.

Tait JF, Brown DS, Gibson DF, Blankenberg FG & Strauss HW. (2000). Development and characterization of annexin V mutants with endogenous chelation sites for (99m)Tc. *Bioconjug Chem.* Vol.11(No. 6):918-925.

Tait JF, Smith C & Blankenberg FG. (2005). Structural requirements for in vivo detection of cell death with 99mTc-annexin V. *J Nucl Med* Vol.46(No. 5):807-815.

Taki J, Higuchi T, Kawashima A, Tait JF, Kinuya S, Muramori A, Matsunari I, Nakajima K, Tonami N & Strauss, HW. (2004). Detection of cardiomyocyte death in a rat model of ischemia and reperfusion using 99mTc-labeled annexin V. *J Nucl Med* Vol.45(No. 9):1536-1541.

Taki J, Higuchi T, Kawashima A, Tait JF, Muramori A, Matsunari I, Nakajima, K, Vanderheyden JL & Strauss HW. (2007a). 99mTc-Annexin-V uptake in a rat model of variable ischemic severity and reperfusion time. *Circ J.* Vol.71(No. 7):1141-1146.

Taki J, Higuchi T, Kawashima A, Fukuoka M, Kayano D, Tait JF, Matsunari I, Nakajima, K, Kinuya S & Strauss HW. (2007b). Effect of postconditioning on myocardial 99mTc-annexin-V uptake: comparison with ischemic preconditioning and caspase inhibitor treatment. *J Nucl Med* Vol.48(No. 8):1301-1307.

Thimister PW, Hofstra L, Liem IH, Boersma HH, Kemerink G, Reutelingsperger CP, Reutelingsperger CP & Heidendal GA. (2003). In vivo detection of cell death in the area at risk in acute myocardial infarction. *J Nucl Med* Vol.44(No. 3):391-396.

Tokita N, Hasegawa S, Maruyama K, Izumi T, Blankenberg FG, Tait JF, Strauss HW & Nishimura T. (2003). 99mTc-Hynic-annexin V imaging to evaluate inflammation and apoptosis in rats with autoimmune myocarditis. *Eur J Nucl Med Mol Imaging* Vol.30(No. 2):232-238.

Veinot JP, Gattinger DA & Fliss H. (1997). Early apoptosis in human myocardial infarcts. *Hum Pathol* Vol.28(No. 4):485-492.

Vriens PW, Blankenberg FG, Stoot JH, Ohtsuki K, Berry GJ, Tait JF, Strauss HW & Robbins RC. (1998). The use of technetium Tc 99m annexin V for in vivo imaging of apoptosis during cardiac allograft rejection. *J Thorac Cardiovasc Surg* Vol.116(No. 5):844-853.

Wang F, Fang W, Zhang MR, Zhao M, Liu B, Wang Z, Hua Z, Yang M, Kumata K, Hatori A, Yamasaki T, Yanamoto K & Suzuki K. (2011). Evaluation of chemotherapy response in VX2 rabbit lung cancer with 18F-labeled C2A domain of synaptotagmin I. *J Nucl Med* Vol.52(No. 4):592-599.

Wencker D, Chandra M, Nguyen K, Miao W, Garantziotis S, Factor SM, Shirani J, Armstrong RC & Kitsis, RN. (2003). A mechanistic role for cardiac myocyte apoptosis in heart failure. *J Clin Invest* Vol.111(No. 10):1497-1504.

Zhao M, Zhu X, Ji S, Zhou J, Ozker KS, Fang W, Molthen RC & Hellman RS. (2006). 99mTc-labeled C2A domain of synaptotagmin I as a target-specific molecular probe for noninvasive imaging of acute myocardial infarction. *J Nucl Med* Vol.47(No. 8):1367-1374.

Zhou D, Chu W, Rothfuss J, Zeng C, Xu J, Jones L, Welch, MJ, & Mach RH. (2006). Synthesis, radiolabeling, and in vivo evaluation of an 18F-labeled isatin analog for imaging caspase-3 activation in apoptosis. *Bioorg Med Chem Lett* Vol.16(No. 19):5041-5046.

11

Dosimetry for Beta-Emitter Radionuclides by Means of Monte Carlo Simulations

Pedro Pérez[1], Francesca Botta[2], Guido Pedroli[2] and Mauro Valente[3]
[1]*Agencia Nacional de Promoción Científica y Tecnológica*
Universidad Nacional de Córdoba
[2]*Medical Physics Department, European Institute of Oncology*
[3]*CONICET, Universidad Nacional de Córdoba*
[1,3]*Argentina*
[2]*Italy*

1. Introduction

Nowadays, there are interests as well as active investigations devoted to the study and application of radiolabeled molecules able to selectively target and irradiate tumoral cells during nuclear medicine procedures. With this kind of pharmaceuticals, spatial activity distribution with extremely non-uniform characteristics may be assessed in patients. Actually, this feature constitutes precisely the main advantage in view of maximizing the discrimination between affected and healthy tissue. The mentioned situation constitutes the main motivation for the present work. In this sense, the chapter is focused on nuclear medicine dosimetry pointing out the main features about how to implement Monte Carlo (MC) approaches to this aim.

Nowadays, from a general point of view, therapies with radiopharmaceuticals using beta-emitter radionuclides are growing significantly and very fast. Beta-emitters can be emitters of β^- or β^+ radiation. Commonly, β^+ emitters, like ^{18}F are used for imaging techniques, whereas β^- are mainly used with therapeutic purposes, to deliver high dose rate on tumors. Therefore, β^- emitters are usually those of more interest for dosimetry.

During nuclear medicine procedures, radiopharmaceutical activity distribution may be determined by means of different modalities. Nowadays it is mainly assessed using imaging techniques but otherwise it is also possible to infer it [Stabin (2008)]. This information is then incorporated in the treatment planning system in order to obtain an estimation of the dose distribution. More specifically, patient-specific dose distribution owing to alpha, beta and/or gamma emitters can be calculated starting from activity distribution by means of either direct MC simulation or analytical methods.

On the other hand, patient-specific dosimetry requires anatomical information, which shall be further considered as input for establishing mass distribution during MC computations. Patient anatomical information can be suitably extracted from typical non-invasive imaging techniques, like computed tomography (CT) or magnetic resonance imaging (MRI).

Many studies have been performed by means of MC applications in Nuclear Medicine up today, both in the imaging field, and regarding dosimetry calculations [F. Botta & Valente (2011), Zubal & Harrel (1992), H. Yoriyaz & dos Santos (2001), M. Ljungberg & Strand (2002)].

Numerous Monte Carlo codes have been benchmarked and used for different purposes in radiation transport including nuclear medicine imaging and dosimetry. Some examples are MCPT code of Williamson (1988), EGS4 code (Luxton and Jozsef, 1999), GEANT4 code (Agostinelli, 2003) and MCNP4 code (DeMarco et al 2002b, Bohm et al 2003). The more recently developed PENELOPE (PENetration and Energy Loss Of Positrons and Electrons; photon simulation was introduced later) Monte Carlo code 2001 (Salvat et al 2001) uses cross-sections from the up-to-date EPDL97 dataset, and thus takes advantage of the latest improvements in cross-section libraries [R.D. Stewart & Strom (2001), A. Sánchez-Crespo & Larsson (2004)].

Although several MC codes are available allowing to transport photons and electrons in user-defined geometries, it should be mentioned that there two codes particularly useful for voxel dosimetry applications, named EGS4 and MCNP [E.B. Bolch & Watson (1999)].

As a particular and non common approach this chapter will discuss how to implement MC simulation in nuclear medicine by means of the PENELOPE code.

The proposed method along with the developed computation system allow to introduce as input data different types of images -both metabolic and anatomical- commonly used for nuclear medicine diagnostic, like CT, MRI, SPECT, gamma camera and PET. This capability arises from the incorporation of dedicated routines for reading and interpreting the "Digital Imaging and Communication in Medicine" (DICOM) information code, therefore significantly simplifying input data handling processes aimed to specific-patient absorbed dose distribution calculation. In this sense, suitable combination of metabolic and anatomical imaging techniques provides relevant information helpful when attempting reliable and accurate specific-patient dosimetry. When considering all together the mentioned potential advantages of the proposed method along with the implementation of dedicated voxelization techniques, it would be expected that it may constitute an important tool for daily treatment planning by means of MC simulations for specific-patient dosimetry assessment.

The estimation of dose from a distributed source is an important aspect of the application of labeled monoclonal antibodies to targeted radiotherapy. A major contribution to the dose arises from beta particles. The source may be described mathematically by a function giving the activity concentration at each position in the source. The dose produced at a specific site may then be calculated as the linear superposition of contributions from each volume element in the distribution treated as a point source. The dose produced by a point source of isotropic unit activity is known as dose point kernel [Prestwich WV (1985)] (DPK). Due to its significant importance and largely proved benefits and convenience for dosimetric purposes, carefully characterization of DPK has always received significant interests and efforts, therefore extended discussion will be presented about DPK calculation by means of MC techniques.

In summary, it would be desirable to assess a suitable and reliable method helpful for patient-specific treatment planning calculating full stochastic radiation transport by means of MC methods. Therefore, once the calculation system is already developed, it should be carried out careful and rigorous verifications of certain parameters which can point out the reliability of the proposed method.

In this sense, considering that the main goal of this work consists on performing dosimetry for beta-minus radiation therapy and according to the significant importance of beta DPK in nuclear medicine dosimetry, this quantity may be taken as a suitable parameter to check the feasibility of the proposed MC code. With the aim of simplifying, it is established from here that DPK will be referred as beta-DPK unless it will be explicitly specified.

2. Monte Carlo methods and nuclear medicine

2.1 Monte Carlo radiation transport simulation

Radiation transport, including absorption and scattering processes are determined by the Boltzmann transport equation. However, it is hard to apply and to analytically solve Boltzmann equation within non-homogeneous media or regions consisting of complex boundaries. Actually, it is well known that Boltzmann equation can be analytically solved only in few cases consisting on oversimplified situations, that would strongly differ from real clinical situations. Therefore, numerical methods have been proposed for solving Boltzmann equation in complex situations performing full radiation transport by means of stochastic methods. The MC techniques belong to the most important group within this category.
Physically, the evolution of an electron-photon shower has an intrinsic random nature, so MC methods provide a convenient alternative to deal with transport problems [Salvat (2009)].
On the MC method for radiation transport, the "life" of each particle is seen as a random sequence of free paths that end with an interaction event where the particle suffers any kind of interaction. Generally, the "interaction event" refers to any change in the particle quantum state and it can arise from the change of its movement direction, the loss of energy or the production of a secondary particles. The interaction type depends on the kind of actual particle along with the medium where it is moving by random processes because of its nature.
In order to point out main characteristics about how to handle with MC codes with the aim of performing nuclear medicine dosimetry, it has been selected to work with the PENELOPE main code. The fundamental motivations for using PENELOPE relays on its suitability of electron and photon transport along with the relevant characteristic of providing open source routines (written on fortran 77 language). The general considerations described below could be similarly implement on any general purposes MC main code.

2.2 The PENELOPE Monte Carlo code

The PENELOPE v.2008 is a MC algorithm and computer code for the simulation of coupled electron-photon transport. The simulation algorithm is based on scattering models that combines numerical databases with analytical cross section models for the different interaction mechanisms and it is applicable to energies (kinetic energies in the case of electrons and positrons) from a few hundred eV to approximated $1GeV$. Photon transport is simulated by means of the conventional detailed method. The simulation of charged particles (electron and positron) transport is performed by means of a mixed procedure. Hard interactions, with scattering angle θ or energy loss W greater than preselected cutoff values θ_c and W_c , are simulated in detail. Soft interactions correspond to scattering angle and energy loss less than the corresponded cutoffs θ_c, W_c and these interactions are considered by means of suitable mechanisms for simulation condensation, mainly based on multiple scattering theories, like Mollier theory. The user can select the cutoff parameters quite large looking for speeding up the calculation considerably, but it should be preliminary carefully studied the ranges for each parameter that may produce non-negligible alterations in the final scores. A characteristic feature of the here presented simulation code is that the most delicate parts of the simulation are handled internally; electrons, positrons and photons are simulated by calling the same subroutines. Thus PENELOPE makes the practical simulation of electrons and positrons as simple as that of photons (although simulating a charged particle may take a longer time).
One of the main advantages of the latest version of PENELOPE (PENELOPE v. 2008 package) regards the improvements for inner shells ionizations by electron and positron impact, which are described by using a numerical database of total cross-sections for K, L and M

shells derived from the theory described by Bote and Salvat (2008). It was also included photon polarization effects in Rayleigh and Compton scattering, as well as refinements in the modeling of Rayleigh photon scattering and of inelastic collisions of electrons and positrons. These improvement would provide significantly better description of charged particle transport and energy deposition.
In this study, PENELOPE v. 2008 MC code has been considered for use in nuclear medicine dosimetry assessment as well as treatment planning approach when possible. During the last years, PENELOPE has been widely employed for different studies by physicists on the radiation transport field [J. Asenjo & Sánchez-Reyes (2002), S.J. Ye & Naqvi (2004), J. Sempau & Salvat (2004), Bielajew & Salvat (2001), J. Sempau & Fernández-Varea (2001)], therefore supporting the selected choice.

2.3 Dose Point Kernel

The Dose Point Kernel can be defined considering an extremely simplified model of a monoenergetic isotropic point source emitting electrons which move outwards within an homogeneous medium and slow down continuously according to a stopping power function $S(E)$ [W.V. Prestwich & Kwok (1989)]. If the source energy is E_0, therefore the distance r from the origin, at which the source is located, is related with the remaining energy $E(r)$ by:

$$r = \int_{E(r)}^{E_0} \frac{dE}{S(E)} \tag{1}$$

The CSDA Range (R_{CSDA} also called r_0 by other authors) satisfies

$$R_{CSDA} = \int_{0}^{E_0} \frac{dE}{S(E)} \tag{2}$$

Then, the absorbed dose per source transformation in a spherical shell is:

$$D(r) = \frac{S(E(r))}{4\pi\rho r^2} \tag{3}$$

The specific absorbed fraction is given by

$$\Phi(r, E_0) = \frac{S(E(r))}{4\pi\rho r^2 E_0} \tag{4}$$

It can be shown that $\Phi(r, E_0)$ satisfies the constraint

$$\int_0^{\infty} 4\pi\rho r^2 \Phi(r, E_0) dr = 1 \tag{5}$$

It is convenient to introduce a dimensionless quantity to represent distance as the fraction of the CSDA range, asigning:

$$x = \frac{r}{R_{CSDA}} \tag{6}$$

The scaled electron DPK is defined through the relation

$$F(x, E_0) = 4\pi\rho r^2 R_{CSDA} \Phi(r, E_0) \tag{7}$$

It will be useful to introduce a new quantity satisfying

$$\int_0^{\infty} F(x, E_0)dx = 1 \tag{8}$$

And therefore, according to the simplified model, the scaled DPK becomes, from Eq. (7)

$$F(x, E_0) = \frac{R_{CSDA} S(E(x, R_{CSDA}))}{E_0} = \frac{S(E(x, R_{CSDA}))}{< S >} \tag{9}$$

where the track average stopping power ($< S >= E_0/R_{CSDA}$)has been introduced. In this sense, it could be possible to interpret the scaled DPK as the ratio of the stopping power at a particular point along the electron track to the average stopping power over the entire track.
It is also customary to use radial distributions of dose around isotropic point sources of electrons or beta-emitters in an infinite water medium, so called dose DPKs, as the basis of many calculations of dose from various distributions of beta sources.
In fact, DPKs have proved to be adequate and remarkable useful for several dosimetric purposes in nuclear medicine. Actually, DPKs are commonly used for daily applications and calculations when some approximations may be acceptable, like non high tissue inhomogeneity around the emission point.
Contrary to monoenergetic sources, for the case of beta-emitting radionuclides it will be necessary to calculate the DPK as resulting from a spectrum of electrons. The spectrum associated with beta-decay may in general be written as:

$$n(E) = \sum_{i=1}^{N} \beta_i n_i(E) \tag{10}$$

which represents a decomposition into N groups, each of which has a branching probability of β_i and end-point energy E_i. Also associated with each group is an average energy

$$< E_i >= \int_0^{E_i} E n_i(E) dE \tag{11}$$

given that the spectral distribution $n_i(E)$ is normalized to unit area.
The specific absorbed fraction associated with i^{th} beta-group is given by

$$\Phi_i(r) = \int_0^{E_i} \frac{E_0}{< E_i >} n_i(E_0) \Phi(r, E_0) dE_0 \tag{12}$$

and from the Eq. (9) it follows that

$$4\pi\rho r^2 \Phi_i(r) = \int_0^{E_i} \frac{E_0}{R_{CSDA} < E_i >} n_i(E_0) F\left(\frac{r}{R_{CSDA}}, E_0\right) dE_0 \tag{13}$$

A scaled DPK for a beta group may also be introduced. To this end a scaled distance is defined as the fraction of the CSDA range for an electron with energy E_i . Designating the latter r_i , then the scaled DPK for i^{th} beta group becomes

$$F_i(x) = 4\pi\rho r^2 r_i \Phi_i(r) \tag{14}$$

where $x = r/r_i$. Scaling the distance in this manner differs from the suggested by Berger, who uses the 90% point. It has the advantage, however, of using a quantity that is more readily available, the CSDA range.
As indicated before, calculation of the DPK requires the evaluation of the CSDA range. In order to accomplish this task approximations have been employed. As first approach, it may

be useful to look for databases containing relevant and required information, like *Stopping Power and Range Tables for Electrons* which may be available from the National Institute of Standards and Technology[1]. A good recommemdation is that database values should be compared with the corresponding data used by the MC code (it can be assessed using the Table subroutine in the case of the PENELOPE v. 2008 code). In he case of PENELOPE v. 2008, it can be seen that NIST tabulated data and PENELOPE database values present negligible differences. Therefore, CSDA ranges required for shell thickness calculations can be derived from internal MC database or NIST tables without distinction.

On the other hand, in order to establish the corresponding dose delivering shell thicknesses in the case of isotope emission spectra, it may be considered the approximation of treating an isotope spectrum as monoenergetic source with an effective energy (E_{Eff}) associated with the average (properly weighted according to the actual spectrum) energy of the whole emission spectrum. Due to the fact that shell thicknesses depend upon source energy, once material is given, it becomes clear the motivations for introducing and determining E_{Eff} in order to assess some effective or equivalent energy value with the aim of calculating the corresponding shell thickness for the DPK calculations.

As a consequence of this assumption, the corresponding shell thickness for the k-isotope (R_{CSDA}) can be calculated from the relation:

$$R^k_{CSDA} = R_{CSDA}\left(E^k_{Eff}\right) \quad (15)$$

where $k = {}^{90}Y, {}^{131}I, {}^{89}Sr, {}^{153}Sm, {}^{177}Lu, \ldots$ and E_{Eff} is computed according to:

$$E^k_{Eff} = \frac{\sum_{i=1}^N p_i E_i}{\sum_{i=1}^N E_i} \quad (16)$$

Where N is the number of channels of the k-isotope energy spectrum and p_i and E_i are its weight and energy respectively. It can be seen, as reported in Table 1, two examples of the calculated E^k_{Eff} and R^k_{CSDA} along with the corresponding graphic sketch (Figure 1) outlining how E_{Eff} may be estimated. Radionuclide emission spectra were extracted from the NIST database tables[2].

Isotope	E^k_{Eff} calculated $[keV]$	R^k_{CSDA} used $[cm]$
^{90}Y	936.9	0.4029
^{177}Lu	138.9	0.0246
^{89}Sr	583.6	0.2182
^{153}Sm	231.3	0.0565
^{131}I	188.2	0.0407

Table 1. R_{CSDA} used and E^k_{Eff} calculated for different isotopes.

2.4 Dedicated subroutines based on Monte Carlo techniques

The Monte Carlo method has been successfully applied to radiation transport problems in clinical dosimetry. The method is particularly useful for complex problems that can not be solved analytically and/or deterministically or when measurements are not practical.

[1] http://www.nist.gov
[2] Idem 1.

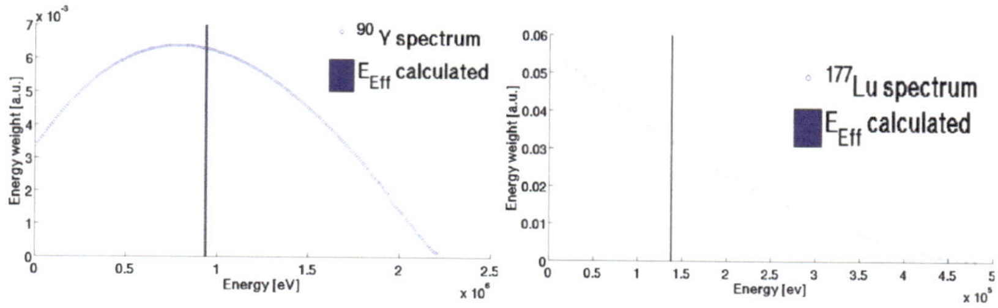

(a) (b)

Fig. 1. ^{90}Y and ^{177}Lu spectra compared with its E_{Eff} calculated.

The accuracy of Monte Carlo simulations strongly depends on the accuracy in the probability density functions, and thereby the material cross-section libraries used for radiation transport calculations.

The PENELOPE parameter E_{abs} determines -for each simulated material and transported particle type- the energy threshold for particle absorption, defining the energy value below which transport is no longer simulated and residual energy is assumed to be deposited locally. The lowest possible E_{abs} value is $100eV$ according to manual recommendations based on the lower energy ($50eV$) in PENELOPE v. 2008 database.

With the aim of performing radiation transport for dosimetric purposes, the first step may be the design and development of a code devoted to the DPK calculations, which may basically consist on a main program able to allow the user to set up the energy or the spectrum to be radiated by the point source centered in a geometry defined by concentric spheres defining shells of thickness $R_{CSDA}/40$ (the corresponding R_{CSDA} for each material is calculated for the actual or effective energy for monoenertic sources or radionuclides, respectively). Due to phisical properties of charged particles, it may be enough to tally DPK up to $1.5R_{CSDA}$. Finally, the material for which the DPK needs to be investigated along with the corresponding simulation parameters may be adjusted by the user in the input file.

The geometry file can be obtained from a dedicated user-designed program devoted to set up the R_{CSDA} obtained from MC or reliable databases. Once the user provides R_{CSDA} the program will automatically generate the corresponding file according to internal PENELOPE requirements for simulation geometries.

Preliminary simulations are performed to achieve E_{abs} parameter values in order to optimize computation process assessing suitable balances between statistical errors and the CPU computation times. Therefore, after exhaustive examinations, absorption cutoff values of $100eV$ (minimum recommendable by PENELOPE developers) have been considered for emitting sources of energies lower than $100keV$ (*i.e.* $5keV$, $10keV$, $20keV$ and $50keV$) whereas cutoff values of $1keV$ have been set for emitting sources with energies equal or higher than $100keV$ (*i.e.* $100keV$, $200keV$, $500keV$, $1MeV$, $2MeV$ and $5MeV$).

As example from the preliminary simulations devoted to achieving suitable absorption energy cutoff valued, it can be mentioned that in the case of the $100keV$ monoenergetic source, it was found a maximum difference in the DPK of 0.16% when changing cutoff value from $1keV$ to the minimum possible of $100eV$, which may be taken as negligible. However, the situation is significantly different when dealing with low energy emitting sources. DPK differences up to 5% may be found when changing absorption cutoff values from $1keV$ to $100eV$ in the case of $5keV$ monoenergetic source.

As reported in Figure 2, it can be shown that DPK curves do not exhibit strong differences when calculated for 100 or 1000eV considering emission energy of $100keV$.

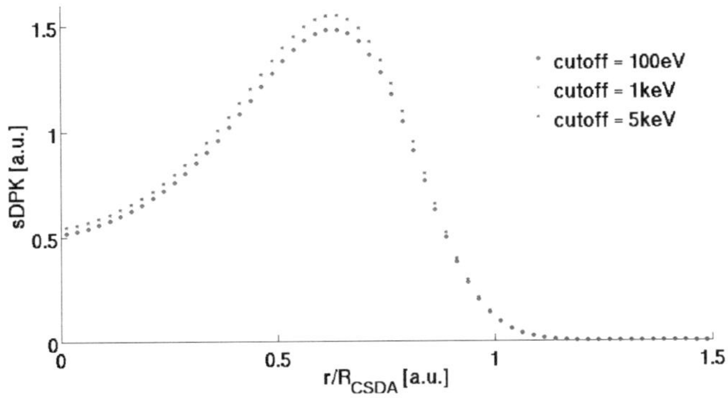

Fig. 2. Total sDPK curves for different cutoffs ($100eV$, $1keV$ and $5keV$)

2.4.1 Monte Carlo DPK calculation

It is considered a punctual source (spectral or monoenergetic) centered in a water sphere divided in many shells. Shell thicknesses are defined according to $R_{CSDA}/40$ and dose delivered within each shell is tallied using the developed MC code system, based on physics from PENELOPE v. 2008.
In addition, dedicated subroutines have been introduced in the MC main code with the aim of computing separately the different contributions to the total absorbed dose. Suitable distinction may be made between primary and scattering components, considering scattering contribution as arising from all energy depositions belonging to non primary particles.
Also, it is necessary to establish an optimal number of showers to be simulated in view of optimizing the compromise between short CPU calculation time and accurate enough results. In this sense, it may be useful to carry out preliminary calculations with different number of showers to assess a suitable choice, according to Figures 3 and 4, for example. In base of these figures it may be suggest that 10^7 primary showers would be an acceptable selection. Actually, it should be usefull to add that according to this choice the CPU time is not longer than 8 hours for a typical microprocessor on a standard PC.

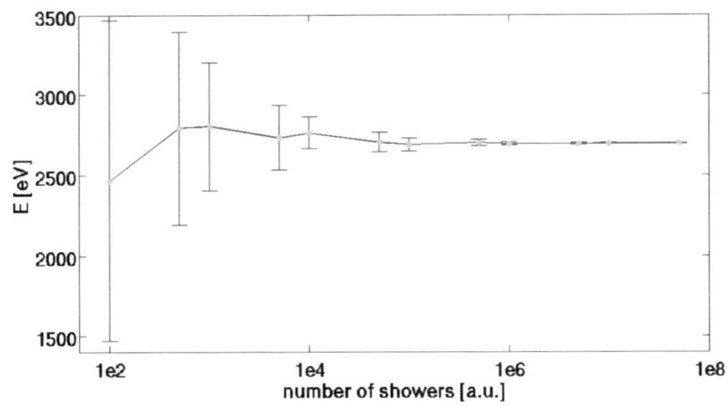

Fig. 3. Convergence analysis of the 15th shell for different numbers of initial showers tallying deposited energy along with uncertainties calculated as three standard deviations.

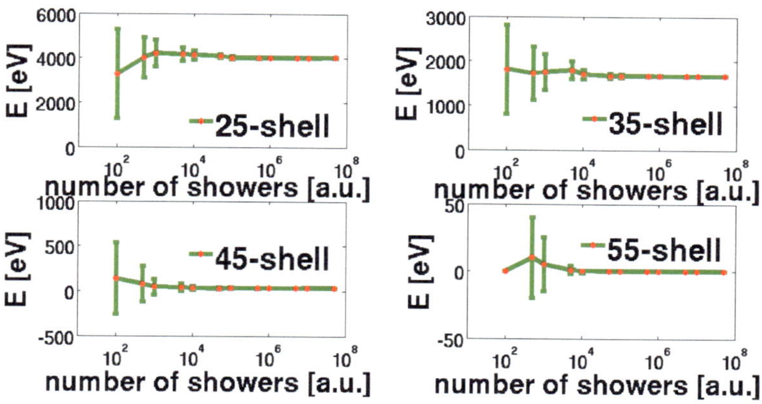

Fig. 4. Convergence analysis for the 25th (a), 35th (b), 45th (c) and 55th (d) shell. Error bars correspond to 3σ, *i.e.* 99.9% of confidence.

The distinction between the scattering and the primary contributions by the developed code is assessed by "marking" or "painting" each particle on the main code distinguishing energy deposition arising from primary or scattered particles. It should be emphasized that this subtlety is able because of the great -actually absolute- aperture of PENELOPE as an open source code. Technically, this aim can be accomplished by adding a special new parameter in the particle quantum state along with the inclusion of suitable flags during particle tracking. With this tool it becomes possible to obtain the dose delivered by each particle while discriminating each kind of contribution.
Therefore, dose contributions calculation is on-run performed and separated files are generated for total, primary and scattering dose delivering tallied at each shell.

2.4.2 Monte Carlo direct simulation on patient images

The first step consists on developing a code capable of reading and interpreting patient-specific medical images in order to use them as input data for further computation with the simulation code.

2.4.2.1 Geometry voxelization in Monte Carlo methods

According to typical medical imaging techniques, the most commonly found image storage formats consist on space voxelization. In this sense, it would be desiderable to have at disposal some mechanism devoted to interpret and handle voxelized information in order to perform patient-specific dosimetry calculations. If the MC package does not provide a voxelization toolkit, it would be useful and/or necessary that the user may implement some dedicated voxelization technique in order to allow the use of patient-specific data from DICOM images within the simulation. The role of the voxelization technique regards the interpretation by the simulation code of the patient data in order to provide the corresponding inputs for simulation geometry and mass distribution. Some MC main codes provide voxelization capability with user distribution, but unfortunately this is not the case of PENELOPE v.2008. Therefore, it was necessary to develop a dedicated program for patient data upload. This aim was accomplished by considering patient geometry as a tensor whose elements correspond to a patient image voxel and therefore its material and mass density may be inferred from CT calibration, which provides the Hounsfield (CT) index vs. electronic density.

Once patient geometry is already voxelized, 3D energy and dose deposition are tallied at each voxel.

2.4.2.2 Input data files from DICOM images

DICOM is a commonly used imaging file format in almost all medical imaging fields, particularly in nuclear medicine. For the purposes of the present work it was developed a specific code for reading these image files and further convertion to suitable ascii files able to be introduced as input for the developed radiation transport code.
One comfortable way for reading and interpreting DICOM images is available in the MATLAB® environment. The implemented method consists on exploiting the useful MATLAB package called "dicomread" that allows the user to read DICOM files as 3D tensors. The obtained tensor is used to generate a suitable array which elements refer to the information at each voxel in the DICOM file. This array is further uploaded as input ascii data providing the required patient-specific radiation transport properties for MC simulations.

2.4.2.3 Metabolic & anatomical patient-specific input data

As described above, analogous treatments apply for uploading DICOM functional or anatomical images. Patient anatomy is used to define simulation geometry and physical properties may be inferred by means of suitable calibrations or implementing some *"ad hoc"* criterion consulting expert physicians. On the other hand, functional images, like SPECT or PET are used to provide activity spatial distribution and knowing the corresponding infused radionuclide spectrum, it may be possible to use this information as simulation radiation source. Combining both of these imaging techniques as simulation inputs, it would be possible to assess reliable patient-specific dosimetry.
The DICOM functional images provide the activity information which is interpreted by the code to establish the source distribution and its activity everywhere.

2.4.2.4 Specific-patient dose distribution calculation

Once input data are already uploaded by means of the developed subroutines aimed to converting DICOM images into simulation geometry and radiation source, it becomes possible to perform the corresponding MC simulation to the actual patient-specific situation. As reported in Figure 5, the DICOM images are successfully interpreted to establish both a N-material (four different materials in the reported example, namely: compact bone, soft tissue, air and lung have been selected as a simplified first approximation) patient-specific geometry. In addition, activity intensity and spatial distribution are also satisfactory interpreted and combined with the corresponding anatomical data show a suitable definition of the patient body as a virtual phantom for MC calculations.

2.5 Radiobiological models

Once 3D dose distribution is assessed, radiobiological considerations can be derived by applying the adequate models with this aim.
Most calculations of the biological effect of radiation on tumors assume that the clonogenic cell density is uniform even if account is taken of non-uniform dose distribution. Anyway, after implementing some methodology for to identifying tumor/normal tissues on patient images it will be necessary to introduce a model capable of assesing *Tumor Control Probability* (TCP) on the tumor [Dale (1988),D.J. Brenner & Sachs (1995),M. Guerrero (2004)] and *Normal Tissue Complications Probability* (NTCP) over the normal tissue and organs closed to the treatment region [V.A. Semenenko (2008),L.A. Dawson & Haken (2002)].

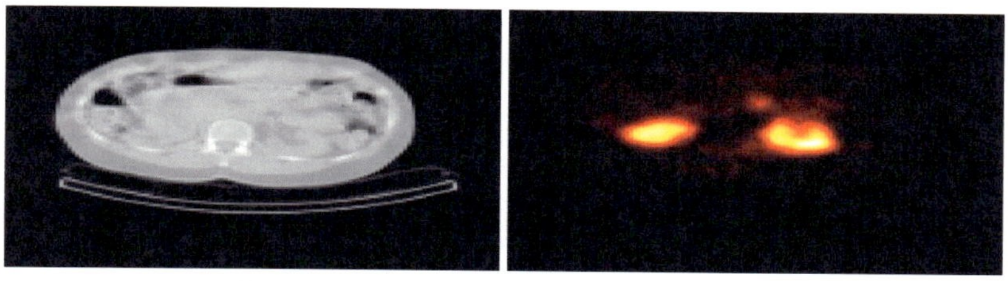

(a) (b)

Fig. 5. CT (a), and SPECT (b) images showing both a transversal cut of the geometry and the activity information.

Over the two past decades, the linear-quadratic (LQ) model has emerged as a convenient tool to quantify biological effects for radiotherapy. Therefore, just for didactics purposes ilustrating how to proceed for implementing radiobiological calculations, the LQ model will be taken as example. From a general point of view and without interest on going deeper, it should be mentioned that the LQ model provides a simple method to calculate the cell survival fraction (SF), and on its consequences it is possible to see a reliable measure of the TCP.

Assuming the Poisson statistics to survival cells and considering the control probability of the tumor as the probability of having them death, it can be assessed the LQ model, assuming a dose D homogeneously distributed over a homogeneous tumor, establishes that the SF is given by the relationship

$$SF = e^{-\alpha D - \beta D^2} \tag{17}$$

where α and β are empiric biological parameters associated to the probability of breaking DNA helix. The α parameter represents the probability to induce a double strand break in DNA helix with a single energy deposition, whereas the β parameter represents the probability to have two single strand breaks with two separate energy depositions, one on the first DNA helix, the other on the second one, which are close enough -both spatially and temporally- to combine together producing the same effect of a double strand break, *i.e.* a lethal (non reparable) damage.

Also, eq. (17) considers SF and it is defined by the equation,

$$SF = \frac{N_s}{N_0} \tag{18}$$

where N_0 refers to the initial quantity of tumoral cells and N_s to the survival tumoral cells. Then, the TCP is given by the equation

$$TCP = e^{-SF} = \exp\left(-e^{-\alpha D - \beta D^2}\right) \tag{19}$$

Whereas NTCP formulation is considered by the interpretation of empirical clinical data, since the organ behavior cannot be easily described by equations, and also the sparing of a normal tissue is not simply linked to the number of surviving cells, but also to the maintenance of its functionality, which depends on the organ architecture.

The Lyman-Kutcher-Burman (LKB) [V.A. Semenenko (2008), Z. Xu & Jiang (2006)] model proposes that the NTCP may be assessed by

$$NTCP \equiv c(u) = \frac{1}{\sqrt{2\pi}} \int_{\infty}^{u} e^{-t^2/2} dt \tag{20}$$

where

$$u = \frac{D - TD_{50}}{m \cdot TD_{50}} \tag{21}$$

when conditions are assumed as in the LQ model for the TCP calculations, m is a dimensionless correction factor and TD_{50} is the dose, over all the tumor, for that NTCP is equal to 50%. And it is possible to characterize $c(u)$ as

$$\begin{aligned} c(u) &= \frac{1}{2} \exp\left(\kappa u - \frac{\kappa^2 u^2}{2}\right) \qquad for \quad u < 0 \\ c(u) &= 1 - \frac{1}{2} \exp\left(\kappa u - \frac{\kappa^2 u^2}{2}\right) \qquad for \quad u \geq 0 \end{aligned} \tag{22}$$

where κ is a dimensionless parameter approximated by 0.8154.

3. Application of patient-specific dosimetry system

According to dosimetry calculation purposes, DPKs are all what is needed to calculate dose distributions in homogeneous media starting from activity distributions by simply means of analytical convolution. However, it can be shown that in cases of inhomogeneous media, these analytical methods may not provide accurate enough results for dose distribution calculations, as expected.

Therefore, this section will present some results about the calculation of DPK both for monoenergetic and spectral β^- sources within homogeneous as well as inhomogeneous media with the aim of pointing out the corresponding differences.

In addition, results for preliminary dose maps along with TCP and NTCP calculations for patient-specific images will be reported, the last ones will be considered as examples of the wide range of possibilities in radiobiology offered by the versatility of the implemented calculation system based on 3D dose distribution.

3.1 Monoenergetic beta-emitting sources scaled DPK

Beta-minus monoenergetic sources were simulated and their sDPK were calculated for initial primary particles energies of $5keV$, $10keV$, $20keV$, $50keV$, $100keV$, $200keV$, $500keV$, $1MeV$, $2MeV$ and $5MeV$. The obtained results are shown in Figures 6 and 7.

As mentioned, the implemented calculation code incorporates dedicated routines devoted to quantify the different dosimetric contributions. Figures 8 and 9 show some obtained results for the total sDPK along with the corresponding separation between the primary and scattering contributions for different monoenergetic sources.

In addition, it is interesting to report the relative contribution from scattering component to the total sDPK at different distances, as shown in Figure 10.

3.2 Spectral beta-emitting sources Dose Point Kernels

With the aim of preliminary benchmarking the capability of the developed calculation code in the framework of clinical implementation of beta-minus radiolabeled therapy, sDPK at different energies were calculated for homogeneous media. Therefore, some of the most

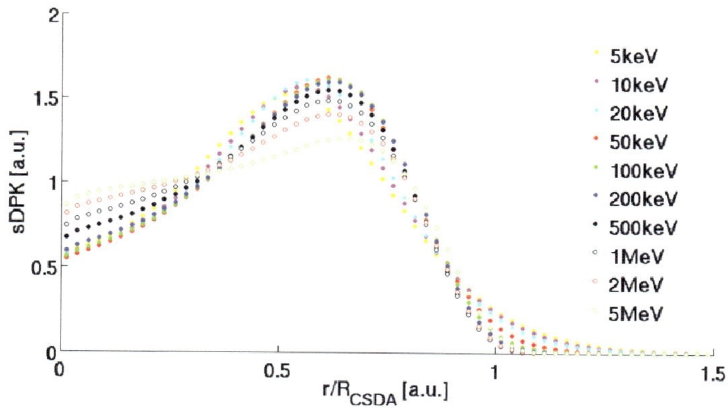

Fig. 6. sDPK calculated for all the monoenergetic beams simulated.

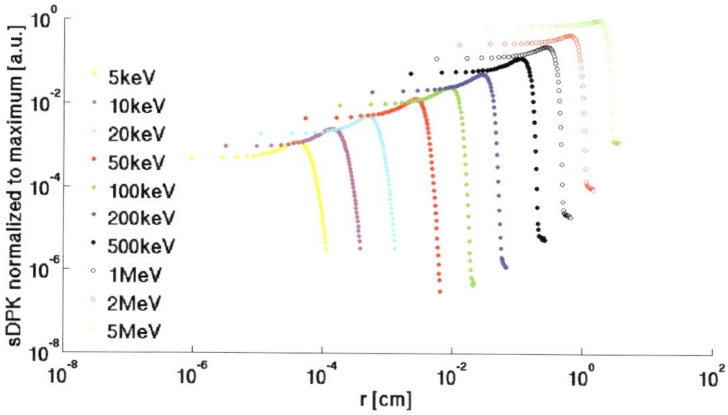

Fig. 7. All monoenergetic beams simulated on log-log scale normalized to maximum, expressed in length units [cm] highlighting differences for a wide range of emission energies.

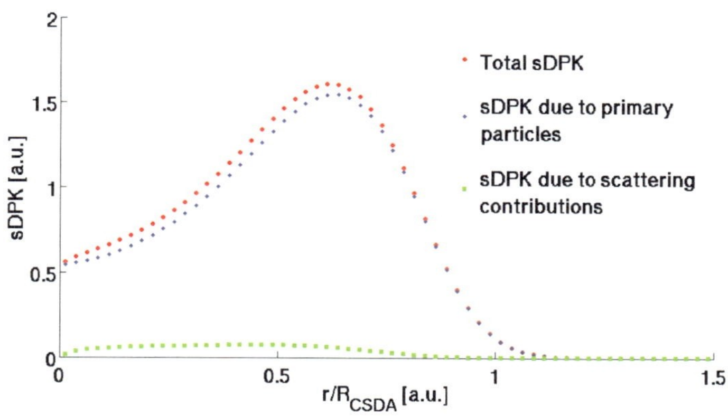

Fig. 8. sDPK for 100keV showing total, primary and scattering contributions.

commonly used radionuclides for targeted radiotherapy treatments have been studied with the developed calculation code. The obtained results for ^{90}Y, ^{131}I, ^{89}Sr, ^{153}Sm and ^{177}Lu are reported in Figures 11 and 12.

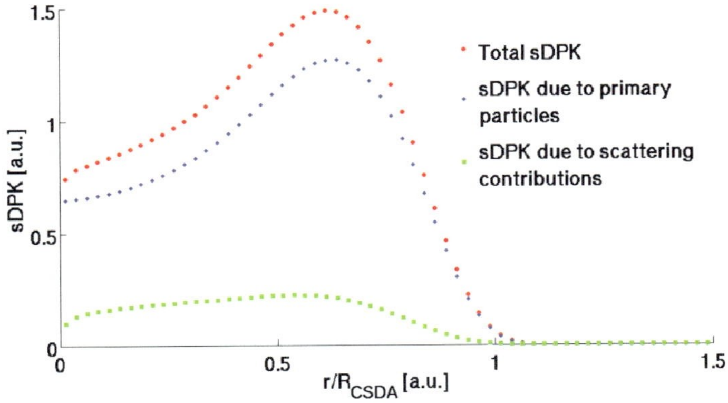

Fig. 9. sDPK for $1MeV$ showing total, primary and scattering contributions.

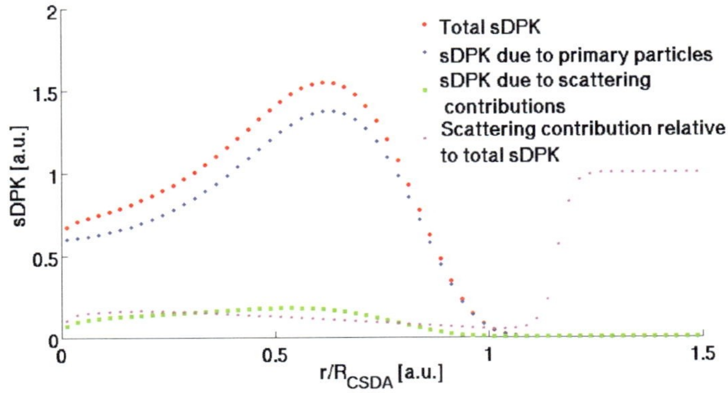

Fig. 10. sDPK along with relative scattering contribution for $500keV$ monoenergetic source.

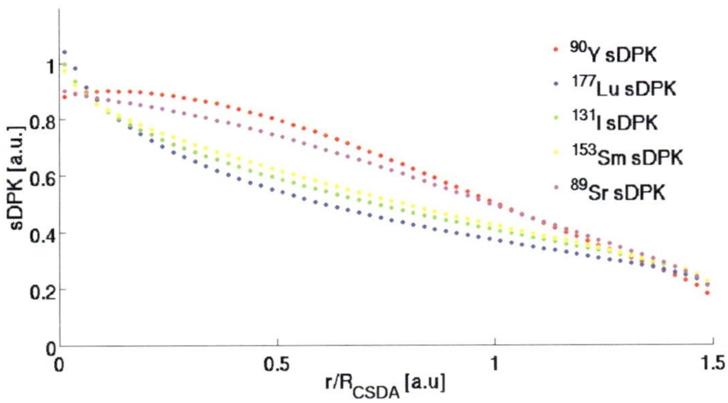

Fig. 11. Total sDPK for different β^- radionuclides.

In the case of radionuclides, the different contributions to the total delivered dose have been assessed by means of an analogue procedure to that of the monoenergetic sources.
Figures 13 and 14 report the obtained results for the contributions to total sDPK allowing to appreciate qualitative different behaviours according to each radionuclide.

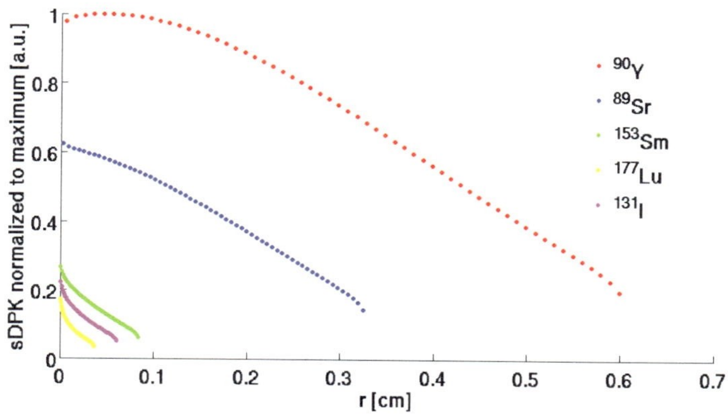

Fig. 12. Total radionuclide DPK normalized to global maximum pointing out the differences in penetration capabilities.

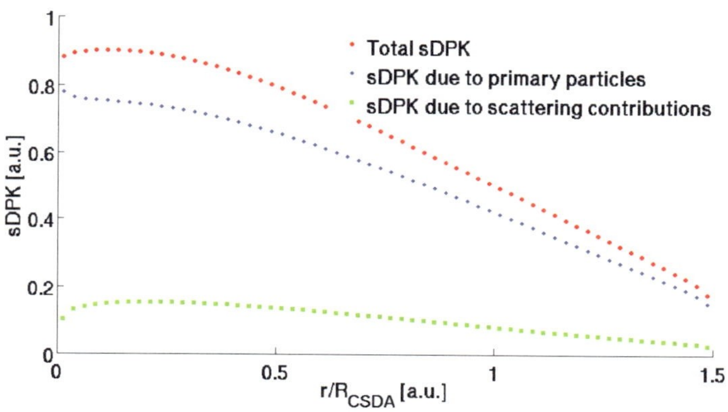

Fig. 13. Different contributions to the ^{90}Y sDPK.

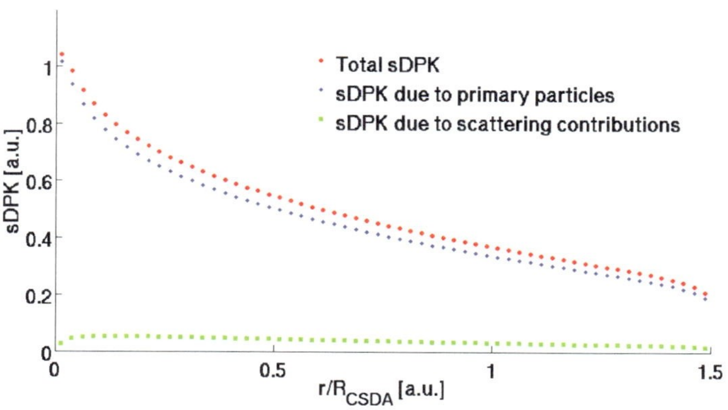

Fig. 14. Different contributions to the ^{177}Lu sDPK.

3.3 Scaled Dose Point Kernels for non water-equivalent media

As mentioned above, it is commonly found in clinical applications the requirement of considering different materiales for patient dosimetry. In this sense, it may be useful to

investigate the effect on sDPK due to the consideration of irradiated media constituted of materials typically used in clinics other than water or normal soft tissue.
In order to show the capability of the developed calculation code to perform radiation transport in different materials, two typical clinical tissues have been selected for this investigation. Bone (defined according to International Commission on Radiation Units and Measurements, ICRU) and lung (International Commission on Radiological Protection, ICRP) tissues have been considered because they represent somehow the extreme cases in typical clinical situations. Figures 14 and 15 report he obtained sDPK calculated over bone and lung spheres for $100keV$ and $500keV$ sources. As a consequence of the sDPK suitable dimensionless length normalization, it has been obtained that the sDPK qualitatively preserve the same shape disregarding of the specific considered medium.

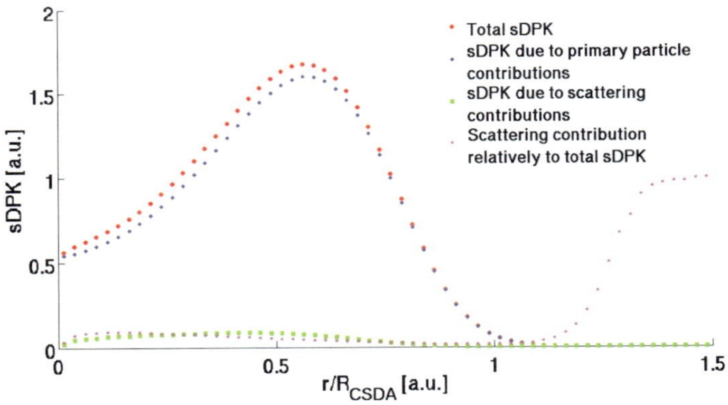

(a)

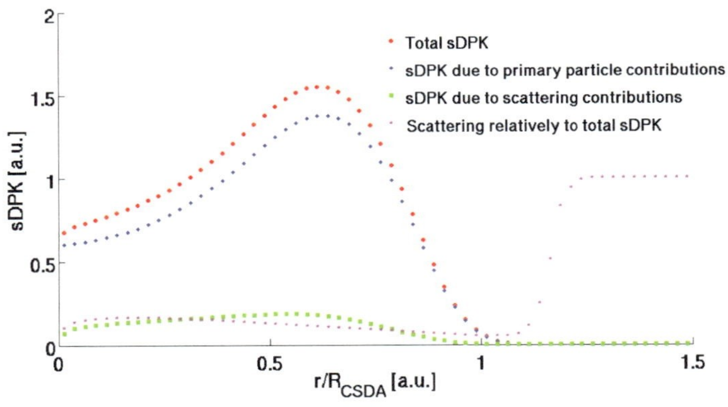

(b)

Fig. 15. Contributions to the sDPK calculated for $100keV$ (a) and $500keV$ (b) centered at a bone and lung spheres, respectively.

3.4 Scaled Dose Point Kernels on inhomogeneous media

In order to highlight the effects of inserting an inhomogeneity in the calculation of the sDPK different situations have been suitably designed and investigated. Water has been selected as

reference medium and bone or lung inhomogeneities have been introduced considering wide ranges of inhomogeneity thickness and relative position within the irradiated sphere.
Figures 16 and 17 report the obtained results for the above described cases. It can be appreciated that, at least *a priori*, it seems to be an anomalous behaviour at the interfaces between different materials. It has been obtained that this "peculiar" situation is always found for all the considered cases independently of inhomogeneity type, thickness or relative position.

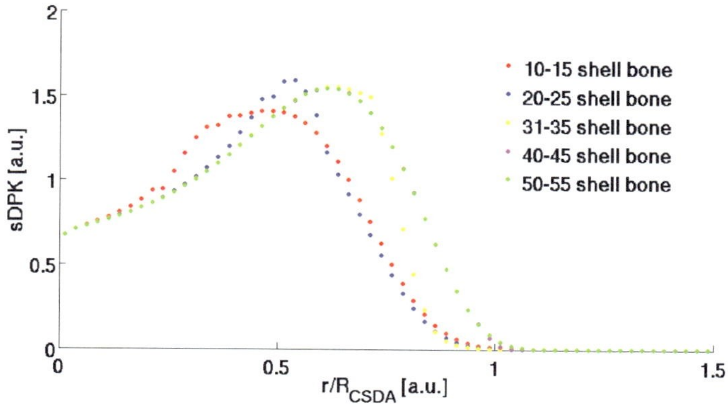

Fig. 16. sDPK corresponding to different relative positions of a 6-shell ($\frac{6}{40} \cdot R_{CSDA}$) thick bone inhomogeneity.

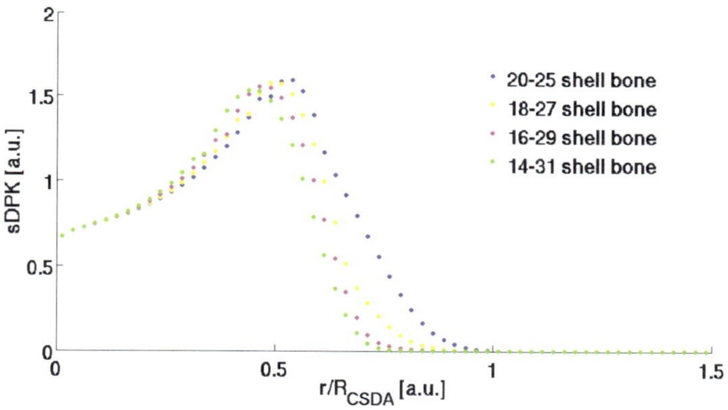

Fig. 17. sDPK corresponding to different bone inhomogeneity thicknesses.

3.5 Patient-specific dose distribution along with TCP and NTCP calculations

Once both the anatomical and metabolic images were already uploaded to the developed calculation code it became possible to perform the corresponding patient-specific dosimetry establishing the desidered radionuclide and corresponding activity. As example of the proposed method in practical cases, dual SPECT-CT images have been used to carry out the simulation. Dose distribution calculations have been performed for different beta-minus radionuclides, as reported in Figure 18 for ^{131}I.
Although relative dose distribution have been presented, it should be emphasized that once the source activity is established, it becomes possible to determine the corresponding number

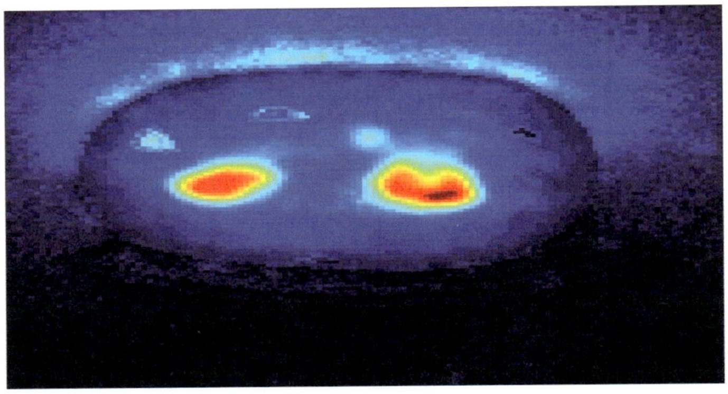

Fig. 18. Relative dose distribution on virtual patient irradiated by ^{131}I.

of primary showers and therefore obtaining straightforwardly the corresponding absolute dose distribution. This information will be necessary for the calculation of radiobiological quantities.

The 3D absolute dose distribution constitutes the basic required information for implementing suitable algorithms devoted to estimate the TCP and NTCP. As mentioned previously, the linear quadratic model has been implemented for TCP estimation. As example of how to proceed, it has been arbitrary taken a total infused activity of 1mCi and typical values for the LQ radiobiological parameters have been used according to the literature, namely $\alpha = 0.12Gy^{-1}$ and $\beta = 0.0137Gy^{-2}$ given a relationship of $\alpha/\beta = 8.7591$. Figure 19 reports the obtained TCP distribution for the slice of interest.

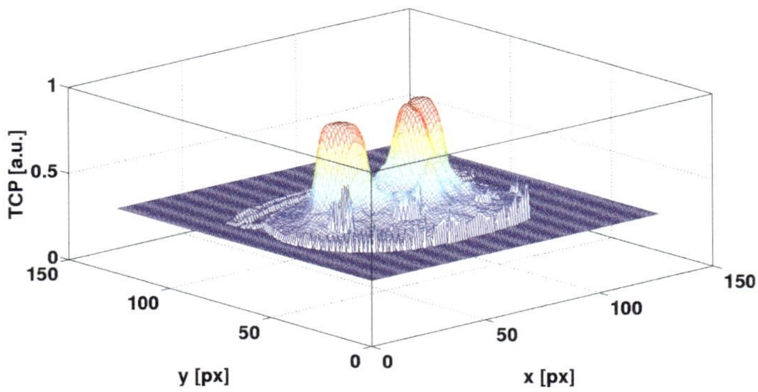

Fig. 19. TCP for the slice of interest obtained for $1mCi$ activity delivered by ^{131}I.

However, it is necessary to remark that in real clinical situations TCP and NTCP estimation will require the implementation of some mechanism dedicated to the identification of normal/tumor tissue regions in order to proceed with the assigment of the corresponding radiobiological parameters. Actually, TCP evaluations have to be applied to tumor region, whereas NTCP evaluations apply to normal organs, each having different radiobiological parameter values. Once the previous step is accomplished the calculation method is performed following the procedure described above.

Similarly, it can be proposed some model for calculating the NTCP. With the aim of highlighting the required procedure, typical radiobiological values for the LKB model have been extracted from literature [G. Luxton & King (2008)], namely $TD_{50} = 24.5$ and $m = 0.18$. The obtained NCTP distribution is presented in Figure 20.

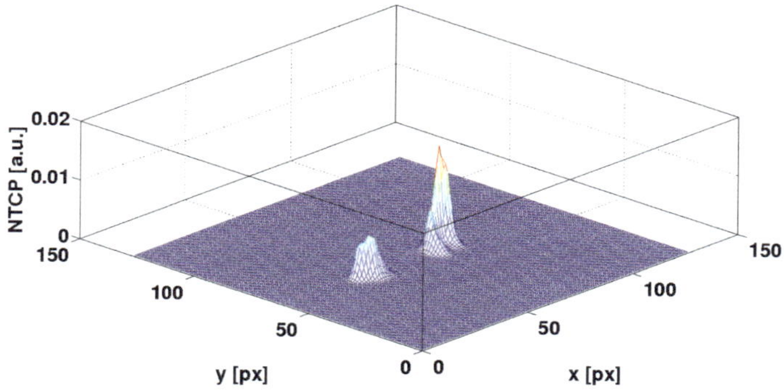

Fig. 20. NTCP for the slice of interest obtained for $1mCi$ activity delivered by ^{131}I.

4. General overview and final remarks

The adequacy of the developed radiation transport simulation code based on PENELOPE v.2008 for nuclear medicine and focused on beta-emitters dosimetry has been preliminary investigated checking the consistency of the results expected when considering electron transport in the energy range from $5keV$ to $5MeV$.

In this sense, dose point kernels have been calculated for several monoenergetic and spectral sources including the most commonly used radionuclides for typical nuclear medicine therapies.

Contrary to other works, it was considered the R_{CSDA} range for both monoenergetic and spectrum sources, instead of the X_{90} parameter used commonly on spectrum sources. Therefore it could be not straightforward to compare the obtained results for radionuclides with those reported by other authors. However, it does not constitute a significant drawback because comparisons can be performed for monoenergetic emission sources, which may help for assessing the reliability and accuracy of the proposed method.

It is interesting to comment about the obtained results for sDPK when inserting inhomogeneities. It has been found that non negligible abrupt changes appear in sDPK curves poducing remarkable discontinuity on the sDPK derivate. This behaviour may make difficult or actually avoid adequate analytical calculation of sDPK, as could be the case of realistic clinical situations. In this sense, it constitutes one of the main advantages of developing and implementing MC methods devoted to reliable radiation transport computation.

Technical features of simulation process have been studied in detail including convergence of representative observable mean values and standard deviations. In view of the specific requirements for most of the calculation performed in this work, it has been found that 10^7 primary showers seems to be a convenient and suitable compromise between calculation time and accurate enough results.

Regarding the investigations about the separation and characerization of the different contributions to the total absorbed dose, it should be mentioned that the main contribution comes from primary radiation, as expected. Although clearly non negligible, scattering contributions are always significantly lower than the primary component to absorbed dose. In addition, it has been shown how to obtain the different dose contributions at different positions and therefore obtaining that relative importance of scattering component varies significantly according to the tally position. Furthermore, the relative balance between primary and scattering contributions has shown to be dependent upon the physical properties of specific considered material.

Nevertheless, in the case of monoenergetic sources it has been obtained that the relative greater importance of the scattering contribution occur at distances larger than the R_{CSDA} and it could be inferred that the same may happen for radioisotopes.

It can been concluded that a characterization of primary and scattering contributions to the total absorbed demand significant efforts. However, the importance of investigating about this would be relevant for further radiobiological studies, because they can take advantage from the characterization of dose components for assessing improved results including LET-weighted dosimetry. When dealing with beta-minus emitters the relative impact of performing LET-weighted dosimetry could be somehow negiglibe becuase of the almost constant LET depence on electron kinetic energy within the range of clinical interest. However, on the other hand, implementing this kind of procedures could be really important for alpha-emitters dosimetry due to the involved high LET values and variations between energy fluence and particle type associated to primary and scattering components.

When considering different absorbing media, like lung or bone, it has been obtained that sDPK show qualitatively the same behaviour found for water. Therefore, it seems possible to propose that sDPK could be satisfactory assessed by analytical methods whenever considering homogeneous media. Furthermore, exhaustive analysis and investigations about the precedent results, which have not been discussed in this work, may suggest that simplified models based on linear scaling of stopping powers could provide acceptable conversion between different biological materials. This scenario may strongly improve calculation comfortability for analytical methods. However, it should be emphasized that MC methods would always provide more accurate and reliable results. Actually, MC methods should be strongly recommended when dealing with complex situations, as may be a realistic patient-specific dose distribution calculation.

In addition, it is important to remark that this MC direct simulation on patient images can be very useful and convenient in some selected cases, like the presence of inhomogeneities, whereas in case of homogeneous tissue simple methods due to their less demanding requirements (especially in terms of computation time) even providing results with accuracy more than adequate. In addition, poor image (anatomical or metabolic) resolution may strongly affect MC calculation, which may be taken as a possible drawback of the proposed method.

Significant improvements regarding CPU calculation time may be assessed in some situations appropriate for suitable approximations allowing deterministic computation, but it is out of the scopes of this work. Otherwise when dealing with homogeneous tissues, analytical methods will be more adequate than MC simulations, preserving MC techniques as the most reliable and recommendable method, at least up today, for accurate dosimetry in presence of inhomogeneities.

Summarizing, this work presented a suitable and useful description about the main features involved in the development and implementation of Monte Carlo techniques for nuclear medicine purposes. A general overview of nuclear medicine dosimetry and radiation transport concepts has been presented. In addition, simplified and detailed explanations have been provided about how to design and elaborate dedicated Monte Carlo subroutines for nuclear medicine purposes.

Several application examples have been added considering typical clinical situations in order to support the exposed concepts and procedures.
As result from the proposed method, it was possible to characterize the scaled dose point kernel, as an important parameter of common daily use in nuclear medicine practice. In addition, the computation of sDPK has been also used for taking advantage of preliminary assessment of reliability and accuracy of the performed dosimetric calculations with the developed code.
The developed simulation code adapted for nuclear medicine radiation transport and dose delivering has been successfully integrated and complemented with dedicated algorithms devoted to patient image reading and interpreting for both anatomical and metabolic patient-specific medical images. Therefore, as example of the potentiality of the developed calculation system, it was shown how to estimate realistic dose distributions computed over reliable patient-specific virtual phantoms using activity information from SPECT DICOM images and the geometries and materials obtained from CT DICOM images. Furthermore, dose volume histograms (DVH) as well radiobiological quantities, like TCP and NTCP can be straightforwardly determined once 3D absorbed dose is already calculated. In base on the obtained performance, it should be emphasized that, after further rigorous tests and benchmarkings, the proposed calculation system would be able to provide accurate and reliable information enough to suggest its consideration as a suitable and useful tool for routine dosimetric calculations.

5. References

A. Sánchez-Crespo, P. & Larsson, S. (2004). Positron flight in human tissues and its influence on pet image spatial resolution, *European Journal of Nuclear Medicine and Molecular Imaging* Vol. 31(No. 1): 44 – 51.

Bielajew, A. & Salvat, F. (2001). Improved electron transport mechanics in the penelope monte-carlo model, *Nuclear Instruments and Methods in Physics Research Section B: Beam Interactions with Materials and Atoms* Vol. 173(Issue 3): 332 – 343.

Dale, R. (1988). Radiobiological assessment of permanent implants using tumour repopulation factors in the linear-quadratic model, *British Journal of Radiology* Vol. 62(No. 735): 241 – 244.

D.J. Brenner, L.R. Hlatky, P. H. E. H. & Sachs, R. (1995). A convenient extension of the linear-quadratic model to include redistribution and reoxygenation, *International journal of radiation oncology, biology, physics* Vol. 32(No. 2): 379 – 390.

E.B. Bolch, L.G. Bouchet, J. R. B. W. J. S. R. H. A. E. B. A. S. C. & Watson, E. (1999). Mird panphlet no. 17: The dosimetry of nonuniform activity distributions - radionuclide s values at the voxel level, *The Journal of Nuclear Medicine* Vol. 40(No. 1): 11S – 36S.

F. Botta, A. Mairani, G. B. M. C. A. D. D. A. F. A. F. M. F. G. P. G. P. & Valente, M. (2011). Calculation of electron and isotopes dose point kernels with fluka monte carlo code for dosimetry in nuclear medicine therapy, *Medical Physics* Vol. 38(No. 7): 3944 – 3954.

G. Luxton, P. K. & King, C. (2008). A new formula for normal tissue complication probability (ntcp) as a function of equivalent uniform dose (eud), *Physics in Medicine and Biology* Vol. 53(No. 1): 23 – 36.

H. Yoriyaz, M. S. & dos Santos, A. (2001). Monte carlo mcnp-4b–based absorbed dose distribution estimates for patient-specific dosimetry, *The Journal of Nuclear Medicine* Vol. 42(No. 4): 662 – 669.

J. Asenjo, J. F.-V. & Sánchez-Reyes, A. (2002). Characterization of a high-dose-rate 90sr-90y source for intravascular brachytherapy by using the monte carlo code penelope, *Physics in Medicine and Biology* Vol. 47(No. 5): 697 – 711.

J. Sempau, A. Sánchez-Reyes, F. S. H. O. b. T. S. J. & Fernández-Varea, J. (2001). Monte carlo simulation of electron beams from an accelerator head using penelope, *Physics in Medicine and Biology* Vol. 46(No. 4): 1163 – 1186.

J. Sempau, P. Andreo, J. A. J. M. & Salvat, F. (2004). Electron beam quality correction factors for plane-parallel ionization chambers: Monte carlo calculations using the penelope system, *Physics in Medicine and Biology* Vol. 49(No. 18): 4427 – 4444.

L.A. Dawson, D. Normolle, J. B. C. M. T. L. & Haken, R. T. (2002). Analysis of radiation-induced liver disease using the lyman ntcp model, *International journal of radiation oncology, biology, physics* Vol. 53(No. 4): 810 – 821.

M. Guerrero, X. L. (2004). Extending the linear-quadratic model for large fraction doses pertinent to stereotactic radiotherapy, *Physics in Medicine and Biology* Vol. 49(No. 20): 4825 – 4835.

M. Ljungberg, K. Sjogreen, X. L. E. F. Y. D. & Strand, S. (2002). A 3-dimensional absorbed dose calculation method based on quantitative spect for radionuclide therapy: Evaluation for 131-i using monte carlo simulation, *The Journal of Nuclear Medicine* Vol. 43(No. 8): 1101 – 1109.

Prestwich WV, Chan LB, K. C. . W. B. (1985). Dose point kernels for beta-emitting radioisotopes, *Proceedings of the fourth international radiopharmaceuzical dosimetry symposium*, US Department of energy, Oak Ridge, pp. 545–561.

R.D. Stewart, W.E. Wilson, J. M. D. & Strom, D. (2001). Microdosimetric properties of ionizing electrons in water: a test of the penelope code system, *Physics in Medicine and Biology* Vol. 47(No. 1): 79 – 88.

Salvat, S.; Fernández-Varea, J. . S. J. (2009). *PENELOPE-2008: A Code System for Monte Carlo Simulation of Electron and Photon Transport*, Nuclear Energy Agency.

S.J. Ye, I.A. Brezovich, P. P. & Naqvi, S. (2004). Benchmark of penelope code for low-energy photon transport: dose comparisons with mcnp4 and egs4, *Physics in Medicine and Biology* Vol. 49(No. 3): 687 – 397.

Stabin, M. (2008). *Fundamentals of nuclear medicine dosimetry*, Springer Science+Business Media.

V.A. Semenenko, X. L. (2008). Lyman-kutcher-burman ntcp model parameters for radiation pneumonitis and xerostomia based on combined analysis of published clinical data, *Physics in Medicine and Biology* Vol. 53(No. 3): 737 – 755.

W.V. Prestwich, J. N. & Kwok, C. (1989). Beta dose point kernels for radionuclides of potential use in radioimmunotherapy, *Journal of Nuclear Medicine* Vol. 30(No. 10): 1036 – 1046.

Z. Xu, S. Liang, J. Z. X. Z. J. Z. H. L. Y. Y. L. C. A. W. X. F. & Jiang, G. (2006). Prediction of radiation-induced liver disease by lyman normal-tissue complication probability model in three-dimensional conformal radiation therapy for primary liver carcinoma, *International Journal of Radiation Oncology Biology Physics* Vol. 65(No. 1): 189 – 195.

Zubal, I. & Harrel, C. (1992). Voxel based monte carlo calculations of nuclear medicine images and applied variance reduction techniques, *Image and Vision Computing* Vol. 10(Issue 6): 342 – 348.

12

Skeleton System

Rongfu Wang
Peking University First Hospital
China

1. Introductions

Bone and soft tissue disease is kind of detrimental disease and the precise diagnosis and timely therapy is also the clinical doctors' object of a prolonged endeavour. This chapter will introduce the diagnostic and therapeutic methods of bone and soft tissue diseases with nuclear medicine techniques.

The singular advantages of skeletal scintigraphy are high sensitivity in detecting early disease and its ability to survey the entire skeleton quickly and reasonable expense. Most broadly, the uptake of skeletal seeking radiotracers depicts osteoblastic activity and regional blood flow to bone. Any medical condition that changes either of these factors in a positive or negative way can result in an abnormal skeletal scintigram.

Radionuclide distribution has played an important role in understanding normal bone metabolism, in addition to the metabolic effects of pathologic involvement. Radionuclide imaging of the skeleton is being used with increasing frequency in the evaluation of abnormalities involving bones and joints. Several studies have demonstrated that different information can be obtained by radionuclide bone imaging compared with radiography and blood chemistry analysis. Innovations in equipment design and other advances, such as single-photon emission computed tomography (SPECT), positron emission tomography (PET), positron emission tomography/computed tomography (PET/CT), positron emission tomography/magnetic resonance imaging (PET/MR) and hybrid SPECT/CT have been incorporated into the investigation of various musculoskeletal diseases.

The first part of this chapter introduces the mechanism of skeletal radionuclide imaging, which also reviews part knowledge of skeletal anatomy and physiology. The remainder of the chapter discusses radionuclide imaging of the bones and joints, with an emphasis on the applications of the imaging procedures, and the radionuclide therapy of some bone tumors.

2. Mechanism and technique of skeletal radionuclide imaging

Bone scintigraphy is one of the most common investigations performed in nuclear medicine and routinely used in the evaluation of patients with cancer for suspected bone metastases and in various benign musculoskeletal conditions. The uptake of radiotracers in bone is associated with local osteoblastic activity and regional blood flow. More radiopharmaceutical is delivered to hyperemic areas. Either increased blood flow or increased osteogenesis for many types of lesions results in higher tracer uptake than in unaffected or normal parts of the skeleton.

The accumulation of radionuclide in bone is related to both vascularity and rate of bone turn over. Increased blood supply to an area of bone result in increased activity in a blood-pool image (obtained immediately after radiopharmaceutical administration).

The localization of various bone imaging agents is related to exchange with ions in the bone. The process of exchange of an ion native to bone for a labelled, bone-seeking ion is termed heter-ionic exchange. Calcium phosphate is the main inorganic constituent of bone; however, calcium is also found in the form of carbonate and fluoride. Calcium is located in microcystals of hydroxyapatite. Analog elements of calcium, such as strontium-85 (^{85}Sr), are believed to exchange with the calcium. Flurorine-18 (^{18}F) exchanges with hydroxyl ion in the hydroxyapatite. The accumulation of labelled phosphate compounds is probably related to the exchange of the phosphorus groups onto the calcium of hydroxyapatite. Although these mechanisms are not completely understood, the principle of bone imaging is fairly basic. Calcium analogs or phosphate compounds have a low concentration in blood and tissues, and this will supply a good bone-to-soft tissue background ratio.

Radiopharmaceuticals used for bone imaging sometimes can localize in soft tissue areas, demonstrating not only calcification but also infarction, inflammation, trauma, and tumor. The portion of any radiopharmaceutical that does not accumulate in bone and tissue or stays in the circulation is eliminated from the body by various routes, depending on the radiopharmaceutical. ^{85}Sr can be concentrated in the gastrointestinal tract for several days. ^{18}F-fluoride (^{18}F-NaF) and phosphate scans labelled with technetium-99m (^{99m}Tc) demonstrate activity in the kidneys and bladder, since these agents are excreted through the urinary tract.

2.1 Radiopharmaceuticals

Because of different radiopharmaceutical defining the imaging type, it is necessary to introduce some tracers widely used in clinical departments. Radiopharmaceuticals are classified into three goups; single photon emitting agents, positron emitting agents and therapeutic radiopharmaceuticals according to the radiation types.

2.1.1 Single photon emitting agents

SPECT, which is short for single photon emission computer tomography, is the most widely used equipment in departments of nuclear medicine. There are lots of different kinds of single photon emitting radionuclides, however not all of them are suitable for skeleton imaging. The most widely used radionuclide is technetium-99m (^{99m}Tc).

Technetium-99m is a metastable nuclear isomer of technetium-99, symbolized as ^{99m}Tc. Technetium- 99m emits gamma rays which can be detected by SPECT. It is well suited to the role because it emits readily detectable 140 keV (excitation energy) gamma rays, and its half-life for gamma emission is about 6 hr. The short half life of the isotope (in terms of human-activity and metabolism) allows for scanning procedures. The following table (table 1) summarizes its nuclear physics characteristics.

The agents are composed of radiation emitter and chemical or biologic molecules. The Tc-99m-labelled skeletal radiopharmaceuticals are distributed rapidly throughout the extracellular fluid space. For example, ^{99m}Tc-methylene diphosphonate (^{99m}Tc-MDP) is the most famous tracer of skeletal imaging, ^{99m}Tc (V)-2, 3-dimercaptosuccinic acid (^{99m}Tc (V)-DSMA), and ^{99m}Tc-sestamibi (^{99m}Tc-MIBI) are also used in skeletal and soft tissue tumors imaging.

Nuclide symbol	Z(p)	N(n)	isotopic mass (u)	half-life	Decay mode(s)	Daughter isotope(s)
	excitation energy					
^{99m}Tc	43	56	98.9062547(21)	6.0058 hr	IT (99.99%)	^{99}Tc
	140.5 keV				β^- (.0037%)	^{99}Ru

Table 1. The nuclear physics characteristics of radionuclide ^{99m}Tc

Upon intravenous injection, the uptake of ^{99m}Tc-MDP appears to be related to bone metabolic activity and to skeletal blood flow. ^{99m}Tc-MDP exhibits a specific affinity for areas of altered osteogenesis. The adsorption is believed to occur primarily to the mineral phase of bone, with little biding to the organic phase. The uptake is significantly higher in amorphous calcium phosphate than in mature crystalline hydroxyapatite, which helps explain the avidity of the tracer for areas of increased osteogenic activity. Localized areas of decreased skeletal accumulation of ^{99m}Tc-MDP may be seen in areas of reduced or absent regional blood flow (i.e. bone infarction) and in areas where the skeleton has been destroyed to the point that no bone matrix elements are present for uptake to occur.

^{99m}Tc (V)-DSMA and ^{99m}Tc-MIBI are usually used in seeking tumors in soft tissues. Also there are reports on the ^{99m}Tc (V)-DSMA scintigraphy as a monitor in the response of bone disease to vitamin D3 therapy in renal osteodystrophy and ^{99m}Tc (V)-DSMA whole body scan in detection of metastases in thyroid medullary cancer.

Gallium-67 (^{67}Ga) is also a single photon emitting radionuclide; it is an iron analogue which avidly binds to iron-binding proteins. It competes for iron sites in transferring and is absorbed by lysosomes and endoplasmic reticulum of white blood cells. It has been used in the evaluation of unknown original fever, chronic inflammations, detection and localization of osteomyelitis and/or disk space infection, etc. The excitation energy of ^{67}Ga is 93.3 keV (36%) and has a life time of 3.26 days. ^{67}Ga scintigraphy has been used to determine the treatment response in soft tissue tumors, such as osteosarcoma.

Thalium-201 (^{201}Tl) is another single photon emitting radionuclide, it has been used in many different SPECT imaging protocols such as myocardial perfusion imaging, skeleton imaging, tumor positive imaging, parathyroid imaging combined with pertechnetate, etc. ^{201}Tl decays by electron capture and gamma emitter with subsequent gamma emission of 68.9 to 80.3 keV (94%) and has a life time of 3.04 days.

Although the role of ^{201}Tl scintigraphy for staging the disease of bone tumor and differentiation of benign from malignant lesions is limited, it has provided important information on the management of patients with bone tumors. ^{201}Tl scintigraphy reflects the disease activity after treatment and it should be used to determine the treatment response and for early diagnosis of recurrence in bone soft tissue tumors.

2.1.2 Positron emitting agents

PET, which is short for positron emission computed tomography, is the most advanced equipment in the field of nuclear medicine even in the area of image science. Lots of kinds of positron emitting radionuclide have been used in practice, such as ^{18}F, ^{11}C (carbon-11), ^{15}O (oxygen-15), ^{13}N (nitrogen-13), etc. The most widely used radionuclide is fluorine-18 (^{18}F) and carbon-11 (^{11}C). The ^{18}F radiolabelled and ^{11}C labelled skeletal radiopharmaceuticals are used in PET imaging, which reflect the bone metabolism. The following table (table 2) summarizes their nuclear physics characteristics.

Nuclide symbol	Z(p)	N(n)	isotopic mass (u)	half-life	Decay mode(s)	Daughter isotope(s)
	excitation energy					
Fluorine-18 ^{18}F	9	9	18.0009380(6)	109.7min	Positron	^{18}O
	0.6335 MeV				β-	
Carbon-11 ^{11}C	6	5	11.011433(10)	20.33 min	β+	^{11}B
	0.96 MeV					

Table 2. The nuclear physics characteristics of positron radionuclide ^{18}F, ^{11}C

^{18}F-2-fluoro-2-deoxy-d-glucose (^{18}F-FDG), ^{18}F sodium fluoride (^{18}F-NaF) and ^{11}C-choline PET imaging is also called bone metabolic imaging. Here we will mention ^{18}F-FDG and ^{18}F-NaF imaging. ^{18}F-FDG (2-fluoro-2-deoxy-d-glucose) is a glucose analogue with a fluorine atom replacing a hydroxyl group in the C-2 position of d-glucose. ^{18}F exchanges with the hydroxyl (OH) ion in the hydroxyapatite. Although the mechanisms are not completely understood, the principal of bone imaging is fairly basic. Radiopharmaceuticals used in bone imaging can localize in soft tissues, demonstrating not only calcification but also inflammation, trauma, and tumor.

2.1.3 Therapeutic radiopharmaceuticals

In the area of therapeutic nuclear medicine, there are lots of applications of different kinds of radiopharmaceuticals. For example, sodium of ^{32}P-phosphate is an FDA-approved radiopharmaceutical indicated for treatment of polycythemia vera, chronic myelocytic leukemia, chronic lymphocytic leukemia, and for palliation of metastatic bone pain. Chromic ^{32}P-phosphate is suspension of ^{32}P used for intracavity installation for treatment of peritoneal or pleural effusions caused by metastatic disease. Phosphorus-32 decays by beta-emission with a half life of 14.3 days. The major toxicity noted is significant marrow suppression in approximately one third of patients receiving this radiopharmaceutical.

Iodine-131 (^{131}I) is the important therapeutic radiopharmaceutical, as a capsule or a solution for oral administration, which decays by beta- emission with subsequent gamma emission of 364 keV (82%) and has a life time of 8 days. Iodine-125 (^{125}I) delivers a higher radiation dose to the patient due to the half life of 60 days and ^{125}I seeds have been used in the therapy of solid tumors.

In skeleton nuclear medicine, some radionuclides are chosen as an effective way for treating the bone pain caused by the bone metastases. ^{89}Sr-chloride (Metastron) has been approved by the FDA for relief of bone pain in cases of painful skeletal metastases. The compound behaves biologically like calcium and localizes in hydroxyapatite crystal by ion exchange. Strontium uptake occurs preferentially at sites of active osteogenesis. This allows primary bone tumors and areas of metastatic involvement to accumulate significantly higher concentration of strontium than surrounding normal bone. ^{89}Sr decays by beta- emission with a half life of 50.6 days.

Another two radiotherapeutic agents, ^{186}Re-HEDP and ^{153}Sm-EDTMP are also used in the area. ^{186}Re decays by beta- and gamma emission with a half life of 90.6 hr and ^{153}Sm decays by beta- emission and has a half life of 46.3 hr. Both of these beta-emitting radionuclides are complex with bone-seeking ligands, which localize by chemisorption. The duration of response is 1-12 months. The main toxicity of these radiotherapeutics is mild transient bone marrow suppression.

2.1.4 Precautions

In pediatric cases the physiology and metabolism is different from adults' and the uptake of radiopharmaceuticals vary greatly, for example the bone uptake in children is up to 80% compared with that of adults at up to 40%. The pediatric dose of radiopharmaceuticals is calculated based on the standard weight method (the pediatric dose=(patient weight in kg×standard adult dose)÷70kg) or body surface area methods. With ^{99m}Tc labelled radiopharmaceuticals, we suggest a 24 to 36 hr breast feeding delay, and ^{67}Ga based products for a 72 hr delay.

In pregnant women, the nuclear medicine examinations are forbidden.

2.2 Technique of skeletal radionuclide imaging

After the radiopharmaceuticals prepared, an emission computed tomography is needed. Tomography is the process of producing a section or slice in a picture of an object. The emission computed tomography (ECT) can produce a picture of the distribution of radiopharmaceuticals administered to the patient. At present the widespread used ECT are SPECT and PET.

2.2.1 Technique of skeleton SPECT imaging

By far the most popular SPECT consists of a rotating Anger camera, which equipped with a large field of view detector, mounted on a 360-degree rotation gantry. Multipledetector SPECT has increased the diagnostic sensitivity and lessened the acquisition time. In skeletal imaging protocols we often chose a low energy and high resolution collimator.

2.2.2 Technique of skeleton PET imaging

PET is one of the exciting tomographic techniques, and provides functional information of blood flow and metabolism. As a positron meets a free electron in the tissue, annihilation occurs and the two 511keV annihilation photons are detected by coupled opposing detectors in coincidence. PET is more sensitivity than SPECT, and differs from SPECT by "electronic collimation".

2.3 Appearance of normal skeleton scintigram

According to the different imaging objects, the nuclear physician chose the proper protocols. Generally speaking, the imaging type are divided into whole body scan, local static bone scan, local bone tomography, dynamic bone scan (i.e. three phase imaging: blood flow phase, blood-pool phase, and delay scan). The whole body bone scan is the most widely used scintigraphy, which reflects the whole skeleton situation.

The appearance of the normal skeletal scintigram should be clear, symmetric and uniform and the uptake of joints, junctions, and scapulas increased. In some older patients the image may have a globally poor quality. The normal image can change dramatically among infancy, childhood, adolescence and mature adulthood. In adults, growth center activity normally becomes equal to activity in adjacent bone, on the contrary more radioactivities in growth center than adjacent bone in childhood. Tracer uptake is greatest in the axial skeleton (spine and pelvis), and relatively less intense uptake in the extremities and skull. The kidneys are routinely visualized in normal subjects and should have less intensity than the adjacent lumbar spine because the urinary system is the excretion pathway of the radiopharmaceuticals. If the kidneys show equal or greater intensity, a renal abnormality or concomitant drug therapy should be suspected. Here shows a normal skeleton scintigram (Figure 1).

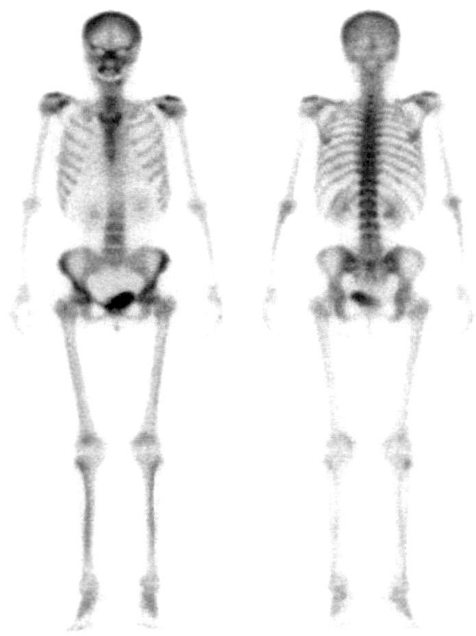

Fig. 1. Normal skeletal scintigram shows the symmetric and uniform activity absorption in anterior and posterior image.

A number of normal variants must be recognized for correct interpretation. Here we list some possible conditions as below.
①Bilaterally increased radionuclide concentration may be normal.
②The anterior aspect of the mandible may appear as a "hot spot" on lateral views of the skull.
③The laryngotracheal cartilages are usually seen in adults probably related to some degree of calcification.
④The thyroid gland can be visualized because of avid accumulation of unbound pertechnetate.
⑤Some mild diffuse asymmetry in paired joints is commonly seen in adults especially in shoulders and correlates with handedness.
⑥Some asymmetry is frequently seen in the sacroiliac joints, and this should be interpreted with caution in patients with scoliosis.

3. Applications of skeletal radionuclide imaging

It is definite that the skeletal radionuclide imaging can present the information of blood flow and osteogenesis of regional area once. There are various abnormalities in skeletal radionuclide imaging, whatever the defects or increased uptake of radionuclide; they can manifest some clue of the lesions. We conclude some abnormal results as below, and describe the details as follow based on the clinical applications.

①Asymmetric focal areas of increased or decreased activity: basically, this type of abnormality can happen in almost every scintigram. Focal increased activity can be associated with more blood flow (caused by hyperaemia, such as trauma, inflammation, etc) and active of osteogenesis (such as bone metastases of prostate cancer).
②"Super scan" is another scintigraphic pattern, with good bone-to-soft tissue background ratio, bone uptake showing brightly, absent or faint visualization of kidney and bladder, an increased uptake in the axial versus appendicular skeleton (appendicular skeleton, distal extremities, facial bones, subtle asymmetries of the rib, skull vault, and proximal long bones, and no soft-tissue uptake apparent at normal intensities). In some patients with breast cancer or prostate cancer the entire axial skeleton becomes diffusely and rather uniformly involved with metastatic disease (Figure 2).

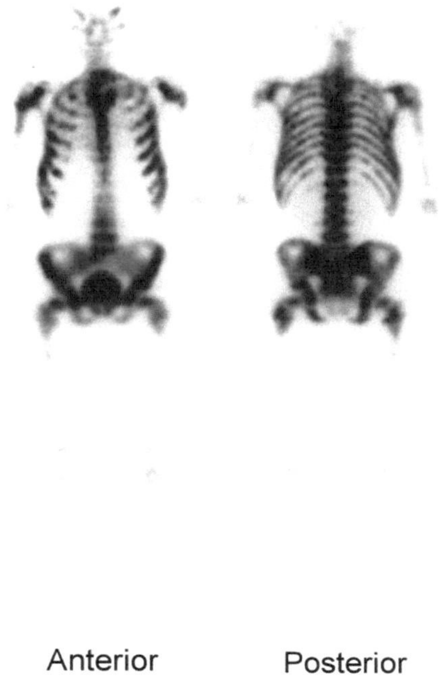

Fig. 2. A patient diagnosed as prostate cancer, the whole body bone scan with ^{99m}Tc-MDP showed "super scan": absent visualization of kidney, increased uptake in the axial versus appendicular skeleton and no soft-tissue uptake apparent at normal intensities.

③Cold areas, which means diminished activity or none distribution of activity, is indicative of osteonecrosis, osteoporosis, osteomalacia, multiple myeloma, radiation or steroid therapy, end-stage cancer patients with diminished metabolism, renal cell carcinoma, thyroid cancer, anaplastic tumors, neuroblastoma.
④"Donut" sign is the typical scintigram of osteonecrosis of the femoral head. The cold area within the femoral head is highly specific and is the earliest scintigraphic evidence of avascular necrosis. Over a period of weeks to months, increased uptake represents revascularization and repair surrounds, and eventually replaces the region of photopenia. The central region of photopenia with surrounding zone of increased uptake is termed as "donut" sign (Figure 3).

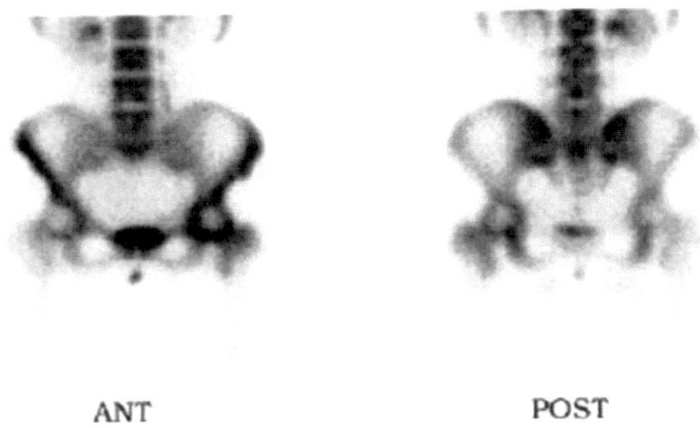

Fig. 3. The image showed "donut" sign in bilateral femoral head (worse in left side than right side), which is the diagnostic evidence of femoral head necrosis resulting from long-time use of dexamethasone.

⑤No uptake in focal areas: patients receive radiation therapy, bone infarct, avascular necrosis, metal prosthesis, bone infiltrated by tumor, poor venous return, edema in extremity may seen cold spot in focal area.
⑥Three phase bone imaging: it is one of the types of imaging protocols, and can help the qualitative diagnosis of some skeletal diseases, such as increased uptake in flow, blood pool, and delays in osteomyelitis cases; increased uptake in flow and blood-pool with mild or no uptake in delays in cellutitis; increased activity in and around joints in flow, blood pool, and delays in arthritis; increased vascular flow, blood pool, and delays focally in primary malignant tumor (Figure 4); increased blood pool and delays, focally intense in benign primary tumor.

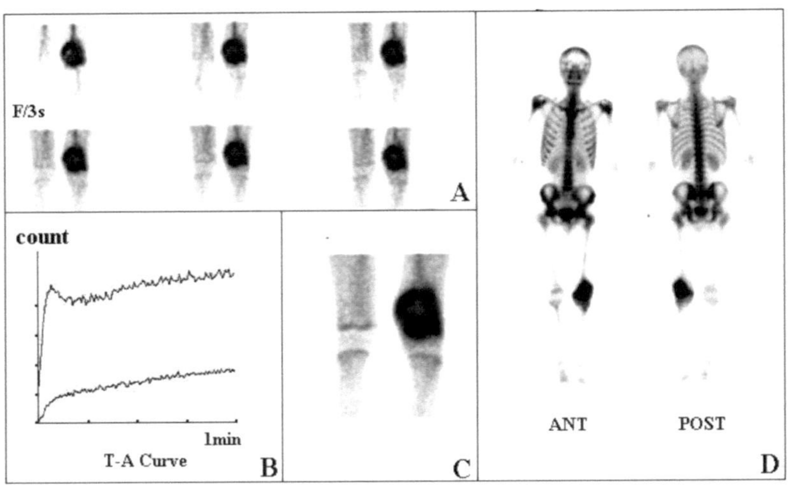

Fig. 4. Three phase bone imaging showed increased activity in left distal femur in blood flow phase (A), blood pool phase (C), and delayed phase (D). Malignant bone tumor: blood supply obviously increased in blood flow phase, vascular extension can be seen. Irregular tracer accumulated in soft tissue, in blood pool phase. Hot spot accumulation can be found on bone in delayed phase. In this case the patient was diagnosed as left femur osteogenic sarcoma by pathological proven finally.

3.1 Metastatic diseases

The most common clinical application of skeletal imaging is in evaluating patients with extraskeletal primary malignancies for the presence of metastatic disease and staging metastatic disease. In many patients the presence of extent of skeletal metastasis directly influences treatment decisions and prognosis. Bone imaging plays an important role in treatment of bone pain and pathological fracture which are common management problems in patients with skeletal metastatic disease.

Anterior and posterior images of the whole body scan are generally obtained. Metastases to bone are common in several primary malignancies, including lung, breast, and prostate carcinomas (Figure 5-6). Metastases to the spine are difficult to detect radiographically, since loss of approximately 50% of the mineral content of the bone must occur before lytic lesions are detected. The usual scintigraphic pattern of skeletal metastatic disease is multiple focal lesions throughout the skeleton, with the greatest involvement generally in the axial skeleton. The area of abnormal radiopharmaceutical deposition represents the edge of the metastatic deposit where osteoblastic repair is attempted.

As metastatic lesions grow in the marrow space, the surrounding bone remodels through osteoclastic (resorptive) and osteoblastic (depositional) activity. The relative degrees of bone resorption and deposition elicited are highly variable among the different types of tumors and sometimes even different locations for the same tumor. The relationship between the two remodelling processes determines whether a metastatic deposit will appear as predominantly lytic or sclerotic or will exhibit a mixed pattern radiographically.

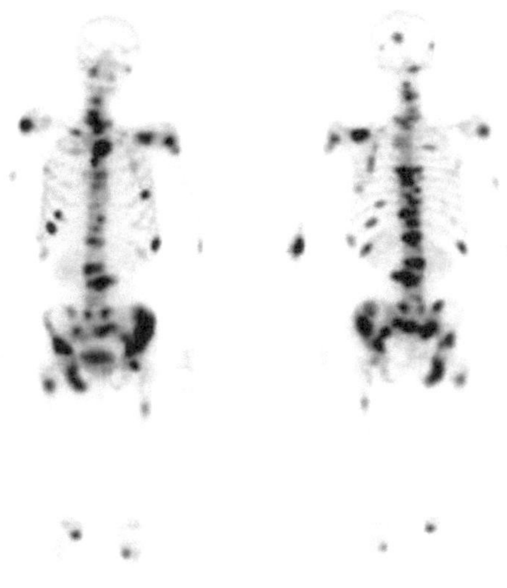

Fig. 5. The image showed multiple hot spot in skull, vertebrae, ribs, pelvis, femur, etc. Combined with the history of prostate cancer and night bone pain, it was concluded as bone metastases of prostate cancer.

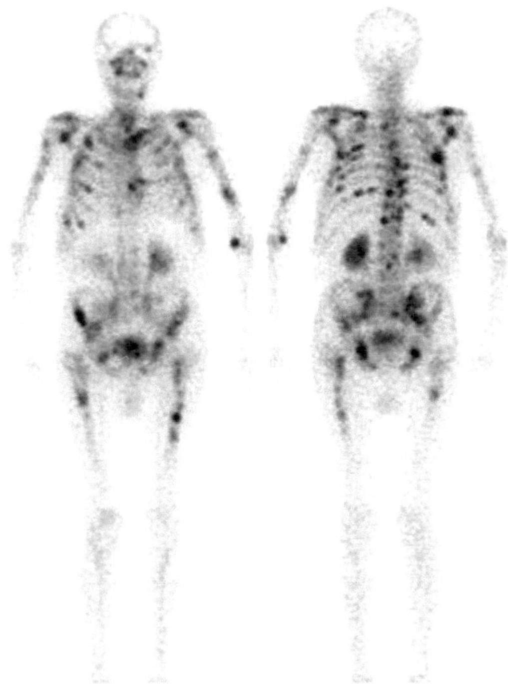

Fig. 6. The image showed multiple focal lesions in bone of patient with breast cancer.

False negative scans have been related to several factors. If the skeleton is diffusely involved with metastatic disease, the focal nature of the lesions might not be apparent. Metastatic lesions may have no associated osteoblastic activity and thus may not be detected by bone scan or may be detected as a photon-deficient area.

3.2 Primary malignant bone tumors

Bone scanning is also used for the evaluation of primary bone neoplasm. Usually the patient has already had radiographs of the primary tumor, but the bone scan offers additional information of that area. The extent of the abnormality on the bone scan is generally not much different from the radiographically apparent lesion. The value of bone scanning in patients with primary bone malignancy lies in the detection of the disease elsewhere.

Uptake of bone-seeking radiopharmaceuticals in primary bone tumors is avid and frequently striking. PET imaging with FDG is being explored for primary bone tumors. FDG uptake correlates with tumor metabolism. Scans can be helpful in localizing sites for biopsy and in assessing response to preoperative radiation and chemotherapy.

^{99m}Tc-MIBI have been used for sarcoma imaging to determine whether tumors are low or high grade and to assess response to therapy. As with FDG, high-grade tumors show higher uptake. Successful radiation therapy or chemotherapy is associated with decreasing uptake. Studies of primary tumor have led to at least one important observation about skeletal tracer uptake. Many tumors elicit marked hyperemia. The increased blood flow is not restricted to the tumor itself but affects the entire watershed distribution of regional flow, most characteristically involving an entire extremity (Figure 7).

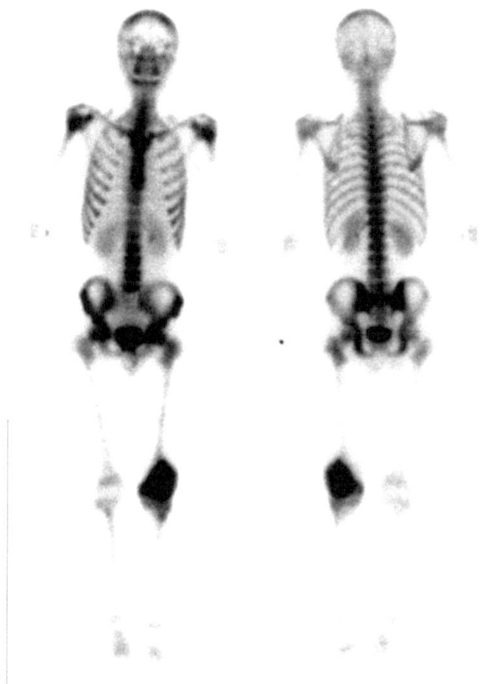

Fig. 7. Anterior and posterior whole body scintigram of a patient with osteosarcoma in the left distal femur. The degree of tracer accumulation in the lesion is striking. Note also the "watershed" phenomenon with increased tracer accumulation in all of the bones of the left lower extremity above and below the lesion. The increased blood flow induced by the osteosarcoma results in increased tracer delivery to the entire limb.

Another primary malignant disease commonly involving bone is multiple myeloma (MM). MM is really a disease of the red marrow space, and the most frequently involved skeletal structures are the vertebrae, pelvis, ribs, and skull (Figure 8). On skeletal scintigram the only finding in MM may be osteopenia. Unless an associated fracture or a focal lesion such as a plasmacytoma is present, skeletal scintigrams are often normal. MRI is an excellent modality for evaluating the marrow space for areas of involvement.

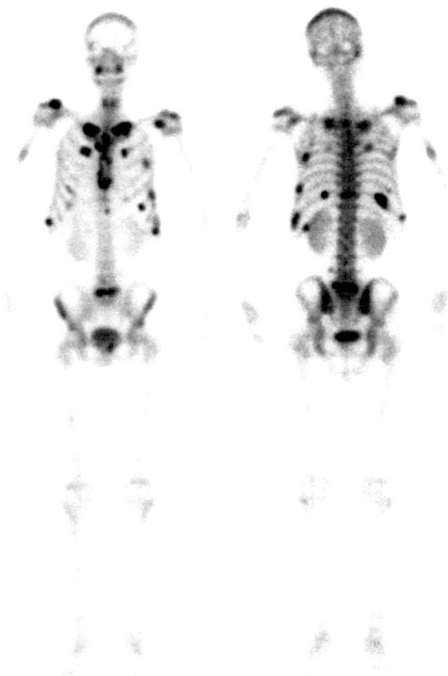

Fig. 8. Multiple myeloma, showed multiple focal accumulation of radioactivity in bone.

3.3 Benign bone tumors

Skeletal imaging is highly sensitive for detecting osteoid osteomas (Figure 9), which can be difficult to find by standard radiography, especially in the spine.

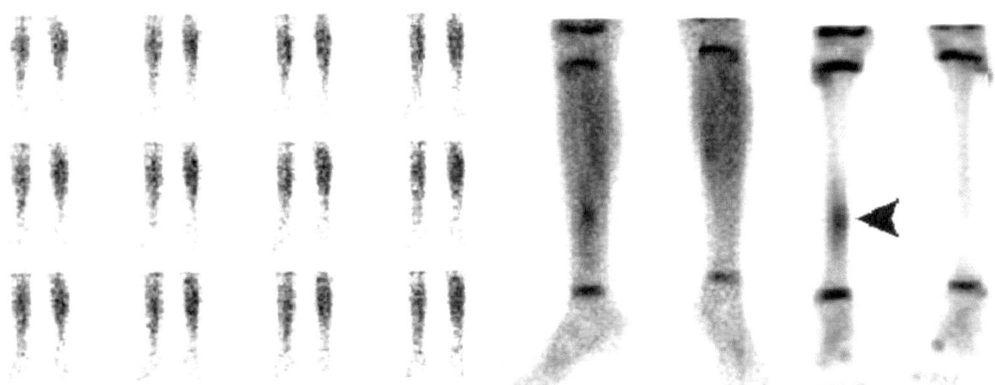

Fig. 9. Three phase bone scan (bottom row) of a 13 years old boy with history of pain and swelling in the right shin. The swelling was localized to the mid shaft of right tibia. Plain x-ray revealed a large area of sclerosis in the mid shaft of right tibia. Bone scan showed normal blood flow phase, high soft tissue uptake in the blood pool phase and a double density hot lesion in delayed image over the mid-shaft of right tibia. Surgical excision of the tumor resulted in total relief of symptoms. Histology confirmed the diagnosis of osteoid osteomas.

3.4 Trauma and athletic injuries

Skeletal trauma is common and presents both an opportunity and a problem in skeletal scintigraphy. As we known, the first choice for suspected bone fracture is radiography, which shows the fracture line and type clearly. But SPECT bone imaging has its own advantages in some aspects. SPECT is a useful adjunct in the course of process such as stress fracture. Normal bone is constantly remodelling, bone resorption and deposition are balanced. When the skeleton is placed under stress the rate of remodelling increases, and that will result in change of activity in bone scintigraphy,

The time a fracture takes to return to normal scintigraphically depends primarily on its location and the degree of damage to the skeleton.

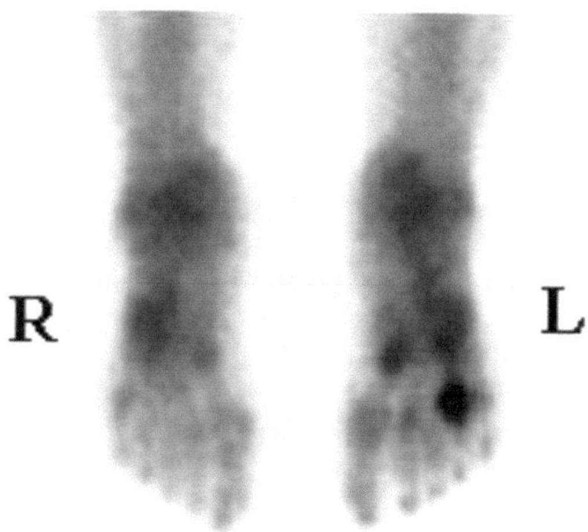

Fig. 10. Occult fracture of the left foot 4th toe, which can not be detected by radiography.

3.5 Osteomyelitis

In addition to being used in the evaluation of malignant disease involving the skeleton, radionuclide bone imaging is helpful in the assessment of several other non-malignant processes, such as patients with suspected osteomyelitis and diskitis. Acute hematogenous osteomyelitis typically begins by seeding of the infectious organism in the marrow space.

A three-phase bone scan is performed by acquiring a rapid blood flow sequence of images over the interested area during agent injection. Early images (blood flow phase) are important in evaluating inflammatory processes. Flow images are performed 40 to 60sec and 2 to 4 sec for each frame. Blood pool images are then immediately obtained for totally 300 to 500 kcounts without moving the patient, and delayed images are taken as necessary. Both osteomyelitis and cellutitis can cause early increased radioactivity accumulation due to an increased vascular response to the affected area. The third phase is routine scanning at 2 to 3 hr after injection. Sometimes there will be a forth phase that can be added 24hr delay. Osteomyelitis demonstrates focally increased activity in the involved bone on both the blood-pool and routine images (Figure 11). Since the use of bone imaging for detecting osteomyelitis, it has been found that several patients do not subsequently develop the typical radiographic changes because the early treatment prevents the development of radiographic abnormalities.

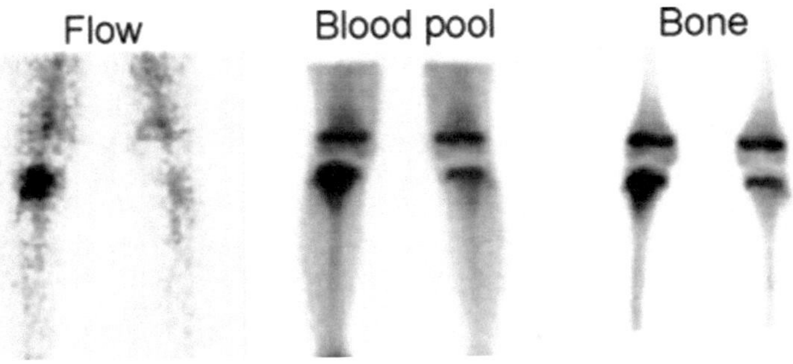

Fig. 11. Plantar view flow image show increased perfusion to the right proximal tibia. Blood-pool image also demonstrate abnormal accumulation in the same area. Delayed image have persistent radiopharmaceutical collection consistent with osteomyelitis. Focal hyerperfusion, focal hyperemia, and focally increased bony activity in the proximal right tibial metaphysic are the classic findings of osteomyelitis.

3.6 Metabolic bone diseases

A number of metabolic conditions can result in marked abnormalities on bone imaging. Although these do not represent important clinical indications for bone imaging, they may be encountered incidentally in other applications, most importantly during metabolic skeletal survey. Hyperthyroidism, primary hyperparathyroidism, renal osteodystrophy, osteomalacia, and hypervitaminosis D all can result in generalized increased tracer uptake throughout the skeleton that has some features in common with the "supers can" seen in metabolic disease(Figure 12). These features are described before, such as increased

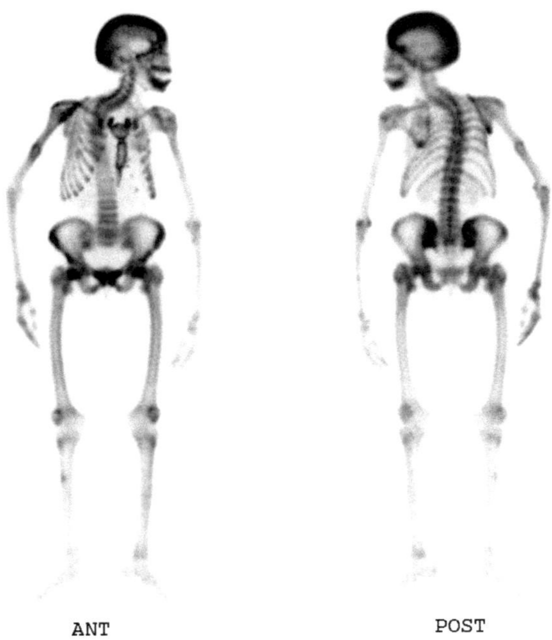

Fig. 12. Supers can in metabolic disease from the patient with hyperparathyroidism

skeleton-to-soft tissue ratio and faint or absent visualization of the kidneys. Increased skull activity, involvement of the long bones of the extremities, and increased periarticular uptake are features that distinguish scan in these conditions from the supers can of metabolic disease.

3.7 Bone marrow disorders

Non-invasive imaging techniques have been used in the past for visualization the functional activity of the bone marrow compartment. Imaging with radiolabelled compounds may allow different bone marrow disorders to be distinguished. These imaging techniques, almost all of which use radiolabelled tracers, such as ^{99m}Tc-nanocolloid, ^{99m}Tc-sulphur colloid (^{99m}Tc-SC), ^{111}In-chloride, and radiolabelled white blood cells (^{99m}Tc-WBC), have been used in nuclear medicine for several decades. The results support that the radiolabelled agents can be alternatives to bone marrow scan.

4. Radionuclide therapy of skeletal tumors

Metastatic bone cancer is a common complication of malignant tumor. It is reported that 20%-75% of cancer patients has developed bone metastases according to necropsy results. Malignant bone pain is still a challenging clinical problem. Pain due to bone metastases will greatly decrease the patient's quality-of-life because of patient's gradual deterioration, local body dysfunction, and mental and physical collapse. Recently, there are several reports on therapy of painful bone metastases by radiotherapy or anticancer drugs showing therapeutic efficacy. The studies, however, were generally heterogeneous trials involving stage of diagnosis, radiopharmaceuticals dosage, combination with other therapeutic modalities and methods of pain assessment. In addition, there are few reports on the study of comparison of radionuclide therapy with chemotherapy for evaluating the therapeutic effectiveness of the patients with painful bone metastases.

4.1 Radionuclide internal-radiation therapy

Radionuclide internal-radiation therapy of severe bone pain due to multiple skeletal metastases has recently achieved successful stage in nuclear medicine, which has been much considered and widespread used. In this chapter we described the principle of treatment of painful disseminated skeletal metastases, therapeutic approaches, evaluation of effective treatment according to our clinical experience in routine clinical treatment and its future applications.

^{89}Sr-chloride (Metastron) has been approved by the FDA for relief of bone pain in cases of painful skeletal metastases. The compound behaves biologically like calcium and localizes in hydroxyapatite crystal by ion exchange. Strontium uptake occurs preferentially at sites of active osteogenesis. This allows primary bone tumors and areas of metastatic involvement to accumulate significantly higher concentrations of strontium than surrounding normal bone. ^{89}Sr decays by beta- emission with a half life of 50.6 days. The conventional dose of ^{89}Sr-chloride is 148 MBq (4mCi), and can be reinjection after three months if necessary. Before administration, a blood regulation test should be checked.

Another two radiotherapeutic agents, ^{186}Re-HEDP and ^{153}Sm-EDTMP are also used in the area. ^{186}Re decays by beta- and gamma emission with a half life of 90.6 hr and ^{153}Sm decays by beta- emission and has a half life of 46.3 hr. Both of these beta-emitting radionuclides are complex with bone-seeking ligands, which localize by chemisorption. The duration of response is 1-12 months. The main toxicity of these radiotherapeutics is mild transient bone marrow suppression.

4.2 Radionuclide seed implantation

Radionuclide seed such as ^{125}I 、^{103}Pd 、^{198}Au implantation has been used in lots of clinical departments. Mostly ^{125}I seeds (Figure 13) have been chosen as the proper one. Iodine-125 delivers a higher radiation dose to the patient due to the half life of 60 days and ^{125}I seeds planted have been used in the therapy of solid tumors.

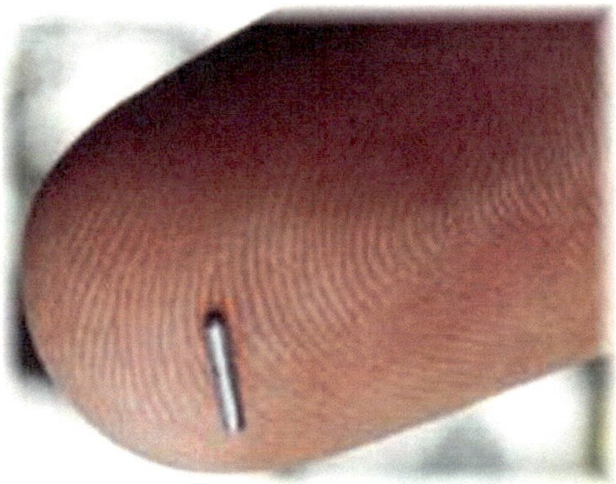

Fig. 13. ^{125}I seed is used in the therapy of solid tumor by implantation.

5. Recent advances of skeletal radionuclide imaging and therapy

It's well-known that the skeletal radionuclide imaging and therapy will have a prospective development in novel radiopharmaceuticals of skeletal imaging (^{18}F-NaF) (Figure 14) and therapy (heavy ion Carbon-11 and boron neutron capture therapy (BNCT)) and advanced nuclear medicine equipments such as SPECT/CT, PET/CT and PET/MR. In routine clinical practice, a variety of new radiopharmaceuticals have been introduced in recent years. There are three commercial radiopharmaceuticals of Samarium-153-ethylenediaminetetramethylene phosphonic acid (^{153}Sm-EDTMP), Rehnium-188-(Sn)-hydroxyethylene diphosphonate (^{188}Re-HEDP) and Strontium-89 chloride ($^{89}SrCl_2$). $^{89}SrCl_2$ is still the most widely used agent due to a longer physical half life ($T½$ = 50.5 days) and a pure beta-emitter playing an important role in radionuclide internal radiation therapy. ^{188}Re-HEDP ($T½$ = 16.9 hr) obtained from ^{188}W-^{188}Re generator is cheap and convenient in clinical practice routine, with scintigraphic imaging of gamma rays in order to perform individual dosimetric studies, but ^{188}W-^{188}Re generator must be imported from other countries. ^{153}Sm-EDTMP developed by our country is one of the radiopharmaceutical therapeutic agents and has relatively ideal physical, chemical and biological properties similar to ^{188}Re except of slightly longer have-life ($T½$ = 40.4 hr). The 0.103-Mev gamma ray is suitable for imaging in vivo distribution. The benefit of the favourable clinical experience with ^{153}Sm-EDTMP has been reported in several multicenter trials.

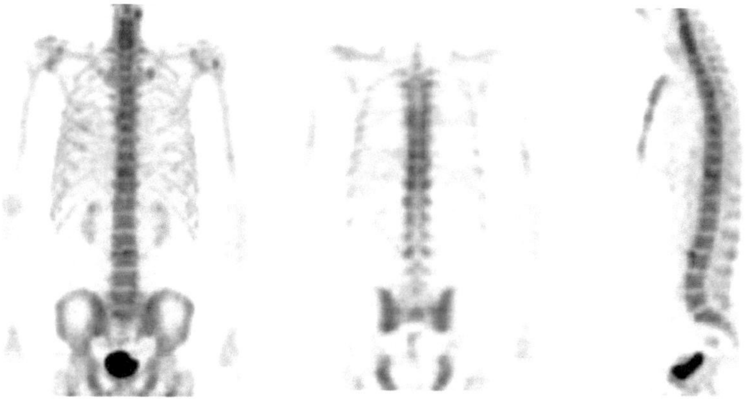

Fig. 14 Normal image of ^{18}F- Fluoride PET（a: 3D projection imaging b: coronal slice iamging: c: sagittal slice imaging）

6. Conclusion

It is important to resolve the problems on skeletal and soft tissue tumors for clinicians to seek for new diagnostic and therapeutic radiopharmaceuticals. Although rapid developments of medical science and great progress have been made recently, there are still some limitations. The clinical applications of radionuclide tracing technique in diagnosis and treatment of skeletal and soft tissue tumor is attached importance to clinical physicians with widely using the technique in clinical routine practice and continuing development of nuclear medicine.

7. References

[1] Herzog H, Pietrzyk U, Shah NJ, et al. The current state, challenges and perspectives of MR-PET. Neuroimage, 2010 , 49(3): 2072-2082.

[2] Wang Qiang, Wang Rong-fu. A novel molecualr imaging technique of PET/MR. China Med Device Information, 2011, 17(4): 4-7.

[3] Wang Rong-fu. Molecular Functional Diagnosis and Targeted Therapy in Tumor. J Oncol, 2010, 16(6):421-422.

[4] Wang Rong-fu. Progress and Application of Molecular Functional Imaging with Radionuclide Tracing Techniques in Oncology. Contemporary Medical Imaging, 2010, 8(1):19-22.

[5] Wang Rongfu. Prospect of clinical application of radionuclide imaging and radiotherapy in skeletal and soft tissue tumors. Chi Cancer Clin, 2007, 34(19): 1127-1130.

[6] Wang RF, Zhang CL, Zhu SL, et al. A comparative study of Sm-153- ethylenediamine- tetra -methylene phosphonic acid with pamidronate disodium in the treatment of patients with painful metastatic bone cancer. Med Princ Pract (MPP), 2003, 12(2): 97-101.

[7] Wang Rong-fu. Prospect and status of positron radiopharmaceuticals in oncology. J Nucl Radiochem, 2006, 28(2): 65-71.

[8] Ohta M, Tokuda Y, Suzuki Y, et al. Whole body PET for the evaluation of bony metastases in patients with breast cancer: comparison with ^{99m}Tc-MDP bone scintigraphy. Nucl Med Commun, 2001, 229(8): 875-879.

[9] Piffanelli A, Dafermou A, Giganti M, et al. Radionulide therapy for painful bone metastases. Q J Nucl Med, 2001, 45(1): 100-107.

[10] Wang Rongfu. Prospect of clinical application of radionuclide therapy in skeletal and soft tissue tumors(Part I). Chi Med News, 2006, 21(4): 13.

[11] Wang Rongfu. Prospect of clinical application of radionuclide imaging in skeletal and soft tissue tumors(Part II). Chi Med News, 2006, 21(2): 15.

[12] Savelli G, Maffioli L, Maccauro M, et al. Bone scintigraphy and the add value of SPECT in detecting skeletal lesions. Q J Nucl Med, 2001, 45(1): 27-37.

[13] Cook GJ, Fogelman I. The role of positron emission tomography in management of bone metastases. Cancer, 2000, 88(12 Suppl): 2927-2933.

[14] Evan-Sapir E, Mester U, Flusser G, et al. Assessment of malignant skeletal disease: initial experience with ^{18}F-fluoride PET/CT and comparison between ^{18}F-fluoride PET and ^{18}F-fluoride PET/CT. J Nucl Med, 2004, 45(2): 272-278.

[15] Zhang H, Tian M, Oriuchi N, et al. ^{11}C-choline PET for the detection of bone and soft tissue tumors in comparison with FDG PET. Nucl Med Commun, 2003, 24(3): 273-279.

[16] Brenner W, Bohuslavizki KH, Eary JF. PET imaging of osteosarcoma. J Nucl Med, 2003, 44(6): 930-942.

[17] Wang Rong-fu. Application study and development of molecular nuclear medicine. J chin Clin Med Imaging, 2008,19(8): 585-590.

[18] Wang Rong-fu. New technique Application of PET/CT. CT Theory & Application, 18(4): 9-14.

[19] Wang RF. Clinical and positron imaging with coincidence detection. Beijing: Peking Univ Med Press, 2004.

[20] Wang RF. Progress in imaging agents of cell apoptosis. Anti-Cancer Agents in Medical Chemistry, 2009, 9(9): 996-1002.

[21] Ali Sarikaya, Saniye Sen, Sevim Hacimahmutoglu, etc. ^{99m}Tc(V)-DMSA scintigraphy in monitoring the response of bone disease to vitamin D3 therapy in renal osteodystrophy. Annals of Nuclear Medicine, 2002, 16(1): 19–23.

[22] Shahram Dabiri. ^{99m}Tc(V)-DMSA in Detection of Metastases of Medullary Thyroid Carcinoma. Iran J Nucl Med 2006; 14(26): 15-24.

[23] Charito Love, Christopher J. Palestro. Radionuclide imaging of infection J Nucl Med Technol, 2004, 32(2): 47-57.

[24] Wang Rong-fu. Diagnostics of PET/CT in Oncology. Beijing, Peking Univ Med Press, 2008

[25] Ali Agool, Andor W.J.M. Glaudemans, Hendrikus H. Boersma, etal. Radionuclide imaging of bone marrow disorders. Eur J Nucl Med Mol Imaging, 2011, 38(1):166-178.

[26] Sousa Ricardoa, Massada Martaa, Pereira Alexandrea, etal. Diagnostic accuracy of combined 99mTc-sulesomab and 99mTc-nanocolloid bone marrow imaging in detecting prosthetic joint infection. Nuclear Medicine Communications, 2011, 32(9): 834-839.

[27] Ryo Takagi, Yuji Suzuki, Yoshiko Seki,etal. Indium chloride-induced micronulei in in vivo and invtro experimental systems. J Occupational Health, 2011, 53(2): 102-109.

[28] Lou Lawrencea, Alibhai Karim N.b, Winkelaar Gerrit B.b, etal. 99mTc-WBC scintigraphy with SPECT/CT in the evaluation of arteral graft infection. Nuclear Medicine Communications, 2010, 31(5): 411-416.

[29] Zhao Yuan, Wang Rongfu, Liu Pengcheng. Current status and recent advance in ^{125}I seed implantation in the treatment for malignant tumors. J Oncol, 2010, 16(6): 432-431.